Theoretical Epidemiology

ISBN 0-8273-4313-2

90000

9 780827 343139

Theoretical Epidemiology

PRINCIPLES OF OCCURRENCE RESEARCH IN MEDICINE

Olli S. Miettinen, M.D., Ph.D., M.D. (hon.)

Professor of Epidemiology and Biostatistics
School of Public Health, Harvard University
Boston, Massachusetts

Professor of Epidemiology and Biostatistics
Professor of Medicine
Faculty of Medicine, McGill University
Montreal, Quebec

DELMAR PUBLISHERS INC.®

NOTICE TO THE READER

For more information, address Delmar Publishers Inc.
3 Columbia Circle, Box 15-015
Albany, New York 12212-5015

Printed in the United States of America
Published simultaneously in Canada
By Nelson Canada
A Division of The Thomson Corporation

10 9 8 7 6 5 4 3 2

ISBN 0-8273-4313-2

To
K.U., T.S., J.R., S.H.,
and
my students

Preface

This text treats theoretical epidemiology as *the discipline of how to study the occurrence of phenomena of interest in the health field*. Thus it delineates major principles of study design and data analysis in research into the frequency of occurrence of illness and related phenomena in human populations, whether in the community or in clinical situations. Thus it is concerned with the principles of the dominant type of research in applied medical science and in health care administration. Moreover, the principles of research of this type in medicine are not peculiar to the study of illness, health, and health care, nor to studies on humans. They apply equally to statistical research in psychology, behavioral science, technology, and other fields.

The intent is to provide the reader with the necessary theoretical background for dealing with occurrence research in medicine—for thinking about it; for reviewing it; and for conducting it. To this end, the first part of the text deals with the theoretical basis for valid and efficient study design. The remainder addresses data analysis. This latter part deals first with the nature and interpretation of the *results* of data analysis—a topic that is of concern to all investigators, even if the analyses are carried out by statistical collaborators. The rest of the second part is directed to procedures of data analysis, and it is intended mainly for those who aspire to be statistically

self-sufficient in epidemiologic research. Since the intended applications of
this text presuppose understanding as well as knowledge, there is emphasis
on the rationales of the various principles presented.

Even though epidemiologic research is widely regarded as commonsense
activity, a line of research that any physician—even one without statistical
education—is prepared to engage in, its principles have posed a major and
continuing challenge to me over more than two decades of studying the
subject and during a decade and a half of teaching and consulting. A course
text evolved with the early teaching. Revised each year, it grew to be un-
manageably large by 1975. A condensed and updated version was prepared
in 1977. Although various colleagues kept urging their publication, to me
those texts seemed somehow fundamentally unsatisfactory. Indeed, for several years that followed, I taught without any text. Instead, I felt it necessary
to search, even in the class context, for the true essence of epidemiologic
research as a foundation for its principles. This search led to the realization
and conviction that epidemiologic research is *occurrence research*—research into the frequency of occurrence of phenomena of health care interest
among people (and perhaps other units of observation), with measures of
frequency related to their determinants. Thus the epidemiologic concern is
with *occurrence relations*. With this realization it became evident what the
core issues really are: in design, development of the *form* of the empirical
occurrence relation that the study is to produce, formation or selection of
its direct *referent* (the study base), the selection of the strategy of actually
harvesting the base experience in terms of *sampling* design, and so on; in
analysis, the derivation of the chi square or *P*-value not only for the null
situation of no relation but as a *function of the parameter of relation* in the
occurrence relation under study, all statistics of potential interest being implicit in these chi square or *P*-value functions.

Simultaneously with my personal efforts to understand the principles of
epidemiologic research, the field in general has undergone considerable
transformation, mainly as a consequence of a recent rapid increase in the
interest and involvement of *statisticians* in what used to be a physician-
dominated discipline. This progress is manifest in some recent textbooks,
authored by statisticians who have dedicated their careers to the general
conceptual problems of epidemiologic research. Yet the number of modern
texts on this subject remains small, so that the addition of this one does not
seem superfluous, particularly since this text reflects the recent, considerable changes in my conception of the fundamentals of the field.

In the face of this evolution, and the diversity of the prevailing outlooks
in theoretical epidemiology, it should be understood that in some instances
the choice is not a matter of distinguishing between correct and incorrect,
but rather one of intellectual appeal. After all, the patterns of planetary
motion were well understood in terms of Ptolemaic mechanics, even if the
Newtonian outlook is now considered more attractive. On the other hand,
the prevailing epidemiologic outlook today is in many ways intellectually

unsatisfactory, for example, some of the presumed implications of the prevailing commitment to the "frequentist" outlook in epidemiologic statistics (see Sections 9.3.3–9.3.5).

This text is intended to be essentially self-contained. Nevertheless, self-study does present some difficulties. The requisite concentration, reflection, and receptivity of mind may, however, not be unrealistic to expect of someone preparing to address problems that are as challenging conceptually as are those in modern occurrence research in medicine.

O.S.M.

Acknowledgments

More than a decade ago, the World Health Organization, on the recommendations of Mr. Kazuro Uemura and Mr. Thalànayar Sundaresan, commissioned me to develop an epidemiology text. The task proved much more challenging than anticipated, and the end result was only an informal and very tentative course text. This early contribution and show of faith did, however, put in motion the development that ultimately led to the present text.

In the ensuing many years the main encouragement for further development was the enthusiasm of my students. They were participants in the regular advanced courses at Harvard and in the annual International Advanced Course on Epidemiologic Methods organized by the Institute of Occupational Health in Helsinki; and they were students in various other international courses, as well as members of informal study groups studying the course texts in various institutions.

Parallel with this, the thoughtful and sustained encouragement of Mr F. Treville Leger, the editor representing Wiley, has been of great importance for the development of this text.

The most immediate and by far the most important contributions were provided by Drs. Jorma Rantanen and Sven Hernberg. Through their influence, the Institute of Occupational Health in Helsinki provided a setting for writing in the summer months of 1981 and 1982, complete with secretarial help, word processing, statistical computing, and other amenities. For computing collaboration there I am very indebted to Mrs. Tuula Nurminen. Two other colleagues there, Dr. Markku Nurminen and Mr. Timo Partanen, read the first draft and provided valuable suggestions. Subsequently, a similar service was provided by a large number of students and other colleagues. In the final revision stage, after a couple of years of testing the text in various courses, Drs. Chung Hsieh and Markku Nurminen were devoted and most valuable collaborators.

The developmental work with previously unpublished results was supported in part by grant number 5 R 01 CA 06373 from the National Cancer Institute of the United States of America.

For long-term support and encouragement within Harvard I am indebted to Dr. Alexander Nadas, the towering clinician and recognized patron of epidemiologic scholarship in the environment of academic medicine.

O.S.M.

Contents

PART 1   STUDY DESIGN

PART 2   DATA ANALYSIS

APPENDICES

Theoretical Epidemiology

1

The Study of Occurrence Problems in Medicine: Introduction

1.1. THEORETICAL EPIDEMIOLOGY AS THE DISCIPLINE OF OCCURRENCE RESEARCH IN MEDICINE

Epidemiology originally dealt with *epidemics of communicable diseases* only. In this context there developed certain principles of how to study the occurrence—prevalence and incidence—of communicable diseases. Naturally, the occurrence rates were related to various characteristics of persons—age and other determinants of occurrence rates, including suspected causal ones.

A small extension of this original concern was to subsume under epidemiology the study of *endemic* occurrence of communicable diseases, and the occurrence, epidemic or endemic, of noncommunicable (noncontagious) *infectious* diseases.

Major expansion resulted from the observation that the principles of studying the occurrence of infectious diseases could be applied to the study of the occurrence of noninfectious diseases as well. This gave rise to so-called *chronic-disease* epidemiology. The term, a misnomer, refers to noninfectious diseases, chronic and acute, and defects as well as diseases. In other words, infectious-disease epidemiology was extended to the epidemiology of any *illness*, whether infectious or noninfectious, acute or chronic, and whether it be a process of ill-health (disease or *morbus*) or a state of ill-health (defect or *vitium*).

Naturally, students of the occurrence of illness, infectious or not, have taken an interest in the occurrence of various states of *health*, insofar as they may be considered to have potential bearing on the occurrence of illness. Thus, an infectious-disease epidemiologist is concerned, for example, with the occurrence of states of immunity; and the "chronic-disease" epidemiologist is interested in issues such as the occurrence of various levels of blood pressure.

The traditional practice of stratifying epidemiologic problems according to the type of illness has led to prevention-oriented specialties such as cardiovascular epidemiology (preventive cardiology) and cancer epidemiology (preventive oncology). This *illness-centered* outlook is not ideal as a basis for preventive intervention. Thus, preventive cardiology has led to recommendations and programs for lowering cholesterol, but there is reason to suspect that these may result in an increase in the risk of cancer.

A more appropriate basis for prevention is *determinant-centered* epidemiology. Thus, when the focus of research is on nutrition, one studies *all* the health effects of a cholesterol-lowering diet; and even if the merits of such a diet be conflicting among different categories of illness, such research provides for evaluating the overall effect. In addition to the field of nutrition, this outlook is common in toxicology, occupational health, and various other fields.

With each of these two outlooks, epidemiology has traditionally been associated with disease *prevention*, and it has been viewed as a *public-health* science and discipline. Indeed, it has been described as "the basic science of public health." In this spirit, there have been attempts to distinguish between epidemiology and clinical medicine, arguing that the former deals with populations and the latter with individuals. This distinction applies, however, more to health care itself in these two areas than to research in them.

Prevention-oriented epidemiology has given rise to the concept and discipline of *clinical epidemiology*. It deals with the occurrence of states and events of medical concern in the clinical context, that is, among patients under medical care. Analogously with more traditional epidemiology, the focus of such research may be on the occurrence of a particular type of health state or event in relation to its various determinants or, alternatively, on the effects of a particular determinant on the occurrence of various outcomes. Thus, a clinical epidemiologist studies the occurrence of infections among hospitalized patients (nosocomial infections) as opposed to the occurrence of infections among people in the community. Similarly, the clinical epidemiologist studies the occurrence of sudden cardiac death among patients with known coronary heart disease rather than among people with no known heart disease in the community. With the research focus on a determinant of illnesses or related phenomena, the clinical epidemiologist interested in nutrition studies the occurrence of various complications of adult-onset diabetes in relation to diet among such diabetics, instead of the effects of diet on the risk of diabetes and other states and events of health among people at large. Similarly, the clinical epidemiologist may be concerned with the various health effects of a particular type of clinical intervention, medical or surgical.

The discipline of epidemiologic research that has developed in the context of these problems of scientific research in preventive and curative medicine is being increasingly applied to medical problems that are of *administrative* rather than scientific interest. Thus, those concerned with planning and/or evaluating health *education* acquire information on the occurrence of health-related knowledge, attitudes, and behavior in the population at issue, with the rates of occurrence related to their major determinants, known or surmised. Similarly, planners of health-oriented *regulation* require knowledge of the occurrence of the target problem of regulation—an industrial or health-care practice, for example—and of matters that have bearing on the feasibility and reasonableness of its solution by regulatory means. The associated evaluation work is a matter of quantifying the occurrence of compliance with the regulation in relation to potential impediments to the willingness or ability to comply. In the context of administrative research on health *service*, whether an innovation (demonstration project) or a routine (established program or practice), the concerns include the occurrence of various types of need or demand for the service, various response actions by the service, impediments to proper response, and so on. The concern is with frequencies of various occurrences, just as in scientific problems of the epidemiologic type. However, the states or events at issue commonly characterize health care more than health or illness per se, and the units of observation may not be persons but, for example, instances of care action. Most significantly, though, the concern is not with abstract issues of science but with here-and-now administrative problems of health-care action within a particular facility or agency for care (see Section 1.6).

As has been seen, epidemiologic research addresses both scientific and administrative problems of practically all areas of medicine. Thus the subject matter of epidemiologic research is catholic and incoherent and therefore does not constitute a field of knowledge per se. Instead, a multitude of medical sciences and areas of practice embody epidemiologic problems. Hence, cancer epidemiology is a specialty within oncology, malformation epidemiology within teratology, health-care epidemiology within health-care administration, and so on. In this regard epidemiology is akin to morphology, for example—an *aspect of various sciences and other fields* as opposed to a science or other subject-matter field in itself. (This feature of modern epidemiology has remained regrettably ill understood, and so there are journals, societies, and other forums of epidemiology—and academic departments besides—with completely catholic subject-matter coverage, in principle at least.)

The evolution of epidemiologic research has, however, maintained coherence in terms of the generic type of problem. Throughout, epidemiologic research has been concerned with the *frequency of occurrence* of illness and related phonomena (states and events) of health and health care. The *discipline* of such research, that is, the aggregate of *principles* of studying the occurrence of illness and related states and events, including those of health care, in man has also maintained coherence.

These principles are the subject of this text, under the board headings of study design and data analysis. In contrast to epidemiologic subject-matter, these principles constitute *general*, or *theoretical, epidemiology*.

1.2. GENERALITY OF THE EPIDEMIOLOGIC DISCIPLINE

It is apparent that the form of epidemiologic problems is not unique to medicine. There is research into the occurrence of phenomena other than medical ones, and into occurrence problems regarding nonhuman objects in addition to humans. Nor are the principles unique to medicine: the principles of occurrence research in medicine should be directly applicable to the study of occurrence in general, regardless of the nature of the state or event and of the unit of observation. Thus, the one who knows how to study the occurrence of sudden death in humans should know how to quantify the risk of airplane crash in relation to its determinants.

For a clear understanding of this generality it may be helpful to take note of some examples of problems that are *not* of the epidemiologic form.

EXAMPLE 1.1. Although the occurrence of malnutrition is an epidemiologic problem, the occurrence of famine is not. The reason is that malnutrition affects individuals in a population, whereas famine is an affliction of a population in the aggregate, rather than of its individuals. (One might think of a population of populations and thereby reach the epidemiologic formulation.)

EXAMPLE 1.2. The occurrence of individual violence is a problem of the epidemiologic form, but the occurrence of war is not.

EXAMPLE 1.3. In contrast to bankruptcy and frostbite, the occurrence of economic depression (national or global) and of exceptionally cold weather are not problems of the epidemiologic form.

EXAMPLE 1.4. The occurrence of *epidemics*, the focal concern of classical epidemiology—a coherent subject-matter field—is not a problem of the form characteristic of modern epidemiologic research. The scientific issues regarding epidemics are analogous to those of the genesis and spread of cancer in the individual, which are matters more of pathologic mechanisms and processes than of cancer epidemiology. The issues are also analogous to those in recurrent attacks of disease in the individual, epileptic seizures for example, where the focal concern is mechanisms of precipitation. The paradigm for modern epidemiology is not the study of epidemic but of *endemic* occurrence of illness.

Given the applicability of the formal aspects of the epidemiologic discipline of research not only to nonmedical states and events in man but to nonhuman objects as well, and given that epidemiology is not coherent as a science but only as a discipline, it would be good to replace the term ''epidemiology''—which refers to people—with something less specific, but an appealing suggestion has not yet been made. On the other hand it is worth noting that in some ways the principles, and to a large extent the factual content, of the discipline are quite peculiar to *medical* occurrence research, as they are dependent on professional value systems, biomedical and public health facts, ingrained patterns of thought and behavior, and so on. These matters, however, are generally outside the scope of this text.

1.3. OCCURRENCE RELATIONS AS THE ACTUAL OBJECTS: OCCURRENCE PARAMETERS, THEIR DETERMINANTS, AND MODIFIERS OF RELATIONS

It has been noted in the philosophy of science that any science is concerned with *functional relations* of its objects (Friend and Feibleman, 1937). This proposition is quite evidently tenable for epidemiologic objects of research. *Parameters of occurrence*, such as the incidence rate for a particular illness, are not constants of nature. Rather, their magnitudes generally depend on— are functions of—a variety of characteristics of individuals—constitutional, behavioral, and/or environmental. Such relations, even if only remotely credible, are generally the objects of medical occurrence research. For example, one is quite usually interested in learning whether the rate of occurrence of some particular illness depends on (is related to or is a function of) gender—regardless of whether there is any express reason to surmise that it might be.

EXAMPLE 1.5.   The prevalence of any given blood type based on the ABO antigen system, while constant over gender and essentially constant over age, is not a constant of nature. It varies by ethnic groupings, for example. Thus the prevalence must be quantified in relation to—as a function of— ethnic group.

EXAMPLE 1.6.   For the occurrence of various values of blood pressure among people, one descriptive parameter is the median of the pressure. (This is a value such that the prevalence of its exceedance is 50%.) This parameter, again, is not a constant of nature but depends on age and other characteristics of individuals. For the quantitative nature of the age relation of systolic blood pressure, a rule of thumb used to be that it is, in mm Hg, "100 plus age in years." This rule expresses a regression model—a regression function—of the form $P = A + B \times$ Age. In this example, P, the occurrence parameter, is the median of systolic blood pressure, $A = 100$ mm Hg, and $B = 1$ mm Hg/yr.

The characteristics on which the magnitude of an occurrence parameter depends (causally or otherwise) are *determinants* of the parameter. Thus, in the examples given above, ethnic grouping is a determinant of the prevalence of any given blood type, and age is a determinant of the median of systolic blood pressure. "Determinant" has no implication as to causality in science—any more than in everyday locution: the current age of a person is "determined" by his/her year of birth (noncausally), just as the expected outcome of a disease is "determined" by the treatment that is used (causally).

The relation of an occurrence measure to a determinant, or a set of determinants, is naturally termed an *occurrence relation* or an *occurrence function*. These relations are in general the objects of epidemiologic research.

Even though the general inconstancy of occurrence parameters leads to the consideration of occurrence relations, this latter outlook affords only a partial accommodation of the inconstancy, because occurrence relations also vary according to the type of individual. In particular, measures of the degree of relation (Appendix 2) have determinants of their own.

EXAMPLE 1.7. Recall Example 1.6 and the occurrence function for systolic blood pressure therein. That function may apply reasonably well to populations with high consumption of sodium in the diet. However, in primitive populations with no "artificial" use of sodium, there is essentially no age trend in the level of blood pressure among adults. For this reason and others, it seems that sodium consumption is a determinant of the degree of the age relation of blood pressure (reflected by the *slope* of the regression relation). (See Figure 1.1.)

The subject characteristics on which a measure of occurrence relation (Appendix 2) depends—its determinants—are termed *modifiers* of the relation. Thus, the slope of the age relation of blood pressure is modified by sodium consumption (Example 1.7); measures of the age relation of the prevalence of immunity to measles are generally modified by crowding; measures of the age relation of the incidence of breast cancer are modified by gender; measures of the absolute efficacy of screening-and-treatment for tuberculosis are modified by socioeconomic status (because the prevalence of the disease depends on socioeconomic status); measures of the relation of mortality in coronary heart disease to bypass surgery are modified by what vessels are stenosed; and so on.

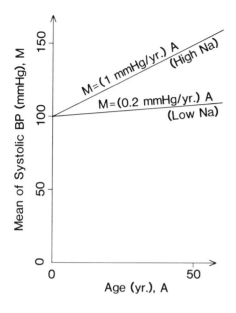

Figure 1.1. Mean systolic blood pressure in relation to age. The parameter of relation— the regression slope—is modified by the level of sodium consumption.

The existence and even the nature of modification can sometimes be surmised on general theoretical grounds. Consider, for example, the relation of the incidence of invasive cervical cancer to screening-and-intervention, as modified by the "background" rate. One would expect, in parsimonious terms, that such a program reduces the prevalence by a fraction that is invariant over the "background" rate, that is, that the preventive fraction is constant over the "background" rate (see Appendices 2 and 3). This means, in turn, that the difference in incidence according to intervention is modified by the "background" rate. This is illustrated in Figure 1.2.

In the context of a causal exposure, it is parsimonious to think of the proportion of people who are causally susceptible as proportional to the proportion of those on whom the illness would not develop in the absence of the cause at issue (see Appendix 3). Again the implication is that the rate difference (or regression slope) as a measure of relation of the parameter of occurrence (cohort incidence, see Appendix 1) to the determinant is modified by the "background" level of the parameter. This is illustrated in Figure 1.3.

A source of modification (of measures of occurrence relation) totally distinct from determinants of the "background" level of occurrence is arbitrariness in the choice of the occurrence parameter. Consider instances in which the "effect" of the determinant is additive with the "background" level of the parameter, as determined by some particular covariate (e.g., age). In these situations the covariate is a determinant of the intercept (the "background" level) but not of the slope (the measure of relation) of the basic occurrence function:

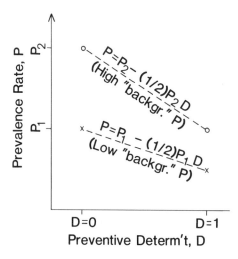

Figure 1.2. Prevalence in relation to preventive intervention, with the rate difference (regression coefficient) modified by "background" prevalence, in the context of invariant preventive fraction ($\frac{1}{2}$).

$$P = A + B_1(C) + B_2(D), \tag{1.1}$$

where P represents the occurence parameter, C the covariate, and D the determinant at issue; for example, P = incidence density of coronary heart disease, C = age, and D = indicator of cigarette smoking (D = 1 for smokers, D = 0 for nonsmokers). Here the intercept of the relation of P to D is

$$A' = A + B_1(C), \tag{1.2}$$

a quantity that depends on the covariate, whereas the slope (B_2) of the relation—the actual measure of relation—is invariant over it. If one con-

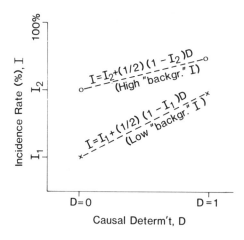

Figure 1.3. Incidence in relation to causal exposure, with the rate difference (regression coefficient) modified by "background" incidence, in the context of absolute effect proportional to the complement of the "background" incidence.

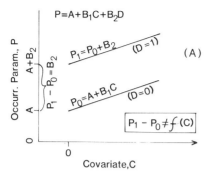

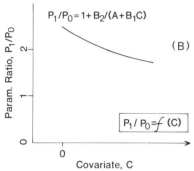

Figure 1.4. Relation of occurrence parameter P to a binary determinant D, with the intercept $A + B_1C$ but not the slope B_2 dependent on the covariate C. For the contrast ($D = 1$ vs. $D = 0$), the parameter difference ($P_1 - P_0$) is invariant over the covariate, but the parameter ratio (P_1/P_0) is modified by it.

siders the ratio of the occurrence parameter P to the value of its "background" level A', the relation shown in Equation 1.1 takes on the form

$$PR = 1 + \frac{B_2}{A'} D, \qquad (1.3)$$

where PR is the parameter ratio P/A'. In this reformulation of the occurrence relation in Equation 1.1, the covariate bears not on the intercept (as in Equation 1.1) but on the slope (through A'). Conversely, additivity with respect to the relative measure of occurrence, PR, means nonadditivity in terms of the corresponding absolute measure, P. This dependence of modification on the choice between absolute and relative measures of occurrence is illustrated in Figure 1.4.

Apart from modification by determinants of the "background" level of the occurrence parameter, and modification that results from the use of an arbitrary measure of occurrence, there is modification that reflects actual interdependence of effects between the determinant at issue and a particular other factor (see Appendix 3).

Modifiers of the relation of an occurrence parameter to a particular determinant are themselves also determinants of that parameter. The concept of modifier in the context of determinants at large results from a hierarchy

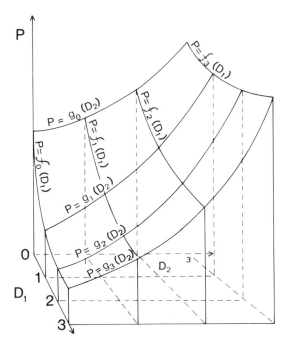

Figure 1.5. Relation of occurrence parameter P to determinants of D_1 and D_2. The relation of P to D_1 depends on D_2, and conversely, its relation to D_2 depends on D_1. The dependence involves the slopes (measures of relation) in addition to the intercepts ("background") levels. The slope variations imply mutual modification: the relation of P to D_1 is modified by D_2, and conversely.

of interests or concerns in any given instance. Thus, when the concern is with the age relation of the incidence of breast cancer, gender assumes a secondary role—that of a modifier of the relation of primary interest. Conversely, if the primary concern is with the gender relation of breast cancer incidence, age is viewed as a modifier of that relation. This interchangeability of roles is illustrated in Figure 1.5.

Determinants of incidence are commonly referred to as *risk factors*. This term is a misnomer. Since the relation of an occurrence parameter to a determinant need not be the result of a causal connection, and since the term "factor" (from the Latin word for doer) suggests causality, "risk factor" is not a proper substitute for "determinant of risk." A proper synonym is *risk indicator*—analogously with "economic indicator," "health indicator," and so on.

The terms "determinant," "risk indicator," and "modifier" refer to subject characteristics (including environmental) without specificity to category or level. Thus, "hypertension" is not a determinant of the risk of stroke; it is a high-risk category—an *indication* of high risk—based on blood pressure as the determinant or indicator of risk.

1.4. DESCRIPTIVE VS. CAUSAL RELATIONS

In medical occurrence research—and presumably in any research of this form—occurrence relations are viewed as either descriptive or causal. In a *descriptive* problem, a parameter of occurrence is related to a determinant without any view to causal interpretation of the relation. Descriptive occurrence relations are of interest for risk assessment or prognosis, diagnosis, allocation of case finding and other services, service evaluation, and other purposes. Etiologic insight and rational intervention, by contrast, rest on information about occurrence relations that may be interpreted in *causal* terms.

EXAMPLE 1.8.   The relation of the incidence (risk) of coronary heart disease (CHD) to age, gender, serum lipid levels, relative body weight, personality, blood type, and other personal characteristics, jointly, is of interest for *risk assessment* as to CHD. This use of the occurrence relation does not require any regard for causality.

EXAMPLE 1.9.   The descriptive relation in Example 1.8 is of consequence also for the *diagnosis* of CHD. But for the latter purpose one is more interested in the *prevalence* of CHD in relation not only to indicators of risk but also to potential *manifestations* of this disease—chest pain, electrocardiographic patterns, and the like. Again, the concern is merely with descriptive relations, not causal ones.

EXAMPLE 1.10.   Prevalence functions are of interest for the allocation of case-finding efforts, again with no regard for causality. In this sense one is interested in the relation of the prevalence of tuberculosis to age, area of residence, and socioeconomic status; the prevalence of venereal disease in relation to occupation; and so on.

EXAMPLE 1.11.   In normative evaluation of health care, actual practices are compared with norms for proper practice. This involves the acquisition of descriptive data. They might deal with the frequencies of various levels of quality (from malpractice to proper) in the treatment of breast cancer, related to type of disease manifestation, type of hospital, and so on. In the context of care for cases of myocardial infarction such data might deal with the duration of hospitalization, related complications, type of hospital, and so on.

EXAMPLE 1.12.   Consider the incidence of complications of the basic disease in adult diabetics in relation to treatment in the sense of insulin vs. no insulin. This relation is of interest in descriptive terms, since it characterizes prognosis in relation to the type of the disease—juvenile (Type I) vs. adult-onset (Type II). In causal terms it is devoid of interest, since the patients receiving the two types of treatment are very different (juvenile and adult-onset, respectively).

EXAMPLE 1.13.   The occurrence of complications in diabetes in relation to type of oral medication is of little or no descriptive interest, but in causal terms this relation is of major interest because it bears on the choice of therapy. Similarly, the risk of stroke or heart attack in hypertensives in relation to drug treatment is of major interest in causal terms but not descriptively. By contrast, the relation of mortality to heroin addiction is of interest in descriptive as well as causal terms.

As noted, descriptive relations bear on such passive matters as prognosis setting and risk assessment, whereas knowledge of causal relations is the basis for interventions, that is, for willful alterations of the outcome through perturbations in the determinant. For this reason, only strong relations are of descriptive interest, while knowledge of even minor causal relations is of value whenever the determinant is subject to ready interventive change. Such a change is particularly easy to accomplish when the determinant of concern is itself an intervention, with the choice between the options based on presumptions about relative benefit-risk characteristics.

1.5. CONDITIONAL RELATIONS: CONFOUNDERS

Causal interpretation of a crude (unconditional) empirical occurrence relation involves the premise that in the absence of the effect at issue there would have been no relation between the outcome parameter and the determinant. For example, the difference in mean blood pressure between treated and untreated hypertensives can be interpreted as a manifestation of the effect of the treatment only insofar as it can be presumed that, in the absence of the treatment effect, the treated would have shown the same mean of blood pressure as the nontreated. Hence, for causal interpretation of an unconditional occurrence relation, all *extraneous determinants* of the occurrence parameter must have suitably balanced distributions between/among the compared categories of the determinant. Thus, in the context of antihypertensive treatment discussed above, distributions by, for example, blood pressure before potential treatment should be similar between the treated and the untreated in order that the unconditional difference in the outcome parameter (mean blood pressure) have causal interpretation.

When an extraneous determinant of the occurrence parameter has imbalanced distributions between the compared categories of the determinant in a causality-oriented study, it is said to *confound* the crude relation, or to be a ''confounding factor'' for the relation under study.

EAMPLE 1.14.   Consider a pair of individuals: one is observing an ''antihypertensive'' diet (low sodium, high potassium, and high linoleic acid) and the other is not. Their difference in blood pressure cannot be viewed as the effect of the diet, unless there is assurance that in the absence of the treatment the two individuals would have had identical blood pressures.

Such assurance is unlikely. In particular, random allocation of the two persons to their respective dietary regimens provides no basis for presuming absence of confounding by the level of "natural" blood pressure.

EXAMPLE **1.15.** Consider two communities: one is subjected to an intervention program directed to blood pressure and the other is not. This is analogous to comparing two persons or two rats; the relative levels of blood pressure on follow-up cannot be interpreted in causal terms. That there are many individuals in each community is not much more relevant than the multicellular character of two compared persons or rats.

EXAMPLE **1.16.** When the treated and untreated series (of individuals or communities—of units of observation) are very large and the allocation of the units to treatment is based on randomization, there is a strong presumption that the occurrence measures for the two series would be essentially identical in the absence of any difference in treatment. Therefore, the empirical relation between treatment and outcome is essentially unconfounded and thus reflects the effect of the treatment.

EXAMPLE **1.17.** Suppose that no randomization is used, but the untreated are matched with those to be treated according to the "baseline" blood pressure. Again, there is no confounding—unless the "natural" course of blood pressure is apt to be different between the two series. In particular, even if these two series have different distributions by some determinant of blood pressure (such as age), this does not mean confounding by those extraneous determinants of the "baseline" level, except insofar as they also are determinants of the course of blood pressure conditional on the initial level.

EXAMPLE **1.18.** Consider focusing not on those *to be* treated but rather on those who *have been* treated for at least 5 years, for example, relative to those with no treatment. Suppose again that the untreated have been matched to the treated according to the "baseline" level of blood pressure. Now there is a good likelihood that the "natural" course of blood pressure would *not* have been similar between the treated and untreated. The reason is that the "natural" course of blood pressure has important bearing on the initially untreated remaining untreated and, differently, on the initially treated remaining under treatment. As a consequence, despite the matching on initial values, the treated, in the absence of the treatment, would likely have had higher "natural" blood pressures than the untreated. Thus, confounding by the indication for treatment—its inception and continuation—could persist.

Where the crude (unconditional) occurrence relation is confounded by a particular covariate, the relation that is *conditional* on that factor is still free of such confounding.

EXAMPLE **1.19.** Suppose blood pressure (BP) is measured for "baseline" values (BP_0) on untreated people, and that treatment is initiated in some of these people. The effect of treatment among the treated at the time of the first follow-up visit cannot be assessed by comparing the treated group as a whole with a representative sample of the untreated, as the respective distributions by the level of "baseline" pressure are different. However, within narrow categories of the latter there is no such confounding.

EXAMPLE 1.20.   Another way of approaching the conditional relation is to fit the regression model $P = A + B_1 (\mathrm{BP_0}) + B_2D$, where P is the mean value of BP on follow-up and D is the determinant at issue—an indicator of treatment ($D = 1$ for treated, $D = 0$ for untreated). The effect of treatment is B_2.

Whereas conditioning by a particular confounder removes confounding by that factor, actual causal interpretation presupposes that such conditioning be applied with respect to *all* confounders. Thus, insofar as an empirical occurrence relation is to be interpreted in causal terms, it must have the structure

$$P = f(D \mid C), \tag{1.4}$$

where P is the occurrence parameter, C is the total set of confounders (C_1, C_2, . . .), f denotes functional relation, and "$\mid$" denotes "conditional on." The meaning of this expression is that the causal relation of P to D is manifest when D is permitted to vary while C remains fixed. The *effect* (see Appendices 2 and 3) of any given category (index category) of D relative to any chosen reference category of it is the *difference* between the respective values of P (value for the index category minus that for the reference category). As the conditioning itself is but a technicality, the fundamental challenge in nonexperimental research on causal relations is one of insight and judgment, one that has to do with the sufficiency of the set of extraneous factors that are being controlled by the conditioning.

In the context of *descriptive* problems there is no general imperative to consider *all* determinants of the outcome as potential confounders. Yet some conditionalities tend to be inherent in descriptive problems as well.

EXAMPLE 1.21.   To say that level of blood sugar is indicative of the risk of degenerative cardiovascular disease is vacuous insofar as it is only a rephrasing of the familiar relation between diabetes and accelerated atherosclerosis. For a relation of the risk of cardiovascular disease to glycemia level to be of prognostic interest, it must be conditional on diabetes status.

EXAMPLE 1.22.   Whereas the relation (if any) of the risk of degenerative cardiovascular disease to height is of prognostic interest unconditionally (in adults), its relation to weight is of interest only conditionally on height.

These considerations indicate that, with descriptive as well as causality-oriented problems, *certain occurrence relations are of interest only condi-*

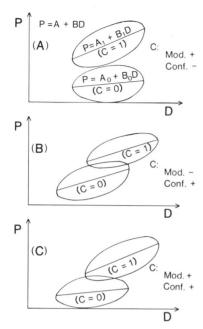

Figure 1.6. Relation of occurrence parameter P to determinant D, with a view to the role of covariate C. (A) C modifies the measure of relation B but does not confound it. If C is ignored, the average (in a sense) of the conditional slopes is obtained. (B) No modification, but confounding. (C) Modification and confounding.

tionally on some other determinants of the occurrence of the outcome at issue. Such other, extraneous determinants of the outcome are referred to as *potential confounders* of the conditional relation of interest. When such covariates have, in the study experience (study base), different distributions between/among the compared categories of the determinant under study, they constitute actual confounders—factors by which the analysis of the empirical occurrence relation must be conditioned in order that it address the causal (conditional) relation of interest.

The distinction between modification and confounding of occurrence relations (Miettinen, 1974a) tends to pose some difficulty for students of epidemiology. The key to understanding is to appreciate that modification has to do with details of the relation of interest, as illustrated by the regression lines in Figures 1.4 and 1.5, regardless of how the study subjects are distributed by the covariate (modifier), whereas confounding represents an impediment for learning about the conditional relation of interest, arising from an association between the determinant and the covariate and the latter's role as a determinant (extraneous) of the outcome. Modification is an aspect of the study object, and one may elect to study it for closer understanding of the relation at issue. By contrast, confounding is not an aspect of the object of study (the occurrence relation); it is to be removed or "controlled."

A graphical illustration of the distinction between modification and confounding is given in Figure 1.6.

There is no necessary relation between the modifying and confounding roles of a covariate. Thus, whether age does or does not confound a relation has no express implication as to whether age is a modifier of the relation to the determinant at issue, and conversely. This basic outlook applies with considerable force to the basic measure of relation, which is a rate difference (Section A.2.2) or, more generally, a difference of means (possibly expressed as a regression coefficient). Rate ratios and other relative measures of relation (Section A.2.2.2) tend to be modified by determinants of the outcome, including confounders.

1.6.   REFERENT OF THE RELATION: PARTICULARISTIC VS. ABSTRACT PROBLEMS

For an occurrence relation to have meaning, one must understand what it refers to, that is, in what realm or domain it is supposed to obtain. In this regard, research problems fall in two broad categories, particularistic and abstract.

In *particularistic* occurrence research the interest is in the occurrence of the phenomenon (state or event) of interest with express and singular reference to a particular population experience, specific in place and time. In medical occurrence research such particularism (spatiotemporal specificity) of the research problem is characteristic of administrative projects directed to description of the health profile of the community being served ("community diagnosis"), description of care utilization, evaluation of programs or practices, and the like. It is not difficult to imagine analogous needs for particularistic research among those responsible for the maintenance of fleets of aircraft, or for administrators of other programs directed to particular populations of subjects or objects.

Naturally, when the object of research is particularistic, the study is conducted in the framework of the very experience of express concern.

In *scientific* research, by contrast, the concern is not with any particularistic experience per se. Such experiences are only exploited to learn about the relation at issue in the abstract (in general), that is, without any spatiotemporal referent. For example, various particularistic research experiences, which are uninteresting per se, have led to the proposition that smoking causes lung cancer—an idea that does not refer to any particular place or time, a relation that for this reason is abstract (general). (Cf. Chapter 3.)

Scientific occurrence problems and results are not general in the sense of having to do with, or applying to, all sorts of persons (as to constitution, behavior, and environment). Thus, the antonym of "generality" in science is not "specificity" but, as pointed out above, "particularism." The aim is always to make the scientific generalizations as specific as possible: the more specific abstract propositions are, the more useful they are for theoretical development and for application. Thus, one is not really satisfied to know that smoking makes lung cancer incidence 10-fold; one is concerned to know the effect specifically for particular types of smoking on particular types of person (as to constitution, behavior, and environment).

Clearly, when the problem is abstract (scientific), the problem itself does not dictate a particular experience for consideration in empirical research; the specification of the experience in place and time is a matter of choice, a question of study design (cf. Chapter 3).

1.7. LEVELS OF STUDY

The point that occurrence research has to do with occurrence relations (Section 1.3) should not be interpreted too ambitiously. It does not mean that the relations are necessarily studied quantitatively, let alone in terms of the *absolute* magnitudes of, for example, the coefficients of such functions as were sketched in Section 1.3. It does not even mean that a relation is studied: the number of determinants in a descriptive occurrence study may well be zero.

1.7.1. Qualitative Exploration and Hypothesis Testing

The most elementary level of viewing an occurrence relation is the *qualitative* one. On this level, the question is *whether* there is a relation between the parameter of occurrence and the *potential* determinant at issue.

In the realm of qualitative questions, the most elementary one concerns the existence of an *unconditional* (crude) relation, a question that ignores all other potential determinants of the phenomenon at issue. On the next level one is concerned with the existence of an association *conditionally* on (within categories of) some other determinants, but still in the framework of purely *descriptive* relations. For example, the question may be whether relative body weight serves as a predictor of the occurrence of heart attack conditionally on blood pressure (which is associated with relative body weight and is also an indicator of the risk of heart attack). Finally, the concern may be with the existence of a *causal* relation. In this context, as has already been suggested (Section 1.5), the challenge is to identify and make allowance for—to condition the relation on—*all* confounders in the situation at issue.

Qualitative questions present a hierarchy also in terms of their origins. Questions may be elementary in the sense of having no express rationale, coming up simply in an exploratory context during a search for relations. Alternatively, a question may be rooted in a *hypothesis*—an idea originating from insight and creativity or simply "suggested" by previous data.

Qualitative questions about occurrence relations need not raise issues of modification. Thus, when Ziel and Finkle (1975) tested the hypothesis that the use of exogenous estrogen is conducive to endometrial cancer, they did not consider modification of the relation, by age even. Their concern was with the very existence of a causal relation, and since that remained in doubt even in the face of their data, it would have been premature to consider modification. They did present *data* on the *magnitude* of the empirical relation in their study base, but the purpose was to address the qualitative question of the existence, in the abstract, of a causal relation. It had bearing on the credibility of confounding as an explanation of the empirical relation. It also bore on the credibility of the data in terms of their ostensible implication—that 50% of endometrial cancer was attributable to the hormone use, even though the relation had not been noticed up to the time of their study.

In qualitative research it is common malpractice to regard *lack* of evidence of modification as evidence in favor of the hypothesis. In point of fact, it does not add to the evidence that the relation was apparent "consistently" in all categories of age, for example. By the same token, the persuasiveness of the overall evidence is not diminished by evidence of modification of the relation according to a covariate.

Another common malpractice is entertaining modification in the absence of not only persuasive evidence for the relation in the aggregate but also any theoretical basis for the relation's confinement to the particular subdomain in which the evidence is (happens to be) strongest (see Section 9.3.3).

1.7.2. Quantification, Relative and Absolute

A level of research more ambitious than the qualitative one is quantification of the relation at issue. It may be viewed in either relative or absolute terms.

In relative quantification the concern is with the *ratio* of the magnitude of the occurrence parameter in any given (index) category of a determinant to that in a chosen reference category. For example, one may wish to quantify the incidence ratio of lung cancer contrasting smokers of two packs of cigarettes per day relative to those who never smoked, without seeking to learn the absolute magnitudes of the incidence rates in the compared categories of smoking (cf. Figure 1.4 and Appendix 2).

The outlook of relative quantification is very popular for three major reasons. First, in certain study situations, only relative magnitudes can be addressed (see Section 4.1). Second, relative magnitudes have the appeal of simplicity: there is only one quantity to consider instead of two, and it is dimensionless even when the absolute magnitudes are not. Finally, relative magnitude is commonly the essential aspect of quantitative interest; even when the absolute magnitudes are on hand, the main interest scientifically tends to be in their relative magnitudes (cf. Appendix 2).

Despite the appeal of relative quantification, there is a need for absolute occurrence relations, particularly in nonscientific contexts such as individualized prognosis-setting (descriptive relation) or individualized prediction of the effect of intervention (causal relation).

In the context of scientific (abstract-general) occurrence relations (see Section 1.6), the quantitative outlook involves a deep problem: the empirical relation generally includes only a small subset of the totality of modifiers of the relation (cf. Section 1.3). Thus, the quantitative pattern in the studied experience is not at all guaranteed to obtain *in general*. Indeed, there is substantial subtlety and difficulty in defining even the *meaning* of the target values of the parameters in the occurrence relation, except in the context of particularistic problems (cf. Section 9.1 and Appendix 5). Therefore, even in the scientific context, technical quantification is closely connected with the (particularistic) study experience itself (cf. Sections 4.1 and 9.1, and Appendix 5); anything beyond that—and such generalization is the real thrust of scientific research—remains judgmental.

PART 1

Study Design

OVERVIEW OF ISSUES OF DESIGN

"Design" means, in general, a vision and stipulation of an end result, as in "the design of a boat," but not a scheme for accomplishing an end, such as that for the construction of a boat defined by the design (blueprint). Both meanings can be given, however, to "study design" in epidemiologic research. Thus, this term can refer to the plan for the *end result* in the sense of the type and quantity of empirical information the study is to yield, and to stipulations regarding the process of securing that information.

Designing the type of end result of an epidemiologic study means making the transition from an informal concept of the research problem to an express definition of the occurrence relation to be studied. This involves design of the following elements:

1. The nature of the occurrence *relation* itself, including:
   a. The *outcome* state(s) or event(s) whose occurrence the study is to address.

21

    b.   The *parameter* in terms of which the population occurrence of that phenomenon is to be characterized in the study.

    c.   The *determinant(s)* (potential or known) to which the occurrence parameter will be related.

    d.   The *time relation* between the outcome and the determinant status.

    e.   *Modifiers* (potential or known) to be considered.

    f.   Potential *confounders* on which the empirical relation is to be conditioned (particularly in the context of causal research).

2.   The *domain* of the empirical occurrence relation, that is, the type of situation for which the occurrence relation is to be studied.

For the outcome itself, as well as for the determinant(s), modifiers, and confounders, the necessary stipulations include:

1.   The conceptual entity.

2.   Its conceptual scale.

3.   The corresponding empirical scale.

As for the domain of study, the aspects that require design consideration are those relevant to the generalizability of the empirical relation, and those affecting validity and/or efficiency of the study (within its domain).

In the design of the study process that is to lead to the type of end result that was designed for the study, the considerations are validity and efficiency alone. With a view to optimizing these two desiderata, design decisions have to be made on the following:

1.   The study *base* itself (the experience to be captured in the study) in terms of:

    a.   Membership of the base population, with the subissues of:

        i.   Eligibility criteria (which also determine whether the base population is a cohort or a dynamic population).

        ii.   Distribution matrix (distribution of the base experience according to the determinants under study, modifiers of the relations, and confounders).

        iii.   Size.

    b.   Duration of the time period for outcome information, and the timing of this period.

2. The approach to harvesting the information in the study base, in terms of the following:

   a. The sampling design (simple census vs. case-referent strategy).

   b. The scheme of information acquisition on the members of the sample(s).

All of these aspects of epidemiologic study design are examined in the chapters that follow (Chapters 2–5 especially).

2

Design of
the Occurrence Relation

2.1. OUTCOME PHENOMENON:
DEFINITIONS, CONCEPTUAL AND EMPIRICAL

Epidemiologic problems of research, as they were defined in Chapter 1, have to do with *occurrence of phenomena* (states or events) among people or other units. Yet the basic problem—the research idea—does not necessarily imply any express definition of even the phenomenon at issue. Thus, that definition can be the first concern in study design. For example, the intent to evaluate the utility of rehabilitation after heart attack does not in and of itself imply what composite of various aspects of health and satisfaction is to be considered as the outcome criterion in the study subjects. Similarly, if an environmental factor is hypothesized to be conducive to degenerative cardiovascular disease, it is not obvious what empirical entity might be used as the index of vascular status in the study.

The key principle in the design of this aspect of a study is the imperative to distinguish between *conceptual* entities and scales on the one hand and their *empirical/operational* counterparts on the other. For the latter, any complex set of empirical items must be translated to an overall, single *index* of the conceptual entity; and when this is not feasible, a minimal set of indices of major *aspects* of the core entity need to be stipulated. These indices (empirical entities) are to be formed, to the maximal extent possible, a priori, in the design phase of the study, and not simply in the analysis and, thereby, in light of the data. Finally, in the formation of the indices, one should seek to avoid undue use of ad hoc indices, that is, *standard* indices should be employed whenever they are deemed reasonably appropriate.

In many instances this is well ingrained in thought and practice.

Example 2.1.   When the conceptual interest is in the occurrence of myocardial infarction, one quite routinely thinks in terms of either "definite" event, "possible" event, or "no" event—that is, an empirical scale (of three possible realizations) that constitutes an index of the underlying, conceptual "truth" (binary). Such a scale summarizes the constituent empirical items— the relevant symptoms, signs, and laboratory findings. Also, standard indices such as the World Health Organization (1958) scale ("criteria") are in common use in this context. The main point is that there is no tendency to use the constituent criteria per se, but only in terms of the summary index, the diagnostic scale, which bears a close relation to the core conceptual scale at issue. In this example, the conceptual outcome-entity is myocardial infarction; its conceptual scale consists of the points "present" and "absent"; and the empirical scale may be that of "definite," "possible," or "no" infarction defined according to the WHO criteria.

In the other extreme, even the core conceptual entity is initially hazy, to say nothing about unavailability of an empirical scale or index of it. Yet the conceptual entity needs to be crystallized and the empirical scale or index needs to be developed as part of the design of the study.

Example 2.2.   In a national collaborative study in the United States, the object was to evaluate the drug Indomethacin (relative to both placebo and surgery) in the treatment of patent ductus arteriosus (PDA) in premature infants. The drug is supposed to close the ductus and, thereby, to stop the shunting of blood from the aorta to the pulmonary circulation, and this is supposed to have desirable secondary effects in various organ systems. On the other hand, the drug may have deleterious effects in terms of the very same, complex set of constituent criteria of clinical course and outcome during the short (1 year) follow-up period of the study. Separate evaluations in terms of each of the component criteria of outcome could have left the overall picture obscure. For the construction of an overall index of outcome, a prerequisite was the development of a proper conceptualization of "the value" of Indomethacin treatment—the core purpose of it. Closing the duct was but the most immediate goal. The outcome at 1 year of age also seemed to fall short of the mark. The ultimate goal, as it was gradually understood, was to improve over-all lifetime health for the baby. Therefore, the principle of aggregating the items of clinical experience in the first year of life became their *prognostic* implication, and the design task was to construct, de novo, a scale of lifetime prognosis for the type of infant under study (as none existed a priori). The scale aggregated all the constituent items into a point on a scale ranging from "excellent" to "poor" prognosis. A point of particular note is that the scale was developed despite considerable uncertainties as to the long-term prognostic implications of the component criteria. In this example, the conceptual outcome entity is utility of life, as it is determined by health-dependent quality and duration; the conceptual scale consists of the possible realizations of "normal" and so on; and the empirical scale is based on a scoring scheme developed specifically for the study. (See Miettinen et al., 1983.)

In instances intermediate between those of the examples given above, it may not be routine nor absolutely necessary to formulate the conceptual entity and the rest expressly, but it is very helpful, nevertheless.

EXAMPLE 2.3. Consider the conceptual entity of body weight. This is unlikely to be of research interest per se. Rather, the concern may be with degree of obesity, the relative quantity of adipose tissue. For this conceptual entity, the conceptual scale might be taken as the proportion of total body weight that is accounted for by adipose tissue. Since this proportion is difficult to measure, one would tend to settle for an index of it. Among the possible indices are several based on weight together with height (see Khosla and Lowe, 1967).

EXAMPLE 2.4. When the concern is with systemic blood pressure as the outcome entity, one usually considers either the systolic or the diastolic pressure, or both of them (separately). By contrast, when dealing with the pulmonary circulation, the custom is to consider the mean pressure instead of the systolic or the diastolic pressure. Moreover, in the latter context, the pressure is not viewed as an entity of interest per se. Indeed, it is rarely used, and when it is, it is viewed as an index of a more relevant entity, namely the resistance of the pulmonary vascular bed (Nadas and Fyler, 1972). In these same terms, one could take the view that on the systemic side research that is said to address blood pressure is actually directed to the conceptual entity of systemic vascular resistance. For this latter entity, the conceptual scale would usually be that of the product of absolute resistance and body-surface area. Insofar as this is how the outcome is conceptualized, measured value of blood pressure is but an index of it in empirical terms. Moreover, one would use neither systolic nor diastolic pressure as the index. Instead, one would aim at measuring the mean pressure, for which a commonly employed index is a weighted average of the systolic and diastolic pressure (with weights of $\frac{1}{3}$ and $\frac{2}{3}$, respectively). Added issues in the definition of the empirical index would be the technique and circumstances of the measurement of the pressure elements.

EXAMPLE 2.5. As yet another illustration, consider research on "diabetic control" [its relation to some particular determinant(s), in diabetics]. This term refers, in general, to the degree of hyperglycemia, commonly measured in terms of the fasting level of blood glucose. Suppose the object of the study is the relation of "diabetic control" to diet. The effect of the daily diet would scarcely be well manifest in the level of *fasting* blood glucose. Instead, the interest is, conceptually, in the typical 24-hour pattern of the glucose level, in the context of the routine diet. This might be thought of in terms of the mean level in the routine course of life. As an empirical index of the circadian mean, the proportion of glycosylated hemoglobin (Hb AlC) would seem to be superior to the fasting level of blood sugar (Gabbay et al., 1977).

2.2. OUTCOME PARAMETER:
PREVALENCE OR STATUS DISTRIBUTION
VS. INCIDENCE OR CHANGE DISTRIBUTION

With the empirical (operational) outcome scale specified, it is possible to characterize the outcome for any given *individual* in the study base, or to identify outcome events when a study base is under surveillance. Next there is a need for a measure, a parameter, to characterize the study base in the aggregate, that is, the experience of a *population* of individuals, with respect to the occurrence of the outcome(s) among its members.

If the concern is with a *state* of the *all-or-none* type, such as immunity to an infection or affliction with cancer, the population focus may be on the *prevalence* of its existence and/or the *incidence* of either its inception (among those who do not have it) or of its termination (among those who have it). Either way, the population frequency of occurrence is expressed as a *rate*. (For a discussion of the concepts of prevalence and incidence, and of the respective rates, see Appendix 1.) In the case of an all-or-none *event,* such as heart attack or death, the concern can be with its incidence only.

An all-or-none state or event is a special case of a *nominal-scale* outcome. The outcome may also be characterized in terms of an *ordinal* scale, with categories such as "none," "mild," "moderate," and "severe;" or it may be expressed on a *quantitative* scale, as in the case of blood pressure. In these more general contexts, the counterpart of prevalence is a cross-sectional *status distribution* of the health characteristic among individuals. Thus, whereas one might consider the prevalence of "hypertension" or "normotension" (e.g., in relation to sodium consumption), which represents distribution on a dichotomous scale, one may, in the very same spirit, consider the distribution of blood pressure in greater detail. This means the consideration of the frequency distribution of blood pressure values in terms of a scale with several categories, that is, the consideration of the prevalence separately for each of several mutually exclusive and all-inclusive categories of blood pressure.

For the examination of cross-sectional status distribution the alternative is the longitudinal outlook—the consideration of *changes* of status over time and the distribution of those changes. The study of changes in this sense is not quite analogous to the study of incidence in cohorts. In cohort incidence (see Appendix 1), the initial state is fixed (every individual is a candidate), and the concern is with events *within* the risk period. In a distribution of changes, even if conditional on a particular initial value analogously with incidence, realizations *at the end* of the period are examined instead of events within it.

The study of prevalence, or status distribution, tends to be unattractive from the scientific point of view. The reason is that a parameter of this type is a reflection—a logical composite—of several component parameters, and the development of insight requires studying those components. As an illustration, consider the prevalence of premalignant skin lesion at a particular age, or the prevalence of hospital-acquired infection in patients still hospitalized a particular number of days after admission. Such a prevalence depends on the following component parameters:

1. The incidence of the condition (specific to time) previous to the time referent of the prevalence.
2. The incidence of cure among cases (according to time of case inception and the time lag since inception).
3. The incidence of fatality among cases (according to time of case inception and time lag since inception).
4. The incidence of termination of follow-up for other reasons, separately for cases and noncases (according to time).

If the magnitudes of these incidence parameters are known, the level of prevalence is known as a consequence.

In the context of a *quantitative* health characteristic, such as blood pressure, there is no general tendency for the study of status distribution (cross-sectionally) to be inferior to the study of change distributions (conditional on initial value, longitudinally), despite the general inferiority of prevalence studies relative to incidence studies (discussed above). There is a need to distinguish between two basic types of situation. One is the case of a stable, chronically active, determinant presumed to exert a cumulative effect; the other is one of a labile determinant presumed to have an acute and reversible effect. An example of the former is diabetes as a determinant of atherosclerosis; the latter is exemplified by diet as a determinant of blood sugar level in diabetes. Consider first the former case, with data obtained at two different points in the process. If the time interval in which the measurements are made (t_1 to t_2) is of short duration relative to that of the antecedent process (t_0 to t_1), at the time of the earliest observation (t_1), the interest is not so much in the change(s) from one observation to another as in their average. By contrast, in the situation of presumed acute effect of a labile determinant, one is interested in changes among repeat observations—in the covariation between changes in the determinant and in the health characteristic.

2.3. DETERMINANT SCALE: VALIDITY OF CONTRASTS

Particularly in scientific occurrence studies directed to *causal* relations, the conceptualization and specification of the scale for the determinant(s) at issue, with a view to the contrasts of interest, constitute important and sometimes challenging problems. The key to successful design of a nonexperimental study in this area, as in general, is the emulation of experimentation (Hill, 1953).

The validity of clinical trials rests on three features:

1. The use of a "placebo" or "sham" treatment for comparison (in "explanatory" trials)—to assure *comparability of effects*.
2. The use of randomization (and possibly also "blocking")—to assure *comparability of populations*.
3. The use of "blinding"—to assure *comparability of information* (and, in part, of effects).

In nonexperimental research the goals of all three of these experimental procedures are pursued by *selectivity* in the formation of the empirical contrast (together with matching of the study base, blinding, and control of covariates in the analysis of the data).

2.3.1. Comparability of Effects

Consider the study of the effect of some exposure, such as may occur in a particular occupation, on the occurrence of a particular illness. Presumably, the experience of an exposed population will be compared with that of a nonexposed one. However, *nonexposure should not generally be taken simply as the absence of the exposure*. Just as in clinical trials the treatment under study is contrasted with a "placebo" or "sham" treatment, exposure in a nonexperimental study should be compared with what may reasonably pass as a corresponding "placebo" or "sham" category—as an appropriate *reference category* of the determinant.

The development of the definition of such a contrast, that is, of the index and reference categories on the empirical scale of the determinant, requires an express conceptualization of what aspect of the index category is under study—as the counterpart of the drug or operation in a clinical regimen (involving various concomitant features whose effects are not under study). Thus, in an occupational study the aspect of interest may be stress in an air controller's occupation, asbestos exposure among insulators, vibration in the case of lumberjacks, or microwave exposure among radar operators. With the factor at issue in the index domain thus specified, one aims at seeing to it that the residual effect of the index category (e.g., occupation) on the health outcome under study is replicated in the reference category. This requirement of *comparability of effects* generally calls for the use of a *subdomain of the nonexposure as the reference category* of the determinant. Those not meeting the criteria for either the index or the reference category fall in a third, "other," category of the determinant.

EXAMPLE 2.6.   In studying the effects of a particular occupation—of a particular *aspect* of it (see discussion above)—the index category of the determinant represents employment in that occupation, naturally. The reference category should generally consist of particular other occupations, chosen expressly with a view to comparability of effects with the index occupation in terms of various extraneous effects of the compared occupations on the outcome(s) under study (cf. Wang and Miettinen, 1982).

2.3.2. Comparability of Populations

The effect of the index category relative to the reference category is manifest in the empirical contrast only insofar as the compared populations, representing these two categories, respectively, are comparable. This *comparability of populations* means that in the absence of differences in effect, the outcomes of the compared populations could be expected to be identical—conditionally on whatever covariates will be controlled in the analysis. When individuals cannot be assigned randomly to the compared categories of the determinant, the empirical categories need to be defined with a view to such comparability of populations.

EXAMPLE 2.7.   Consider the study of the absolute effect of "antihypertensive" drug use as a preventive of stroke. For the determinant scale, the index category—that in which the effect occurs—would be the domain of such drug treatment (as defined) for "hypertension." The reference category would have to be the use of inert substances with indications interchangeable with those for "antihypertensive" drugs in order to assure comparability of populations in terms of "hypertension" of the same degree as that in the index category (cf. Example 1.18). In practice, representation of such a reference category is unlikely to be found.

EXAMPLE 2.8.   Consider the effect (absolute) of reserpine use as a cause of breast cancer. With the use of reserpine for "hypertension" as the index category of the determinant, the reference category could be taken as the use of any other treatment, without reserpine, for "hypertension"—providing that all nonreserpine treatments of "hypertension" can be presumed to be without effect on the risk of breast cancer. The use of this kind of reference category is important insofar as one believes in the evidence suggesting that blood pressure is a determinant of the risk of breast cancer, particularly if "control" of blood pressure in the analysis stage of the study will not be possible. Again, there remains a third, "other" category into which an individual may fall.

In occupational mortality studies comparability of populations means that the compared occupations must have similar forces of job entry and of job exit, insofar as these are related to indicators of risk for the mortality at issue, conditionally on controllable covariates (usually age and gender only).

Failure to appreciate this principle of contrast formation in the field of occupational health is at the root of the problem termed the *healthy worker effect* (McMichael, 1976), that is, the tendency for observed mortality rates in particular occupational populations to be lower than would be "expected" on the basis of national rates (with allowance for differences in the distributions by age and gender, race, and calendar time).

EXAMPLE 2.9.   Consider a population of employees on the payroll of a particular company as of a particular point in calendar time, and its mortality from some particular chronic disease in the ensuing 5-year period. The observed number of such deaths tends to be low relative to that "expected" on the basis of national death rates, even with suitable allowance for the structure of the occupational group in terms of age and gender (see Appendix 4). The main reasons for this are that persons with manifestations of the disease—and thereby high risk of death from it—tend not to seek employment in the company, and that those with the disease who are on the payroll tend to leave the company but not the nation. Thus, the "healthy worker effect" in this example results from *differential selection* into and out of the compared categories of the determinant, with the selection related to indicators of the risk for the health event at issue.

EXAMPLE 2.10.   For nightwatchmen, chronic-disease mortality within 5 years of first employment might be *higher* than would be expected on the basis of national rates, with allowance for age and gender. This "sick worker effect" would again result from differential selection into the compared categories, according to the risk of the outcome at issue.

EXAMPLE 2.11.   Consider evaluation of the preventive efficacy of exercise rehabilitation on patients during the first 6-month period after a myocardial infarction, comparing those who have "complied" with the regimen with those who have not. Suppose the outcome criterion is coronary mortality in the ensuing 1-year period. The migration out of the regimen is likely to be related to poor coronary status, which makes for "healthy complier effect" and renders the two groups incomparable (without adjustment for coronary status, which is infeasible).

EXAMPLE 2.12.   In "hypertension," cardiac arrhythmia, and many other conditions, the highest-risk patients are likely to be the best compliers, exhibiting a "sick complier effect" relative to noncompliers.

The "healthy worker effect"—or any healthy or sick "effect"—is but a monument to habitual malpractice in the formation of contrasts (Miettinen, 1982 c; Wang and Miettinen, 1982), a consequence of epidemiology's intellectual traditions in demography (in addition to the investigation of epidemics and the implementation of sample surveys) as against medical science (for which the paradigms might be pharmacologic laboratory studies and clinical trials). In the face of differential selection forces between/among the compared categories of the determinant, the need is to pursue a better *empirical scale* for the determinant, such that *differential selection* into and/or out of the compared categories would be minimized.

A somewhat different problem of comparability of populations arises in the context of exploring the effects, on current outcome, of *exposures at particular times,* current and past.

EXAMPLE 2.13. The incidence (density) of myocardial infarction in women 45–49 years of age may be of interest with reference not only to current oral contraceptive use but also to use, for example, 1–4, 5–9, and 10–19 years ago (Slone et al., 1981). Suppose the reference category of the determinant scale is taken as that of "never used." The formulation of the corresponding *index* categories involves some subtlety. Consider "current use." If one is studying the effect of current use, the operational category of current users will not do, because they display the effect of past use as well. Instead, the index category needs to be defined as current use *only*—in practice, as current use with no use, for example, more than 1 year ago. In like manner, to study the effect of use 1–5 years ago (relative to "never"), the index category is to be defined as use 1–5 years ago *only,* and so on.

That example illustrates the principle that where the concern is with effects of *exposure in particular subdomains* of time on current incidence, with any given individual potentially exposed in more than one subdomain, comparability of populations may require that the scale of the determinant be based on exposures that occurred *exclusively* in particular subdomains.

EXAMPLE 2.14. For the problem in Example 2.13, a suitable scale of oral contraceptive use might consist of the following categories:

1. Never used (reference category).
2. Current use "*only*" (with no use more than 1 year ago).
3. Past use *only,* 1–5 years ago *only.*
4. Past use *only,* 5–10 years ago *only.*
5. Past use *only,* 10–20 years ago *only.*
6. Other.

This principle of exclusivity of subdomain exposures is not specific to subdomains of *time*, but is completely general.

EXAMPLE 2.15. Consider as subdomains of current cigarette smoking the habits of smoking filter cigarettes and nonfilter cigarettes, respectively. If the interest is in the effect of each of them (relative to no current smoking), it is again necessary, for comparability of populations, to employ the exclusivity principle, and the scale of this determinant might consist of the following categories:

1. No current smoking of any kind (reference category).
2. Current filter cigarette smoking *only*.
3. Current nonfilter cigarette smoking *only*.
4. Other.

Rather than constructing a scale for a single determinant with such exclusivities, it is commonly preferable to think of separate determinants having to do with exposure in particular domains—of history, for example. For a discussion of this, see Section 18.2.1.4.

It is instructive to note that incomparabilities of effects as well as of populations in the construction of the empirical scale of the determinant are matters of *confounding* (see Section 1.5). Thus, comparability of effects means absence of confounding by extraneous aspects of the compared categories of the empirical scale of the determinant, while comparability of populations means absence of confounding by subject characteristics. As for the latter, when those exposed in one subdomain are contrasted to those not exposed in *any* of them, the contrast is confounded by the index group's exposures in the other subdomains—unless the exclusivity stipulation is used in the definition of the scale. If those exposed in a particular subdomain are compared with those not exposed in it, with no other constraints on either category, the possibility of (if not tendency for) confounding persists. Both groups can have exposures in other subdomains, and these are unlikely to be similar, except if the exposure can occur in the index domain only. This latter proviso, when not inherently satisfied in the study situation, is effected through scale construction applying the exclusivity principle.

It is useful to keep these two types of confounding separate, for it forces consideration of the entire range of problems of confounding. In particular, to bring comparability of effects into focus, it is helpful to consider whether randomization—which bears on comparability of populations only—would tend to assure that, with large series, the effect of the agent under study would be manifest in a valid way.

2.3.3. Comparability of Information

When the specification of the empirical scale of the determinant assures absence of confounding, it remains to assure validity in the sense of comparability of information as well. In prospective studies this is a nonissue in the formation of the contrast, insofar as any tendency for incomparability of outcome information can be corrected by blinding. But where blinding is not sufficient, or is impossible, the contrast itself must be such that there is no need for it.

This imperative of comparability of information can constitute a serious problem in nonexperimental studies with the outcome information based on routine documentation. Thus, in a study of occupational mortality, the awareness of the hazard in the index occupation can have bearing on the diagnosis of the illness of concern and on the willingness to attribute deaths to that illness. When this is the case, the reference occupation(s) must be selected with a view to comparability not only of effects and populations but of mortality information as well. Comparison of the index occupation with "the general population," while commonplace, tends to be unsatisfactory with respect to all three aspects of comparability between/among the empirical categories of the determinant (cf. Wang and Miettinen, 1982).

2.3.4. Epilogue

A proper *empirical scale* for the determinant has, then, the following essential features:

1. It consists of mutually exclusive, yet all-inclusive, categories (as does any scale).
2. It involves categories representing the index and reference domains, respectively, of the conceptual determinant of interest (together with possible "other" categories).
3. Its compared categories are mutually comparable, conditionally on whatever covariates can be controlled by matching the compared populations or by analytic procedures. This comparability needs to obtain with respect to the following:
   a. Extraneous aspects of the compared determinant categories themselves, influencing the outcome (comparability of effects).
   b. Extraneous characteristics of the populations representing the compared categories at the determinant—characteristics predictive of the outcome (comparability of populations).
   c. Accuracy of outcome information (comparability of information).

As illustrated, the contrasts on the scale need to be conceptualized a priori to provide for the necessary comparabilities in the design stage of the study.

The *conceptualization* of the scale of the determinant can pose some challenge, even in the absence of any risk of intractable confounding or incomparability of information. Consider a clinical trial as an example:

EXAMPLE 2.16. Recall Example 2.2, dealing with Indomethacin in the treatment of PDA in the premature infant. The esssence of the treatment scheme (Gersony et al., 1983) was as follows: Upon the diagnosis of "clinically significant" PDA, the babies were randomized into two treatment groups—usual medical therapy (UMT) plus Indomethacin and UMT alone (UMT plus "placebo"). This randomization defined Trial A. Where the Trial A therapy failed, a back-up therapy was invoked. If the treatment in Trial A involved Indomethacin, the back-up therapy was surgery. If "placebo" had been used, the baby was allocated randomly to either Indomethacin use or surgery. This randomization defined Trial B. In this phase, failure of Indomethacin treatment led to surgery, just as in Trial A. The point of subtlety here is that, despite the duality of two-treatment randomizations, the study involves a single determinant—the strategy of treatment, with three options:

1. Early use of UMT plus Indomethacin (upon diagnosis of "clinically significant" PDA), with surgical back-up in case of therapeutic failure.
2. Initial use of UMT only, with Indomethacin back-up in case of therapeutic failure, and with surgery as the back-up in case of failure of the Indomethacin back-up for the initial UMT.
3. Initial use of UMT only, with surgery as the back-up.

The randomization in Trial A is the basis for contrasting strategy 1 with the union of strategies 2 and 3, whereas Trial B addresses the relative merits of strategies 2 and 3.

Another example—concerning a nonexperimental study—may add further insight.

EXAMPLE 2.17.   Cardiac function was evaluated in patients operated for tetralogy of Fallot, contrasting those operated in infancy with those on whom the repair was delayed to a later age (Borow et al., 1980). Some of the patients in the latter group had undergone a previous palliative operation. In this study, the contrast of interest is not really that between postoperative patients at the two ages of repair—with confounding by palliative surgery. Instead, it is between the following two strategies of treatment:

1. Direct repair in infancy (no palliation before repair).
2. Repair deferred beyond infancy, with palliation before repair, as needed.

This being the contrast of interest, the asymmetry as to palliative surgery is inherent in the contrast and is not a matter of confounding. Such confounding as is there arises from another aspect of the contrast: instead of comparing those operated on in infancy with those operated on later, one should actually compare those operated on in infancy with those in whom the repair is delayed (strategy 1 vs. strategy 2). In the latter group, also identified as of the time of therapeutic decision (in infancy), only a subgroup survives the palliative surgery and other hazards to undergo the delayed repair.

2.4. RELATION: CROSS-SECTIONAL VS. LONGITUDINAL

Having opted for a particular parameter of occurrence, for example, incidence density or 5-year cohort incidence specific for various ages ($T = t$) in a particular range of age, and having set the scale(s) for the determinant(s) of main interest, the formulation of their interrelation involves an important question of time. The parameter at $T = t$, P_t, could be related to the simultaneous realization D_t of the determinant. In these terms the study would address the *cross-sectional* relation

$$P_t = f(D_t). \tag{2.1}$$

The broad alternative is a *longitudinal* relation, in which realization(s) at some previous time(s) is (are) considered:

$$P_t = f(D_{T<t}). \tag{2.2}$$

In practice, the distinction is not made formally, but with a view to the duration of the process that connects the health outcome to the determinant. Consider, as an example, 24-hour diet history relative to current outcome. With respect to blood sugar level it may be viewed as longitudinal information, whereas in the context of body weight or malnutrition it is cross-sectional.

If the determinant at issue is stable, such as blood type, the distinction between cross-sectional and longitudinal relations is moot.

At the other extreme, if the determinant is very unstable, the distinction is critically important: In the context of chronic etiology, as in the case of alcohol preventing coronary heart disease, there is a need for a broad characterization of the entire period of etiology, and realization at the time referent of the occurrence parameter will not do. When the etiologic period is very short, as in the context of alcohol causing accidents, the time referents of the occurrence parameter and the determinant must be close to each other, an unduly longitudinal formulation being inappropriate.

When the health state influences the determinant in addition to whatever effect the determinant has on the health aspect at issue, cross-sectional relations are of little interest. Examples of such reciprocity include physical exercise as a determinant of body weight or coronary heart disease; and "antihypertensive" treatment as a determinant of blood pressure. In instances like these, a longitudinal relation tends to be more informative, but it, too, may not be interpretable in terms of the one-way relation of interest.

2.5. MODIFIERS: TREATMENT

Decisions about the treatment of modification in a study are closely connected to the stage of knowledge at the time of the study.

Even though the elucidation of modification generally is not of concern in the design of a *qualitative* study (see Section 1.7.1), there is a desire to allocate the study experience to a *domain in which the relation is likely to be most readily apparent*. This need not be the domain of highest "background" level nor that of the largest "effect" (slope of relation). Rather, it is the domain where the "effect" is largest relative to the standard error of its estimate, that is, the domain of minimum coeffecient of variation for the estimate of the measure of association. Thus, as for the "background" level, the preference is for the *lowest-level* domains as long as the pattern of "effects" over the domains is closer to constancy than proportionality to the "background" level.

EXAMPLE 2.18.   Consider the hypothesis that exposure to carbon disulfide increases the risk of coronary heart disease (Hernberg et al., 1970). The exposure occurs in textile (viscose rayon) workers, in whom both genders are well represented. Thus, in designing a study to test this hypothesis, there arises the question of which gender is preferred for the study base. The disease is more common among males, and this might be taken to mean that a male cohort of workers would be more informative than a female cohort of the same size. However, if the effect in terms of the *rate difference is the same* in the two genders, females would be more informative. To see this, suppose a male cohort would be expected to show 100 cases, whereas for a female cohort of the same size the expected (null) number of cases would be 50, with both numbers based on ample reference information. If for the male cohort the empirical number of cases would be 120, the corresponding number for the female cohort would be 70 in the context of identical rate differences. For the male cohort, the chi square test statistic (1 degree of freedom; see Section 11.2) would take on the value $(120^{1/2} - 100^{1/2})^2/(1/4) = 3.6$. For a female cohort, the corresponding value would be $(70^{1/2} - 50^{1/2})/(1/4) = 6.7$. Thus, the evidence from the lower-risk cohort would be expected to be more persuasive. On the basis of coefficients of variation for the effect estimate with male and female cohorts, the conclusion is the same.

EXAMPLE 2.19.   Consider further Example 2.18, now on the presumption that the *rate ratio is the same* in the two genders, that is, that the absolute effect (rate difference) is proportional to the "background" rate. With rate ratio equal to 1.4 for both genders, the typical chi square value from a male cohort would be $(140^{1/2} - 100^{1/2})^2/(1/4) = 13.4$; with a female cohort it would be $(70^{1/2} - 50^{1/2})^2/(1/4) = 6.7$, as before. This suggests that with constancy (nonmodification) of rate ratio, the higher-risk category of the covariate is more informative for any given size of the study base.

As an added consideration, insofar as there are any surmises about the mechanisms of the potential effect and about *causal cofactors* (see Appendix 3), the design would tend to accent the domains in which these would imply *maximal effect* of the determinant under study (conditionally on the background level of the parameter).

When the existence of a relation is already "accepted," the problem is a *quantitative* one: how strong is the relation? The answer generally depends on the type of individual (constitution, behavior, and/or environment), as this influences either the "background" level of the parameter or has implications regarding the pattern of causal cofactors conditionally on the "background" level. Thus, in quantitative research the question of modification usually cannot be ignored. The main options for dealing with it are:

1. Not to study it, but to *describe* the study experience, in the aggregate, as to its distribution by the potential modifiers of concern, using either of the following:
   a. A "naturally" heterogeneous experience.
   b. A restricted, relatively homogeneous experience.
2. To *study* it (making it part of the empirical occurrence relation).

When modification is treated with the seriousness that it really deserves in quantitative research, the options are actually fewer:

1. Not to study it, but to confine the study to a homogeneous subdomain of the potential modifier.
2. To study it—with a design that assures sufficient variability of the modifier (potential or known) to assure reasonable informativeness as to the modification.

The choice between these two options depends on how interesting the modification issue is for the particular relation to be quantified, and how feasible each approach is.

2.6. CONFOUNDERS: IDENTIFICATION IN CONCEPT

As noted in Section 1.5, an empirical occurrence relation may be of interest only insofar as it addresses the relation conditionally on all potentially confounding factors. In the context of designing the occurrence relation, the first issue is the identification of all potential confounders conceptually.

The identification of potential confounders requires keen appreciation of their nature on the level of principle. The essence of confounding was delineated in Sections 1.5 and 2.3. The point of departure was that potential confounders are extraneous factors such that the empirical occurrence relation at issue is of interest only conditionally on these factors.

The most stringent meaning given to this conditionality was that of constancy, that is, that the relation is of interest only as it is manifest within domains defined in terms of narrow categories of each of these covariates— within age–gender categories, for example. An equivalent, yet "looser," meaning is that the relation is manifest when the *distribution* of each of these factors is balanced over the compared categories of the determinant at issue, as in the case of a matched study base. A definitely looser, yet sufficient, condition for "conditional" interpretation is that the *joint* distribution of the entire set of potential confounders be balanced over the compared categories of the determinant at issue.

All this still begs the meaning of "balanced." The ultimate point is that the joint distribution of the potential confounders in the compared categories be such that they imply the same expected frequency of occurrence for the outcome phenomenon of interest (Miettinen, 1976b). Thus, the determinant contrast could be represented by old women in one category and young men in the other—if it is known that these two types of subject have the same expected rate of occurrence for the outcome phenomenon. One final subtlety remains: this identity of expected rate of occurrence is to be thought of in the context of the reference category of the determinant at issue, because if both groups were to represent the index category there could be a difference as a result of modification instead of confounding (Miettinen, 1974a).

It is apparent that the identification of all potential confounders is tantamount to identifying all extraneous determinants of the magnitude of the outcome parameter—a generally infeasible task. Fortunately, it is commonly also unnecessary. As noted in Section 2.3, in experimental research one relies on the process of randomization to balance the entire, unknown set of extraneous determinants of the outcome, as far as subject characteristics are concerned, apart from chance imbalance (chance confounding). In non-experimental research the challenge regarding population comparability is to understand which determinants of the outcome parameter (potential confounders) are such that they directly affect "self-selection" into categories of the determinant under study. It suffices to control these in order that the occurrence relation be conditional on all extraneous determinants—other than extraneous aspects of the determinant in its empirical terms.

The identification of confounders on the level of principle is clearest when the "self-selection" is based on a medical decision. In the study of drug efficacy the treatment contrast is of interest in the domain of a particular indication for the treatment. In this realm the allocation of patients to the compared treatments is a matter of determinants of clinical decision-making, commonly only determinants of the parameter of efficacy outcome such as severity of the indication (Miettinen, 1980; 1983b). Insofar as the decision depends on contraindications for the compared treatments, the typical case is such that these are not determinants of the outcome measure for efficacy. Analogously, in the study of drug toxicity, contraindications are recognizable determinants of some of the relevant measures of outcome but not of others, whereas indications tend not to be outcome determinants at all, so that the studies commonly need not even be confined to the realm of indications (Miettinen, 1983b).

Analogous insights are commonly feasible in the context of studying nonmedical determinants just the same. Thus, when comparing two industrial plants (one implying exposure and the other not) as to the occurrence of lung cancer, one may be reasonably assured that a worker's choice between them, while dependent on area of residence and occupational skills, does not thereby, or otherwise, depend on such relevant characteristics as smoking history. In particular, it is most unlikely that the compared populations would be imbalanced in terms of genetic predisposition to lung cancer, especially if the compared plants are in reasonably close geographic proximity, so as to rule out ethnic differences in the worker populations.

In the other category of confounders—extraneous aspects of the empirical categories of the determinant (Section 2.3.1)—the identification of potential confounders should be guided by appreciation of an unfortunate "law of nature." *Determinants of the risk of illness tend to aggregate their high-risk implications within categories of type of determinant*—industrial, nutritional, behavioral, medical, and so on. Thus, those exposed to a particular toxic substance in industry are prone to be exposed to other such hazards; those with a particular nutritional deficiency are prone to have other deficiencies of nutrition ; those with a particular type of risk behavior are prone to exhibit other risk behavior; and those exposed to a particular hazardous drug are prone to be users of other hazardous drugs. The implication is that a positive *relation known to exist between a health parameter and a particular determinant is prone to be confounded (positively) by extraneous factors within the same genre of determinants.*

With the criteria understood in principle, it is a matter of general *subject-matter knowledge* and familiarity with the particular base that will be used to draw up a list of *potential* confounders. The list can often be reduced by appreciating that the concern is with confounding *conditionally* on the other factors that have already been taken into account.

As the criteria for confounders pertain to the *study base*, successful identification of the set of (potential) confounders to be considered in the study depends on a secure understanding of the base. As a matter of definition, the base of a study is the population experience exhibiting the occurrence relation to be captured by the study (Section 3.1).

EXAMPLE 2.20.   If the exposed (e.g., to carbon disulfide, as in Example 2.18) derive from one particular industrial plant and the reference experience is drawn from another particular plant without the exposure, the study base consists of the union of the follow-up experiences (for outcome) of the two series drawn from the two plants respectively. Thus, if the reference series is matched to the index (exposed) series by age, the age distributions in the determinant contrast (exposure vs. nonexposure) are balanced in the study base; hence, matching of the base will secure lack of confounding in it—by securing balance of the covariate distributions between/among the compared categories of the determinant within the study base.

EXAMPLE 2.21.   Consider further the contrast between the populations in the two industrial plants (Example 2.20), now on the assumption that the two series are not matched by age and have different distributions by this determinant of the outcome. Suppose both series are to be followed over a period of time to observe the occurrence of the event of interest, such as death from coronary heart disease. Suppose further that the strategy is to capture those cases and to draw a sample of the study base (exposed plus nonexposed) as the reference series. This strategy of harvesting the information in the base (Section 4.1) has no bearing on the definition of the base. Thus, even if the reference series (the base sample) is matched to the index series (the set of cases) by age, this has no bearing on the role of age as a confounder (cf. Section 4.3). (The more comprehensive concept of confounding—that of need for conditional analysis, discussed by Miettinen and Cook, 1981—has been rejected in this text.)

EXAMPLE 2.22.   Consider the occurrence of thromboembolism, in women of childbearing age, in relation to ABO blood type. One may approach the problem by first capturing a series of cases of the illness from the domain at issue (women of childbearing age) and classifying them according to the determinant (ABO blood type). It remains to ascertain what the distribution of the determinant is in the study base—some follow-up of women of childbearing age. Whatever it is as to its particulars, chances are that in that population there is no appreciable relation between blood type and age, so that age is not a confounder in the study base. Thus, to explore the blood-type distribution in the base, one might use a series of newborn girls (or boys for that matter). Even though it derives from outside the base, such a reference series does serve as a proxy for a sample of the base itself. And even though it derives from a domain of very different incidence of the illness than does the case series, there is no confounding by age (or gender): in the study base—among adult women—there is no relation between blood type and age, and therefore age does not satisfy one of the two criteria necessary for confounding in the base. If there should be a blood-type difference between adults and newborns, the series of newborns would be an improper proxy for a sample of the actual base (see Jick and Slone, 1969).

Further insight into these matters is given in Chapters 3 and 4.

2.7. CONFOUNDERS: OPERATIONAL IMPERFECTIONS

When confounding is strong, it is important to use accurate measures or indices of the confounders; otherwise the control of confounding will be incomplete. The matter deserves examination in terms of several examples.

EXAMPLE 2.23.   Consider two series of women, quite different in their distributions by socioeconomic status. Suppose they are stratified according to categories of the extent of husband's education. The subseries within any given stratum remain dissimilar as to socioeconomic status, so that confounding persists. The duration of education of the husband is quite an incomplete measure of *his* educational status, let alone *his* socioeconomic status; in any case, his status is an imperfect indicator of the status of the woman at issue.

EXAMPLE 2.24.   If two unmatched series are very different in their distributions by socioeconomic status, matching by neighborhood will not remove the problem totally, as neighborhood of residence is an incomplete index of socioeconomic class. There is variation of socioeconomic status within neighborhoods—and even within spouse pairs and sibships.

EXAMPLE 2.25. The risk of laryngeal cancer shows a positive relation to alcohol consumption, even after control of smoking habits (Rothman and Keller, 1972). The association between alcohol consumption and smoking is strong, and smoking is an extremely powerful discriminator of risk for laryngeal cancer. Therefore, since even the proper theoretical scale of smoking history is difficult to conceptualize for any given purpose, and since smoking history is subject to errors of reporting, it is possible that the association observed between alcohol consumption and laryngeal cancer conditionally on smoking habits is a result of inadequate characterization of those habits.

EXAMPLE 2.26. In the study of side effects of drugs, a rather common confounder is what one might term—following Illich (1976)—the degree of "medicalization" of the patient. A medicalized person—being a relatively heavy consumer of health services—is more likely than others to use various "life-style" or semielective drugs, such as sedatives, analgesics, and "antihypertensives." The likelihood of getting various asymptomatic conditions, such as gall stones, *diagnosed* is also relatively high. Control of this factor through the number of visits to a doctor during the past year will not achieve unconfoundedness. The reason is that the conceptual factor, "medicalization," is a *propensity* for care use, and actual use, over a limited period in particular, is not a good index of it—just as one's number of traffic accidents over the past year is not a good index of propensity for risk-taking.

EXAMPLE 2.27. In studies on the effect of physical exercise on the risk of heart attack, one seeks to control confounding by coronary status in terms of history of angina pectoris (Morris et al., 1973). It seems possible that in the domain of "no angina," cases of severe coronary atheroma are rarer among those engaging in heavy exercise than in sedentary people, because heavy exercise could have brought about anginal symptoms in such cases. By the same token, cases of "angina" in a heavy-exercise group would seem to represent a lesser degree of coronary atherosclerosis than in sedentary people. This problem (perhaps trivial in magnitude) would be avoided, in principle, by the use of a sedentary reference group which occasionally (e.g., once a year) engages in heavy exertion.

As the examples given above illustrate, the translation of conceptual confounders into operational criteria can involve major difficulties, even failures. There are times when critical consideration of these issues leads to the conclusion that a satisfactory nonexperimental study is not feasible; and in these instances, *a nonexperimental study may be worse than none at all*, so that the optimal study size is zero (cf. Section 3.2.3).

An outstanding domain of difficulties of this sort is research into the *efficacy,* or *intended* effects, of interventions (Miettinen, 1980, 1983b; Strom et al., 1983). Interventions are commonly prompted by an indication, a state or event that signifies the prospect of an untoward outcome. Thus, by the very rationality of decisions to intervene, the treated tend to differ from the untreated with respect to their outlooks for the outcome criterion in efficacy assessment; there tends to be *confounding by the indication*—usually such that the treated tend to have less favorable outcome than the untreated.

An added problem in efficacy research is that this confounding by indication is often difficult or impossible to deal with in nonexperimental terms for two reasons. First, the characterization of initial indication is often quite nebulous, even if done with great care. For example, a physician may record "baseline" blood pressures and other clinical findings in considerable detail, but the *patient's* willingness to initiate "antihypertensive" therapy may be influenced by unrecorded aspects of family history, vague symptoms, previous experience with such therapy, and the like. Second, with treatment that is more or less chronic and in its continuation dependent on the apparent response, this *feedback* creates a select set of patients. Their intrinsic prospects with respect to the outcome criteria are not implicit in the initial indication for intervention, and the subsequent indications for continuation tend not to be recorded in a comparable fashion between the compared groups. (cf. Example 1.18.)

These problems in efficacy research are not shared by side-effect research, whether the concern is with drugs, smoking, occupation, or whatever. Selection into these "exposures" tends to be unrelated to the intrinsic risk for the adverse outcome that the unintended effect promotes. Thus, in terms of the crucial problem of confounding, nonexperimental research is generally better suited for the study of unintended effects than the efficacy of particular intervention modalities, practices, or programs (Miettinen, 1980, 1983b).

2.8. DOMAIN OF THE RELATION

The empirical occurrence relation that the study is to capture (as a basis for generalization into the abstract, as discussed in Section 1.6) generally addresses a limited domain only. Examples of explicit constraints of this type for the empirical relation include the following:

1. Relation (causal) of coronary mortality to tolbutamide use *in patients with adult-onset diabetes not requiring insulin therapy* (University Group Diabetes Program, 1970).
2. Relation (causal) of the occurrence of complications of the disease to treatment *in borderline hypertensives* (Veterans Administration Cooperative Study Group on Antihypertensive Agents, 1970).

3. Relation (causal) of prognosis to therapy *in premature infants with PDA* (Gersony et al., 1983).
4. Relation (causal) of the incidence of myocardial infarction to smoking *in young women* (Slone et al., 1978).
5. Relation (descriptive) of the incidence of death to symptoms and histologic type *in patients with Hodgkin's disease treated with MOPP* (DeVita et al., 1980).
6. Relation (descriptive) of the incidence of coronary events to serum cholesterol level *in men with coronary heart disease* (The Coronary Drug Project Research Group, 1970).

In other instances the constraint in the empirical domain is less explicit but equally definite:

1. Relation (causal) of the incidence of endometrial cancer to the use of conjugated estrogen preparations *in human females with intact uterus* (Ziel and Finkle, 1975).
2. Relation (descriptive) of the incidence of coronary events to major indicators of risk *in humans without history of coronary heart disease* (Truett, Cornfield and Kannel, 1967).

The limitation of the domain of study may be inherent in the basic problem of research. For example, problems of treatment efficacy are specific to the type of indication for the treatment. Similarly, a toxicity problem may have an a priori confinement to the domain of subjects with the target organ (e.g., uterus). However, the limitation may be invoked in the pursuit of study validity and/or efficiency (sensitivity) in the absence of inherent limitation of domain in the basic problem of research (Section 2.5).

With the study domain limited in a particular way a priori, the study base is formed within that domain. In this realm the base represents further constraints—in terms of place and time of necessity, and commonly in other ways as well.

Among the added limitations, the one based on the availability of the subjects is of particularly common relevance. When a vast majority of the available subjects represents a particular category of a potential modifier of the relation, for example, one of the two genders, it is wise to limit the study domain to the majority category of the potential modifier (see Example 3.15). Otherwise, a careless reader of the study report presumes that the study result applies, in a direct technical sense, to both/all categories of the potential modifier—even though the bulk of the evidence derived from the majority domain of the (potential) modifier. Even if, for example, both genders were equally represented in the study experience, the overall result does not necessarily apply to both genders but to people of average gender—which is an empty category.

3

Design of
the Study Base

3.1. INTRODUCTION

As noted in Section 1.6, any empirical study has, by definition, some particularistic (spatiotemporally specific) experience as its *base,* and the results of the study apply in a direct, technical sense to that particular experience. The base thus is the direct *referent* of the empirical information. In science, this particularistic referent is uninteresting per se; it is only a source of learning about an abstract occurrence relation—about a function divorced from the particulars of place and time. In scientific research, therefore, specification of the study base is not inherent in the research problem but is a matter of *choice*—an aspect of the design of any empirical research project.

An authoritative committee on the design of epidemiologic studies (Moore, 1960) has proclaimed that

> The ideal epidemiological study would be based on probability samples from a very large population in order to permit generalization from the study group to the larger population with specifiable limits of precision.

This outlook is expressed in numerous other writings on nonexperimental or "quasi-experimental" (Campbell and Stanley, 1963) studies as well. As

46

it addresses the choice of the study base, it reflects recognition of the existence of the choice. Yet it is profoundly in error.

In science the generalization from the actual study experience is *not* made to a population of which the study experience is a sample in a technical sense of probability sampling. Such statistical sample-to-population inference (generalization) is characteristic of particularistic research only—where parameters of a *particularistic population* are the targets of inference. In science the generalization is from the actual study experience to the *abstract*, with no referent in place or time (cf. Section 1.6). Therefore, there is no point in trying to make the study experience a probability sample of a larger segment of particularistic reality. Indeed, in experimental research, which is generally considered to provide the paradigm for nonexperimental approaches (e.g., Hill, 1953), there is no principle to the effect that, for example, the rats in the experiment should ideally be a probability sample from "a very large population" of rats. Rather, it is well understood that the generalization from any experimental experience with a particular group of rats is to the generic, abstract domain of rats of the same kind (or even humans), and that this generalization is founded on judgment (as to the meaning of "same kind") rather than statistical sampling and technical sample-to-population inference.

It follows that in scientific research the study base is properly defined as *the population experience actually captured* ("harvested")—as a basis for learning about the abstract domain that it represents. What larger experience it may be a probability sample of is immaterial for the generalization and, thereby, for the conceptualization of the base. Hill (1953) exhorts those engaging in nonexperimental research to keep "the experimental approach firmly in mind." In the conceptualization of the base population in any nonexperimental study it is very helpful to keep in mind that *in a clinical trial the base is the follow-up experience of the patients actually enrolled in the study*. It helps further to appreciate that this definition remains unchanged even if the experience of such a randomized base is harvested by the strategy of monitoring the base population for the events of interest and then abstracting the data on these cases together with only a sample of the randomized base (cf. Example 2.21 and Section 4.1).

In the design of the study base, the key concerns are the following:

1. Membership of the base population.
   a. Admissibility: definition of the type of individual who is considered suitable for enrollment in the base population (admissibility criteria).
   b. Distribution matrix: rules for actual admissions within admissibility with a view to distributions, in the actually admitted (actual base) population, of the determinant(s), modifiers, and/or confounders.
   c. Size: how large the base population is to be.

2. Segment of the base population's course over time in which one is to consider the outcome phenomenon, that is, the empirical occurrence that constitutes the basis for learning.

3.2. MEMBERSHIP OF THE BASE POPULATION

3.2.1. Admissibility

The occurrence of illness, or of related states or events of health, is manifest in *populations* of individuals (cf. Section 2.2).

The term "population" has two meanings in epidemiology. One of them is that of "cohort," whereas the other refers to a dynamic population. These two types of population are distinguished by the types of admissibility criteria or by their implied types of *dynamics* of membership.

3.2.1.1. Cohort Admissibility

A *cohort* is a particular, "closed" set of individuals, an enumerable set of persons, all experiencing an admissibility-defining *event* in a domain that is restrictive in both place and time. Examples of cohort populations include:

1. Babies born to expectant mothers enrolled into a particular study.
2. People entering military service in a particular geographic area in a particular span of calendar time.
3. People dying in a particular region in a particular span of time.
4. People examined for diagnostic and risk indicators for coronary heart disease in a particular screening program in a particular domain of type of person (Section 2.8), place, and time.
5. People meeting particular criteria for coronary heart disease in that particular program and subdomain.
6. People enrolled into a particular clinical trial, on the basis of having the indication, lack of contraindications, and so on, together with presentation in a particular hospital in a particular span of time (calendar) and consent to participation.
7. People diagnosed at autopsy to have a particular disease in a particular hospital within a particular span of time.
8. People with a particular condition having a second evaluation, for example patients with unoperated ventricular septal defect having a repeat cardiac catheterization, in a particular hospital within a particular span of time.

The general definition implies that cohorts are closed, or *static,* as to membership (the Latin root of the word referring to enclosure). The criteria for membership are met as of a particular point in time, *zero time, t_0,* which tends to be quite individual. In the examples given above the zero times are the time of birth, conscription, death, screening, diagnosis, randomization, autopsy, and second evaluation, respectively. Once a person meets the admissibility criteria, he/she not only becomes a potential or actual member (see Section 3.2.2) of the cohort as of that time but, in the latter case, also remains a member of it for ever after (see Section 3.3).

A cohort's course is said to be *prospective* following the completion of criteria for membership (as of zero time); it is *retrospective* in "negative time," before the membership criteria are met. Thus in the context of the examples given above the cohort experience is prospective as of birth, conscription, death, screening, diagnosis, randomization, autopsy, and second evaluation, respectively. By the same token, the course before those qualifying events is retrospective.

EXAMPLE **3.1.** Axelson et al. (1978) conducted "A cohort study on trichloroethylene exposure and cancer mortality." The mortality of *exposed* people was explored in terms of a cohort, and the reference experience was that of the national dynamic population (of males). The initial cohort included all persons who, by virtue of working with the substance, had taken advantage of the Swedish producer's offer of free urine analysis for it, and on whom the record of such an analysis prior to 1970 was available at the time of the study (ca. 1977). The availability of the records was said to have been restricted by a company decision: "the earlier part of this register was considered 'useless' and therefore destroyed in 1967. Some files escaped however, apparently in a quite arbitrary manner, and are now utilized as the source of subjects in addition to the complete laboratory files available from 1967 on." Thus, initial admissibility into the exposed cohort required, technically, meeting both of the following criteria (hierarchical):

1. Urine analysis is performed in the producer's laboratory before 1970 (presumably because of working with the substance).
2. The record of the analysis escapes destruction in 1967—and all other threats to its availability at the time of the study.

The second criterion, when operating subsequent to the first one, was judged to amount to only random exclusion among those meeting the first criterion—random in the sense of having no relation to the cancer outcome under study. Insofar as this judgment was correct, only the first criterion had substantive relevance, that is, it alone defined the admissibility in substantive terms and, thus, the zero time of the cohort. Without this presumption the zero time could not have been taken to be simply the time of the first urine analysis but, instead, the time as of which the second criterion was met as well. In these technical terms the admissibility could not be satisfied before 1967 and perhaps not even before 1977 (the time of the study). The cohort-defining event in these latter terms was meeting the temporally last criterion, the availability of the record in 1977. This definition of the exposed population implied a particular identifiable and enumerable series of persons— 582 in number. "Since there were only 50 women . . . the women were excluded . . . " (cf. Section 2.8). This left 532 male members in the exposed cohort. That 14 of these were lost to follow-up (retrospective) is, as was recognized by the authors, immaterial to the *membership* of the cohort, but is a small failure in securing *information* on the exposed segment of the study base.

EXAMPLE **3.2.**   Tola et al.(1979) studied "Lung cancer mortality among foundry workers," with the goal of elucidating the particular aspects of foundry work that account for the previously noted excess in such mortality in this occupational domain. "The cohort from which the cases and controls were drawn comprised workers in 13 iron foundries. All male workers with at least one year's employment in an iron foundry were included. The starting point for inclusion in the cohort was set as early as the registers permitted. In some foundries the registers went back to the beginning of 1918. New entries were allowed until December 31, 1972." Thus an individual became a member of the cohort whose experience formed the study base upon meeting all four of the following admissibility criteria (there was no distinction between admissibility and actual admission):

1. Male.
2. At least 1 year of employment in one of the 13 foundries prior to 12/31/ 72.
3. Notation of that employment in the employer's registry.
4. Availability of that record to the investigators at the time of the study.

The authors evidently judged that the fourth criterion constituted no constraint beyond the first two and thus had no substantive bearing on the zero times of the members of the cohort. If the record retention had been judged to depend on the outcome as to lung cancer, it would have been important to appreciate that technically the zero time of the cohort was the time of the study (ca. 1977). (In these terms, the study was based on the retrospective segment of the cohort's experience, the recognition of which alerts one to the possibility of bias in the base experience; see Section 3.4.)

EXAMPLE 3.3.   Patel et al. (1978) studied "Tricuspid atresia: clinical course in 62 cases (1967–1974)," and attempted to relate the course to the position of the great arteries, the status of the pulmonary vasculature, and the strategy of treatment (surgical). For the definition of the cohort, only the following information was given: "The case notes of patients admitted for haemodynamic investigations between 1967 and 1974 were available. . . . Adequate data were available for 62 out of 71 consecutive patients. The remaining 9

patients lived overseas and there were insufficient follow-up data.'' Thus
the admissibility criteria were:

1. Cardiac catheterization with the diagnosis of tricuspid atresia in The
    Hospital for Sick Children, Great Ormond Street (from which the report
    came) in 1967–1974.
2. Availability of postcatheterization information up to the time of the study
    (ca. 1977).

Technically, this means that the patients were admitted only as of 1977. Yet
the authors evidently felt that the second criterion was of no consequence
to the results, considering that they took the cohort to be of size 62 instead
of 71. In these terms, with the premise subject to serious question, the zero
time for the cohort was the time of the catheterization.

EXAMPLE 3.4.   Recall Example 2.17, concerning the outcomes of two surgical strategies in tetralogy of Fallot. Three component cohorts were defined
and compared (as to left ventricular function):

1. One represented patients who had undergone repair before 2 years of
    age.
2. Another represented patients in whom the repair had been performed
    after 2 years of age.
3. The third represented absence of the disease.

Since the choice between the two surgical strategies is a concern in the
context of *infant* patients, it would have been more appropriate to define
the admissibility into the first two cohorts as follows:

1. Diagnosis and repair before 2 years of age (as above).
2. Diagnosis before 2 years of age, but repair deferred to a later age (with
    palliative surgery in the meantime, if needed).

Of the latter cohort, only a fraction would have been available for postoperative catheterization; the remainder would have had no cardiac function
at all, owing to antecedent death consequent to palliative surgery or due to
some other mechanism.

In the face of these potential subtleties in the definition of the zero time
of a cohort, it is a good practice to *remove the judgmental aspect by taking
the zero time to be the actual time of enrollment—by defining it operation-
ally*. The place of judgment, in these terms, is in the assessment of the
validity of retrospective experience of the cohort (Sections 3.3.4 and 3.4.3).

3.2.1.2. Dynamic Population Admissibility

In contrast to cohorts, *dynamic populations* do not consist of particular, static (closed) sets of individuals. They have, instead, turnover of membership over time; that is, their memberships are dynamic (open). The reason is that dynamic populations are defined in terms of qualifying *states,* for the duration of those states, instead of qualifying events, which provide for cohort membership in perpetuity. Thus examples of dynamic populations include the population of a particular town, the catchment population of a particular hospital, the membership of a particular health-insurance plan, and patients in a particular hospital.

The use of dynamic populations is characteristically associated with the use of the case-referent strategy of harvesting the experience (Section 4.1).

EXAMPLE **3.5.** Flodin et al. (1981) conducted "A case-referent study on acute myeloid leukemia, background radiation and exposure to solvents and other agents." The study was restricted to residents of Östergötland during 1972–1978. "The cases were primarily obtained from the Linköping University Hospital register of deaths, and all individuals with acute myeloid leukemia diagnosed during the study period were included." Thus a person was a member of the dynamic study-population (whose experience in 1972–1978 constituted the study base) for the span of time in which this person met the following criteria:

1. Resident of Östergötland.
2. In the event of acute myeloid leukemia, would go to the Linköping University Hospital, would be diagnosed and die there, and would be registered with the diagnosis in the hospital's registry of deaths.

EXAMPLE **3.6.** Ziel and Finkle (1975) discovered "Increased risk of endometrial carcinoma among users of conjugated estrogens." They enrolled all cases of the disease diagnosed at the Kaiser–Permanente Medical Center, Los Angeles, and reported to its cancer registry, in the period from 7/1/70 to 12/31/74. It is evident that they were monitoring the occurrence of the illness in the dynamic population that was the catchment population, for endometrial cancer, of the Kaiser–Permanente tumor registry in Los Angeles in that span of time. Thus the criteria for base admissibility were:

1. Membership in the Kaiser–Permanente plan.
2. Having a uterus.
3. In the event of endometrial cancer, would go to the Kaiser–Permanente Medical Center, with the illness diagnosed and also reported to the cancer registry of the Center.

Since the definition of a dynamic population does not involve any event, there is no inherent reference point for a distinction between prospective and retrospective experiences. A dynamic population has no inherent tendency for change over time; it can remain unchanging—*stationary*—in its profile in the context of its continual renewal over time. In particular, it has no inherent tendency for aging over time, in contrast to cohorts.

3.2.1.3. Admissibility in Population Cross Sections

The study of incidence requires population experience over time, either cohort or dynamic-population experience. The study of changes in health characteristics of individuals, such as blood pressure, also presupposes population movement over time. For this latter purpose, however, only cohort experience can be used.

However, *prevalence—or the distribution of a characteristic—*is manifest without any movement in time, since it has to do with the occurrence of states rather than events. Only the characterization of the status of a series of individuals as of a particular *point* in time is needed. For each individual the characterization refers to a particular instance in time, but those instances may vary among individuals. As a consequence, the prevalence itself, as a population characteristic, need not be "instantaneous." This is, incidentally, completely analogous with the definition of incidence. For example, the observation of 5-year incidence of bacterial endocarditis in patients with structural heart disease does not require, inherently, that the observation of the members of the cohort begin simultaneously in calendar time, in age, in time since diagnosis, or in any other aspect of time. In both prevalence and incidence observations, the individual information has a particular time referent, but the population parameter need not; it may involve, latently, averaging over the individual times of observation.

It follows from the nature of prevalence, and of outcome distribution in general, that it can be studied in a *population cross section* with respect to time. The population so viewed may be either a cohort or a dynamic population. In cross-sectional terms, members of the population, which is moving over time, are examined as of a particular point in time. This point, as was noted, need not be the same, in any sense, for the different individuals in the cross section. Thus, examples of population cross sections include:

1. Members of a cohort at zero time; for example, patients with a particular diagnosis at discharge from a particular hospital in a particular period of time.
2. Members of a cohort at the end of follow-up, the duration of which may be variable.
3. Members of a dynamic population at a particular point in calendar time.
4. Members of a dynamic population as of their respective times of sampling over a period of calendar time.

These examples illustrate the various ways in which a population cross section may be formed. It may be instructive to note that membership in population cross section is defined in a manner quite analogous to that of a cohort: there is an *event* in an individual's life *at the time of which* one is a member of the cross section. In the context of cohorts, there is also a membership-defining event; however, one is not a member of the cohort simply at the time of the event but for ever after. Thus, a population cross section can be thought of as a cohort considered (as to outcome) at its zero time only.

EXAMPLE 3.7. Hänninen et al. (1976) studied "Behavioral effects of long-term exposure to a mixture of organic solvents." In their study, "The exposed group consisted of 102 car painters . . . from all the car painters in Helsinki . . . " and "the nonexposed reference group was chosen from the employees of the Finnish State Railways . . . " in the same region, with both groups active in their respective occupations at the time of enrollment into the study base—at the time of the study (1975). The admissibility criteria were the following:

1. Employment with either one of the 27 car repair garages or the state railways in the Helsinki region at the time of the study.
2. Absence of brain damage attributable to causes other than solvent exposure.

Although these criteria were used to define a population cross section for the purpose of examining distributions of various aspects of *outcome at "baseline,"* they are completely analogous to defining a cohort for the purpose of assessing outcome on follow-up.

3.2.1.4. Base Membership Secondary to Case Selection

Some of the examples given above involve *primary* definition of the study base—which defines, secondarily, the realm of case identification. In others the definition of the base is *secondary* to case ascertainment. In these latter instances, cases are identified from some "registry" (e.g., a hospital) and the base is the experience of the population—generally dynamic—that is the source of those cases.

For the study of occurrence in such a secondary base, a keen appreciation of its definition is necessary. The base is not the population experience from which cases *could* have come to the registry in the observation period; it is that experience, the *totality* of it, from which each potential case, had it occurred, *would* have appeared in the registry (cf. Examples 3.5 and 3.6). Thus, an individual is a representative of the study base at a particular time if, were he/she to become a case at that time, he/she would appear in the registry and *would become a member of the case series* of the study. As noted, the base consists of the *entire* population experience that satisfies this criterion (Miettinen, 1985).

EXAMPLE 3.8. Suppose that cases of an *acute and serious* illness are identified from a particular hospital (over a particular period of time). The corresponding base is the population experience such that, had a case of the illness at issue developed during the study period, it would have been captured through the study hospital as a case in the study. This means, for example, that generally only experience within a *close distance* from the hospital belongs to the base. Moreover, even a member of the local population contributes to the study base only to the extent that he/she is within the catchment region of the hospital during the time of the study. However, local residents' experience within the region does not represent the entire base if nonresidents are included in the case series.

EXAMPLE 3.9. Suppose that the illness is *serious and chronic,* a form of cancer, for example. Now the base experience, for the cases at large, is not limited to the vicinity of the hospital (except if the case series is geographically restricted as to admissibility), particularly if the hospital is famous for its expertise on the illness. But population experience at a considerable distance is part of the base only insofar as the members of that population would seek care in the study hospital in the event of the illness at issue. This restriction on distant experience is not necessarily met by a case's neighbors, siblings, or friends, for example.

EXAMPLE 3.10. Suppose that the illness represents *elective* hospitalization. In this instance, apart from geographic considerations, the study base is restricted to those who, if they were to get the illness, would be hospitalized in the first place. This presupposes medical attention that leads to diagnosis and referral, and it requires willingness, means, and availability for hospitalization. Clearly, the base does not include the entire local "general population," nor are the cases' neighbors, siblings, or friends necessarily members of it.

These difficult issues are discussed further in Section 4.4.

3.2.1.5. *Place and Time in Admissibility*

Admissibility in terms of *place* and *time* in particularistic research is dictated by the research problem itself, but in scientific contexts those coordinates have no intrinsic relevance (cf. Sections 1.6, 3.1, and 9.1). In scientific studies, however, the selection of study base in terms of place and time can be an important indirect means of achieving a desirable base in terms of the distribution matrix and other desiderata. Thus, felicitous choices as to the location of the base in place and time can help secure:

1. For the determinant(s), large variability.
2. For the modifiers to be studied, large variability.

3. For the confounders, limited range.
4. For the "background" level of the outcome parameter, and for other unstudied modifiers, an efficient and/or relevant domain of study.

These features represent desiderata with respect to *information density* in the base and the *generalizability* of the results to domains of high-priority concern.

In addition, the specifications of place and time can have implications, again indirectly, for base desiderata in terms of *harvesting* the information inherent in the base. These have to do with:

1. The quality and thoroughness of the procured information.
2. The unit cost of information procurement, monetary and other.

The quality and thoroughness of information can often be improved by the use of a base whose placement in time is in the future, as viewed from the vantage of the investigator at the inception of the study project. Such a *prospective* base is inherent in clinical trials and other experimental studies, since interventions for the sole purpose of information acquisition have to be planned with a view to research. In nonexperimental research, the use of a prospective base can provide for the procurement of information with accuracy unattainable for retrospective experience. Only if this opportunity actually exists and is utilized is information from a prospective base preferable to that from a retrospective one.

As for unit cost, particularly in terms of the duration of the research project, a prospective base is usually inferior to a historical or *retrospective* one.

In terms of place, the counterparts of those base locations in time are, again from the vantage of the investigator, relatively trivial. The base may be distant in location, or it may be local. Considerations of cost usually favor the latter.

3.2.2. Distribution Matrix

An empirical relation is not distorted by any manipulation of the distribution of the study base according to the elements in the occurrence relation—the determinant, the modifiers, and/or the confounders. For example, the empirical relation of body weight to gender does not depend on the gender distribution in the study base. As validity thus is a nonissue in this context, the design of the distribution of the study base according to those factors— the *distribution matrix*—is governed by efficiency considerations alone.

3.2.2.1. Distribution(s) of Determinant(s)

For a study to yield any information about an occurrence relation, the determinant must vary in the base. By the same token, the informativeness of the base increases with increasing variation of the determinant in the base, and it is maximal when the base shows *maximal variation of the determinant* among its members. This means that, for efficiency, the range of variation should be wide, and also that both extremes within the range should be heavily represented. In experimental studies this principle leads to the *allocation* of the subjects only to the extremes of the range under study, with equal numbers in each extreme ("two-point design"). To learn about the shape of the relation, a third group of subjects may be allocated to an intermediate category ("three-point design"), and so on. *In nonexperimental research the counterpart of allocation or assignment is selection.* This may mean felicitous specification of the base in terms of its general characteristics, place, and/or time, and it may mean selectivity within a particular source population.

EXAMPLE 3.11.   To study whether a particular occupational exposure is a cause of some particular illness, one might seek to enhance the variation of the determinant in the study base by choosing a population—in terms of a particular town, for example—in which both the exposure and the nonexposure are well represented (cf. Axelson's study of mortality in relation to arsenic exposure, 1978).

EXAMPLE 3.12.   Consider a study in which the main concern is with potential teratogenic effects of the embryo's exposure to drugs before or during organogenesis. Suppose mothers are enrolled during pregnancy, so that the history of drug use in early pregnancy is known at the outset. In such a study the final enrollment into the study should be made dependent on that drug use. Top priority, with up to 100% inclusion rate, should be given to those who did use a drug that is of concern and is subject to study. Since the use of any given drug in the critical stage of pregnancy is quite rare, each of the exposed subcohorts can be compared, without appreciable loss of information, with a single, rather small reference cohort of totally unexposed embryos. Thus, only a fraction of the mothers with no drug use in the critical period need to be enrolled. Considering the cost of follow-up, particularly if it extends well beyond birth, such selectivity could enhance the efficiency of the study base to a great extent (cf. Miettinen, 1982b).

EXAMPLE 3.13.   Consider a cohort study on the incidence of coronary heart disease as a function of a number of potential determinants—age, gender, serum lipid levels, blood pressure, smoking behavior, and so on. An initial survey reveals the distributions of these characteristics in the *source population* within which the cohort is to be formed. It shows that the individuals are of overtly different degrees of informativeness. There are the precious individuals with extreme values for all the determinants; there are those with average values for each (save gender); and the majority represent a variety of intermediate constellations of varying degrees of informativeness. Such information, available at the outset, can be used to advantage in the selection of individuals into the actual study base. Given the cost of follow-up, such selectivity could mean major gains in efficiency (cf. Miettinen, 1982b).

Where interest in the details of the occurrence relation throughout the range of a determinant precludes the use of the two-point design or even the three-point design, suggested in the examples given above, the recourse still is not that of settling for the distribution that prevails in the source population of the study base. That the distribution in the source is a "natural" one is no virtue. For example, natural distributions of the Gaussian ("normal") type are never considered worth simulating in experimental research; on the contrary, one would generally prefer the opposite—a U-shaped distribution of the determinant. To the extent that intermediate levels are studied beyond the three-point design, one generally aims at a uniform distribution.

EXAMPLE 3.14.   Recall Example 3.7. The admissible subjects in the source population were not enrolled indiscriminately into the study population. The distribution of solvent exposure among the exposed as well as between the exposed and nonexposed in the study base was the result of express design: "The exposed group . . . was chosen . . . so that subjects with various exposure times would be equally represented." Moreover, the number of subjects enrolled from the reference (nonexposed) category of the determinant was made equal to the number of exposed subjects.

3.2.2.2. Distribution of Modifiers

Factors that are construed as *modifiers,* potential or definite, of the relation under study are approached somewhat differently from the determinants themselves. As was discussed in the context of the design of the function (Section 2.5), modifiers may have bearing on the *choice of the domain* of study without their appearing in the empirical relation at all. For example, if gender is perceived as a potential modifier, the study may be confined to one gender. But when modification by a particular factor is being studied, its *distribution* within the study base should be chosen as deliberately as that of the determinant of most immediate concern. Thus, if gender is a likely modifier and both genders are to be studied, both must have appreciable and more or less equal representation in the base. A lop-sided distribution means insensitivity in qualitative research and imprecision in quantification. It also tends to be misleading: representation of both genders, even if very scanty for one, tends to be construed to mean that the overall result of the study applies to both genders. To avoid this problem, it is advisable to eliminate fringe groups from the study base, even in the analysis stage of the study.

EXAMPLE 3.15.   Recall Example 3.1 concerning a cohort study by Axelson et al. (1978). In the source of exposed subjects, comprising 582 persons, "there were only 50 women with three deaths . . . and only one caused by cancer (ovarial cancer)." For this reason "the women were excluded as not providing much information." These exclusions, late in the study, restricted the conceptual domain of the study (Section 2.8) to the male gender. At a trivial cost in the amount of information the study gained clarity: even a careless reader will understand that application of the results to the female gender is a matter of extrapolation from experience in the male domain. Had the 50 women been included in the base population, along with the 532 men, the actual basis for inference would have been essentially the same— but the careless reader could have thought that the conclusion of "probably no serious cancer hazard" has an appreciable empirical basis for both genders.

As for age, very generally a modifier of occurrence relations, the common practice in clinical trials as well as in nonexperimental studies is to have the distribution in the source population dictate, possibly within a somewhat restricted range, the age distribution of the actual study base. This practice has no model in laboratory research: one does not let the age distribution of the experimental animals in the source of their acquisition dictate their distribution within the experiment itself. When modification by age is to be studied, the basic options should be taken as those of the two-point design (loading the extremes of the range) and the three-point design (with an added, intermediate group). Only extreme scarcity in the availability of subjects can justify letting the distribution of the source population dictate the structure of the study base in regard to a central aspect of the occurrence relation to be studied (cf. Miettinen, 1982b).

3.2.2.3. Distributions of Confounders

Confounders, in contrast to the determinant, and to the modifiers of the effect of the latter, are extraneous to the relation under study. They are considered only in the sense of conditioning, or control, so as to achieve conditional interpretability for the relation (cf. Sections 1.5 and 2.6). Thus, when a factor is considered solely because of its potential for confounding, the basic impulse in study design is to *restrict* its distribution to a homogenous subdomain, such as one gender or a narrow range of age. When this cannot be effected, reduction of the range is of some value, but modification of the distribution ("marginal") within the range is not. The factor has to be controlled in the analysis anyway, and the efficiency and simplicity of the analysis, if stratified, is served by the reduced range; by contrast, the distribution within the range is generally immaterial in these, and other, regards.

3.2.2.4. Joint Distribution

So far, the distribution matrix has been viewed in terms of the univariate or "marginal" (unconditional) distributions of the three types of factor in the argument of an occurrence function. As to their *joint* distribution, the principles of design derive from the fact that categories of the determinant are going to be compared conditionally on both the modifiers and the confounders. The base serves this end ideally if the distribution of the modifier–confounder set is the same for the compared categories of the determinant. Therefore, it is among the goals of base design to maximize such *comparability* over the determinant range under study, particularly if the information in the base is sparse. In experimental studies this is pursued by the use of *randomized "blocks"* instead of "complete" randomization, the result of the "blocking" being that the compared categories of the determinant show identical joint distributions by certain modifiers and/or confounders. In non-experimental research the analogue of "blocking" is *matching:* the base groups in the compared categories of the determiant are made similar as to their distributions by modifiers and/or confounders, using *restricted selection*. Ordinarily, subjects in the category that has the most sparse representation in the source population of the base are admitted without restrictions; subjects from the other categories are drawn selectively, so as to achieve the desired similarity of distributions.

EXAMPLE 3.16.   Recall Examples 3.7 and 3.14, dealing with the effects of solvent exposure among car painters. The distribution of the determinant (as to duration of exposure) in the study base was the result of careful design (Example 3.14). Moreover, the distribution of age—a potential confounder—was made essentially identical between the exposed and nonexposed groups in the base population. Since exposed subjects were scarce, they were enrolled regardless of age. From the ample source of reference subjects (railway workers), members of the base population were selected so as to achieve an age distribution similar to that of the car painters. This selectivity could be effected without any appreciable cost, and its consequence was a gain in the statistical efficiency of the study—analogously with the implication of the randomized blocks—restricted randomization design—relative to the completely randomized design in experimentation.

3.2.3. Size

The size of the study base might be construed, in superficial terms, as the number of subjects or the amount of population time in it. This definition would imply homogeneity of information and unit cost over varying sizes of the base.

This implication is false. It is commonplace in epidemiologic study design to have substantive and/or efficiency preferences as to the determinant scale and distribution matrix; and expansion of the size tends to mean decreasing amount of information per unit size (size efficiency). Thus, within any given source population, the pursuit of more information tends to mean *compromises* as to:

1. The scale of the determinant (Section 2.3): where a smaller base would have been confined to sharply defined index and reference categories, the quest for a larger one tends to mean acceptance of more loosely defined categories.
2. The distribution of the determinant (Section 3.2.2.1): where a smaller base would have reflected the two-point or three-point design, an expanded one may have a distribution determined not by the wishes of the investigator but by the characteristics of the source population.
3. The distribution of a modifier (Section 3.2.2.2): where a smaller base would have been confined to a homogeneous domain of high informativeness and/or research priority, a larger one will extend into less attractive domains.

The contemplation of various alternative specifications of size for the study base involves consideration of their respective degrees of informativeness and cost. These need to be quantified, ideally in such a way that each may be compared, directly and meaningfully, among the contemplated alternatives.

For the quantification of *informativeness,* the first step is to develop a keen sense of the core analysis (Chapter 6). Whether the research problem is viewed qualitatively or quantitatively (Section 1.7), the most essential analysis addresses some parameter. For example, in qualitative research the question commonly is whether a particular rate ratio exceeds unity or, equivalently, whether the corresponding rate difference exceeds zero, conditionally on a particular set of confounders. An equivalent question is whether the coefficient of regression relating the outcome parameter to the determinant is larger than zero. In the context of even such qualitative problems, the essential result is generally an *interval estimate* of a suitable parameter, and this is all the more so in the context of the quantitative studies. What is needed, then, is the computation of such interval estimates corresponding to typical data (hypothetical) under different parameter values, performed separately for various contemplated size specifications.

Those same contemplated size specifications need to be characterized as to the particulars of all *cost*-relevant aspects—not only the size of the base population and the duration of its follow-up, but also its source population(s), ascertainment scheme, and so on.

When all this information is on hand, one may be able to decide that certain options are less cost-effective than particular alternatives to them. For example, the need to invoke added source populations, such as the catchment population of an additional hospital, tends to imply set-up and other costs that can make relatively small base increments associated with such expansion unattractive; one often prefers to extend the follow-up (of the dynamic catchment population) with a limited set of hospitals.

With such inputs, the ultimate choice of study size represents synthesis of the implications of one's best understanding of the precison and cost as a function of the size of the base, together with judgment about the validity of the study and surmise of the utility of the result on the presumption of validity. *On the first, and pivotal, level the decision is a binary one—the choice between zero and nonzero as the size.* Validity considerations alone are often sufficient to imply that zero is the optimal size; anything larger would have the negative consequence of misleading those with incomplete understanding of the lack of validity, in addition to the obvious problem of cost.

As for the realm of nonzero size, *it is but a misapprehension that the optimal size can be determined statistically.* In point of fact, those calculations have the target amount of information as an input; the calculation only specifies the size of the study that would produce the preset amount of information. The target amount of information as the input to the calculation is not the optimal amount. One reason is that the target amount in the statistical calculation is indeed set before the associated size—and thus cost—of the study is known, so that the target is not based on cost–benefit considerations. Another reason is that the impact of even the most promising study is unpredictable: the result is likely to become obsolete, but the timing of this demise is unpredictable in the face of the surprise potential in science, modern warfare, and other areas. There is no escape from the reality that the size of a study in the nonzero range cannot be optimized, statistically or otherwise. One is left to choose the size *judgmentally* in the light of the considerations outlined above.

A practical problem in this area of design is that statistical "sample size determination" tends to be required by groups that judge research proposals. One is to specify "α" or "type I error rate" (the choice is generally either 0.05 or 0.01), and "β" or "type II error rate" (the routine choice is either 0.10 or 0.20) against "Δ" or "the smallest difference worth detecting" (with no routine value). From these specifications it is possible to calculate the corresponding size of the study, given added inputs in terms of some "nuisance parameters," presumed precisions of observations, and so on. One can conform to this requirement in the practice of "normal science" by back-calculating the Δ that corresponds, for example, to α = 0.01 and β = 0.10 in the context of the size that one *judged* appropriate, and then offering this Δ-value as the "smallest difference worth detecting" in a formal "derivation" of the judgmental size.

3.3.   COVERAGE OF RISK PERIOD

3.3.1.   Follow-up of Entry Cohort

The concern with incidence, or with the time course of health characteristics such as blood pressure, often begins as of a particular event in the experience of individuals. Examples of such events include:

1. Birth (or the attainment of some other point in age).
2. Conscription (or some other "life event").
3. The diagnosis of a particular illness (or some other health event).
4. The commencement of smoking (or some other health-relevant habit).
5. First employment in a particular occupation of health concern (or first exposure to some other environmental hazard).
6. Surgery for a particular ailment (or the beginning of some other clinical intervention).
7. Removal of a particular organ (or some other health-relevant change in constitution).

In situations of this kind, the most natural study base is a cohort defined as of the event at issue—an *entry cohort*. A paradigm for such a base is that of a clinical trial, defined as of the inception of the intervention(s). If that paradigm is emulated in the study of the incidence of coronary heart disease as of age 35, for example, the base is the prospective experience of a cohort of 35-year-olds (free of the disease at that age). Similarly, occupational cohorts are defined as of the beginning of the work at issue and followed from that point forward.

With such a cohort, the incidence experience is drawn from the prospective segment of its course over time. Its determinants may be assessed as of the cohort's zero time, from the retrospective experience of the cohort, and/or during its follow-up. In experimental studies the determinant of main interest is not only intentionally perturbed at the cohort's zero time, but its status is also maintained during follow-up. In nonexperimental entry cohorts, however, changes in its status during follow-up are quite commonplace. As a consequence, the "baseline" status as to the exposure or whatever determinant in nonexperimental cohorts needs to be updated during the follow-up.

3.3.2. Follow-up of Oblique Cohort

In nonexperimental studies on incidence, or on changes in health characteristics, the cohort is often defined as of various times within the time period of interest rather than as of its beginning. Such an *oblique* cohort is then followed for an arbitrary period. The incidence information thus obtained tends to be sparse as to the earliest period after the onset of exposure or whatever event of interest. On the other hand, even a short follow-up of an oblique cohort permits the study of incidence long after the event. Long-term follow-up of an oblique cohort leads to an unattractive distribution of follow-up experience.

EXAMPLE 3.17. Consider the study of the incidence of coronary heart disease after 35 years of age, and suppose that a cohort base with only a 5-

year follow-up is used. In terms of an entry cohort, only the interval up to 40 years of age could be studied. By contrast, an oblique cohort, initially 35–65 years of age, would provide information for the age span from 35 to 70 years of age.

EXAMPLE 3.18.   Consider the same problem, but suppose that a 30-year follow-up is planned. An entry cohort would provide, apart from the attrition due to mortality, for even coverage of the age span from 35 to 65 years of age. By contrast, a cohort initially 35–65 years of age would yield very sparse information for the earliest part of this range, whereas for 65 years of age it would be as informative as the entry cohort. After 65 the proportion of the cohort contributing information would taper off, reaching zero at age 95 years.

It is evident that the coverage of a particular range of individual risk time in terms of a cohort base can be achieved through various combinations of the duration of follow-up in that risk period and the distribution of the cohort's zero time in it. One extreme is an entry cohort, formed as of the beginning of the risk period and followed to its end. The other extreme is an oblique cohort, distributed at its zero time over the entire risk period and followed for a minimal duration. For these extremes to be equally informative, the latter must be of much (in the limit infinitely) larger size.

3.3.3. Dynamic Population Coverage

A *dynamic* population provides for the coverage of a particular period of individual risk period, analogously with an oblique cohort, through its *distribution* over that period. However, its information, accruing over calendar time, can be increased at will without any inherent shift in its distribution in individual risk time.

EXAMPLE 3.19.   For the study of the incidence of coronary heart disease after 35 years of age, the base could be taken, for example, as the experience of a dynamic population, in that range of age, of some particular town. Its follow-up over time would entail the institution of whatever arrangements are necessary in order that the population's profile (status and history) as to the risk indicators of interest can be known over calendar time, and in order that for cases of the illness that information will be accessible. This might mean the institution of *periodic surveys* of the population to record, for *all* members, the desired information, given that the histories would not otherwise be obtainable. The other necessary arrangement would be the institution of a registry of the disease events, given that those events would not otherwise be recorded (cf. Miettinen, 1982b). This type of base for an incidence study is depicted in Figure 3.1.

3.3.4. Retrospective Coverage

Finally, incidence in a particular span of individual risk time might be studied on the basis of the *retrospective* experience of a cohort. In such a study,

A. Base

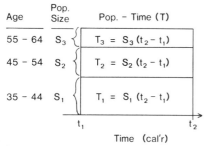

B. Case Registry

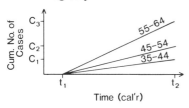

C. RATES: $R_i = C_i / T_i$

Figure 3.1. Dynamic base, covering a particular range of risk time (age) (see Example 3.19).

the zero times for the members of the cohort are subsequent to the beginning of the individual risk period. The cohort's zero times could have an oblique distribution across the interval of interest, or they can coincide with its end.

The retrospective experience of a cohort constitutes a *biased* base for incidence studies whenever previous occurrence of the illness at issue has bearing on the likelihood of becoming a member of the cohort (cf. Section 3.4).

EXAMPLE 3.20. Consider the study of the incidence of subacute bacterial endocarditis (SBE) as a complication of congenital heart disease. Suppose that the base is taken as the retrospective experience of all patients "currently" being "followed" by a particular cardiology service, that is, patients on record as of a particular point in calendar time. Suppose, too, that each patient's experience is considered back to the time that he or she was first seen at the service. Such a base is unbiased insofar as the occurrence of SBE has no bearing on the duration of follow-up by the clinic. This condition is violated by the potential of the event, SBE, for being fatal, and the consequence is a tendency for underestimation of the incidence. Another opportunity for bias to arise is that some patients who would no longer be followed by the clinic are being followed because of the occurrence of SBE. This latter type of connection between the event and membership in the cohort biases the apparent incidence upward.

The potential for bias associated with the use of the retrospective experience of a cohort may be on hand unwittingly, by virtue of a failure to appreciate that a cohort experience thought to be prospective is, in point of fact, retrospective.

EXAMPLE 3.21. Consider the study of the incidence of second primary cancer in patients treated for a first cancer in a particular institution over the past 20 years. One may consider the cohort to be defined as of the treatment for the first cancer, with follow-up from that time forward construed as representing the *prospective* experience of such a cohort. As a practical matter, however, the criteria for membership in the cohort involve not only treatment within the past 20 years but also current existence of a record indicating that such a treatment took place (cf. Section 3.2.1.1). If the records are maintained routinely, this is a nonissue. However, if some records get lost over time, the cohort is actually defined as of the time of the study (cf. Section 3.2.1.1). As a consequence, the experience becomes *retrospective*—and biased if the development of a second primary cancer bears on maintenance of the record, that is, if there is a connection between the outcome event and the likelihood of membership in the "current" cohort. The typical consequence would be an upward bias in the empirical incidence.

3.4. BIASED BASE

The use of a base that is defined by commitment to a particular set of cases involves a risk for bias in the *definition* of the base (Section 3.2.1.4), and so does the use of the retrospective experience of a cohort (Section 3.3.4). There may, thus, be value in an examination of biased base as a topic unto itself, considering that it represents a somewhat subtle and very important concern in study design.

3.4.1. Censorship

For orientation, it may be well to observe that *the experience described in medical journals tends to constitute, in the aggregate, a biased base for learning about any given issue*. The meaning of this is not that the subjects in any given study, or in all published studies combined, are atypical of the subjects to which one might wish to apply the results. Nor does it mean that the procedures, of intervention for example, applied in the published studies are atypical of procedures in that category in general. These limitations of published studies are inherent in scientific research; the concerns in scientific studies are specific, and the particulars of the study situation restrict the domain of generalization instead of making all generalization invalid.

The reason why *any* generalization, however restricted, from published studies tends to be invalid is that studies are not published simply on the basis of how informative they are about the object of study; an added, major consideration is the result itself. Scientific manuscripts are subjected not only to review of merit but to *result-oriented censorship* as well. For the journals to be a forum for unbiased evidence, that is, a basis for valid inference, the sole criterion for the decision to publish would have to be, apart from the topic itself, the informativeness of the study. To this end, the editors would have to take the decision about publicaton on the basis of a manuscript from which the author has blanked out all the actual results, indicating only the terms in which the results would be presented. In epidemiology this would mean, for example, that tables with marginal totals would be shown, with the entries in the body of the table withheld from the editors before the decision about publication. Similarly, all the results-dependent words would be blanked out from the text.

Given the prevailing, institutionally enforced, bias in the medical literature at large, the question of biased base in particular studies could be said to be moot. Why pursue validity for potential components of the aggregate evidence, when the ultimate, published evidence is a reflection of the biases of reviewers and editors anyway? For the cynic the answer is that impeccable validity of the study is likely to reduce the ability of referees and editors to apply censorship. For a true intellectual, the pragmatic question of acceptability is relatively moot; the ultimate issue is the truth itself, even if known to the investigator alone.

3.4.2. Result-Dependent Investigation

Closely related to the bias due to censorship by reviewers and editors is an *investigator's interest in a primary base, conditional on what it seems to show*. Thus, an investigator who explores a particular base with respect to a multitude of issues, and elects to submit for publication the data on a particular issue partly on the basis of what the data seem to show, engages in the same censorship as referees and editors. A truly responsible investigator collects only such data as he/she is also determined to submit for publication, regardless of what those data seem to imply.

Analogous to this result-selective publication from an a priori base is the *formation of the base conditionally on what it is likely to show*. Such a base tends to serve the documentation of the *exceptional,* instead of giving unbiased information about the typical. Generic examples of this include the following:

1. The impression of a remarkable frequency of a particular outcome following some treatment or other exposure may prompt an investigation of the actual rate, which involves documentation of the "denominator" in addition to the "numerator," together with a reference rate. The likely "finding" is a remarkable rate—as a documentation of an *exception* rather than as a basis for inferring the typical rate.
2. The impression that cases of a particular illness show a remarkable frequency of some particular antecedent exposure may prompt an explo-

ration of the exposure rate in the corresponding base experience. Given that the impression was indeed the result of insightful observation, the probe into the base is likely to confirm the impression—of an *exceptional association in the empirical realm*.

3.4.3. Outcome-Dependent Admissibility

Another category of biases in the study base has to do with *errors in the formation of a primary base, independent of what it seems to suggest*. For these biases the basis is *outcome-selective membership* in the base. The characteristic mechanism for this bias is the use of the retrospective experience of a cohort in instances in which membership of the cohort is dependent on experiencing the illness before the membership-defining event (cf. Examples 3.2, 3.3, 3.20, and 3.21). In these instances a study base that is biased with respect to absolute rates of occurrence need not be biased as to rate ratios. For the latter, differential sensitivity according to the compared categories of the determinant, or incomplete specificity is required (Section 5.6).

3.4.4. Outcome-Dependent Termination of Follow-up

Even when membership in the base population is unbiased, individual contributions to the base experience may be biased in incidence studies by virtue of the duration of follow-up being dependent on the outcome. For the end point of follow-up, the only generally unbiased criteria are:

1. The occurrence of the event under study (inception of the illness).
2. The attainment of the end of the individual risk period, whether that period is defined in substantive terms and is therefore variable, or whether it is arbitrarily fixed (see Appendix 1).
3. The end of the study in calendar time.

More specifically, the follow-up is to end on the basis of the particular one of these criteria that is met *first*. Any other criterion for the termination of the follow-up involves the potential for bias, in the sense that the duration of follow-up is outcome-dependent. Again, where such bias is a problem, it need not influence rate ratios; to do so, it has to be dependent on the determinant under study.

4

Design of
Sampling of the Base

4.1. THE CASE-REFERENT APPROACH: FUNDAMENTALS

The study base, as defined, is a segment of particularistic reality. It may be a population cross-section, a segment of the course of a cohort over individual risk time, or a dynamic-population experience over a period of calendar time. Being the empirical realm of outcome occurrence, it constitutes the direct *referent* of the empirical occurrence relation (cf. Section 1.6).

With the base (referent) defined, the next concern is to design a strategy for learning the relevant facts about it. The approach that suggests itself in the context of cross sections and cohort follow-ups is to ascertain the pertinent facts for *each individual* in the base. With a dynamic base there is a clearer distinction between two separate issues. One is the identification of the events and determination of their origins with respect to the subdomains of the base, and the other is the determination of the sizes of the various subdomains of the base, the candidate time (cf. Figure 3.1). Overall quantification of the dynamic base would be based on an ascertainment of its size as a function of time over the observation period. That information implies the average population size in the observation period, and the total candidate time is then the product of the average population size and the duration of the observation period. The sizes of subsegments of candidate time according to age and whatever history or status would be determined in like manner (cf. Figure 3.1).

The duality of fact-finding concerns inherent in the study of a dynamic-population base applies to population cross sections and cohort experiences as well. The need is to determine the two components for each of the rates specific for various categories of the base. The numbers of cases are needed for the numerators. For the denominators needed are the sizes of the respective categories of the study base, either the numbers of individuals (cross-section or cohort follow-up) or the amounts of population time (dynamic-population follow-up). Thus, the rates for the base, specific for the categories of the determinant, indexed by $i = 0, 1, \ldots$, are implicit in two information elements:

1. The total number of *cases, c,* distributed according to the categories of interest, that is, the set of numerator values $c_0, c_1, \ldots$.
2. The total size of the *base, B,* also distributed according to those categories, that is, the set of denominator values $B_0, B_1, \ldots$.

With this information, the rates for the various categories defined according to the determinant can be derived as

$$r_i = \frac{c_i}{B_i}, \qquad i = 0, 1, \ldots, \tag{4.1}$$

regardless of the dynamics of the base.

Given this duality, the question arises as to whether it is reasonable to examine and classify not only all the cases but the entire base as well. An alternative that suggests itself is the execution of two separate tasks:

1. Identification and classification of *all* of the *cases* (or, depending on the overall rate, all noncases), that is, the use of *census* representation of the actual numerator set $c_0, c_1, \ldots$.
2. Drawing a *sample* (of size b) of the *base* (of known size B), again classifying the individuals in the relevant regards, so as to obtain estimates Bb_i/b of the denominator elements B_i. In the context of a dynamic-population base, the concern is to sample population *time* to learn about the relative sizes of its subdomains, but procedurally this, too, is a matter of sampling individuals and classifying them (cf. Miettinen, 1976a).

This *case-base* or *case-referent* (case-"control") representation of the base experience can yield essentially complete information on the base—with considerable advantage in economy relative to the *simple census* approach, in which no sampling is employed.

EXAMPLE 4.1.   Consider again the study of the prevalence of congenital anomalies in relation to exposures in the embryonic period (Example 3.12).

Census representation of the base would lead to a very complex and voluminous data base, whose production would entail great effort and cost. An alternative is to secure all needed information in a timely fashion on data sheets, but *without any routine processing* of those data. Then, the records of cases of anomaly would be processed, together with those of a random *sample* of the entire cohort of newborns. The same strategy can be applied in data editing, starting from the putative cases of malformation.

EXAMPLE 4.2. Recall the dynamic-population study of the incidence of coronary heart disease considered in Example 3.19. The data for all cases in the registry would be processed routinely, but the records from the periodic surveys could be filed unprocessed, without reading the electrocardiographic tracings and so on. The appearance of each new case, however, would lead to processing of all of the case's survey samples and records. In addition, a few reference subjects from the then candidate pool would be identified (based on survey data close in time to the appearance of the case), and for these persons, data from all the surveys up to that time (but not automatically beyond) would be processed.

Sample representation of the base, jointly with the entire set of cases, can provide for quite thorough harvesting of the information in the base, even with a very low sampling fraction. In fact, *practically all the base information is abstracted as soon as the size of the base sample is a small multiple of the size of the case series* (see Appendix 5). This sampling ratio should obtain not only overall but within categories based on the modifiers and confounders considered in the study. If the distributions of the modifiers and/or confounders in the base are very different among the categories of the determinant, that is, in the case of poor comparability in the base (see Section 3.2.2.4) coupled with simple random sampling of it, a relatively larger reference series (base sample), if unmatched to the case series, is needed for thorough harvesting of the information. Commonly, such an imbalance arises from strong confounding in the base by simple characteristics, such as age or gender, or confounding of any strength by a factor measured on a highly polytomous scale.

EXAMPLE 4.3. Consider some occupational mortality study of coronary heart disease, contrasting a predominantly male occupation (index domain) to a set of others (reference domain) that involves equal representations of each gender. Insofar as gender is also a determinant of the risk of the disease, it must be treated as a confounder, that is, the occurrence relation must be made conditional on gender (cf. Sections 1.5 and 2.6). A base sample (simple random) that is, for example, fourfold in size relative to the case series is likely to be overabundant in the female stratum with very few cases; and, in the male stratum the base sample will be only about twice as large as the case series, which implies rather incomplete harvesting of the information available in this stratum of the base—the one in which the bulk of the information resides.

EXAMPLE **4.4.** Suppose genetic influences are being controlled by conditioning the occurrence relation by sibship. In the absence of matching, any given stratum would tend to be represented by either one case with no reference subjects or, conversely, by one reference subject and no cases. In such a situation, each stratum in the analysis is totally empty of comparative information. If full sibships are inherently included in the base and if the sampling fraction for the reference series is *very* high, the siblings of cases would tend to appear in the base sample, and thus the information in the base would be extracted. (A preferable alternative is to match the reference series to the case series by sibship; see Section 4.3.)

This case-referent (case-base or case-"control") approach to the ascertainment of the rates in the base is particularly economical when both of the following conditions obtain:

1. Complete study of the base entails substantial cost (over and beyond the survey or surveilance necessary for case identification and study of the cases).
2. A base sample large enough for near-maximal precision remains a small fraction of the maximal possible sample (census).

The second condition is satisfied in the context of cross-sectional and cohort bases whenever the outcome phenomenon under study is rare in all the base domains of interest. If the base is a dynamic-population experience, a sufficient sample of it is inherently a small fraction of the maximal possible sample.

In the presentation above, the alternative to a census representation of the entire study base was a combination of a census of the cases and a sample of the *base itself* (Miettinen, 1982b; 1985). The customary idea is to sample *noncases*. This distinction applies to population cross sections and to cohorts, but it is a nonissue in dynamic-population studies (Miettinen, 1976a). When there is a difference, it does not favor the case–noncase strategy over the case–base approach (see Appendix 6).

In *particularistic* research, with the base inherent as the *target population* in the research problem (Section 1.6), the case-referent representation of the base is quite analogous to the employment of a census in the exposed domain and only a sample in the nonexposed one. Both types of selective representation, when based on probability sampling, can provide for efficient learning about the a priori base (and referent) of the study—in the technical sense of sample-to-population inference.

In *scientific* research the analogy does not obtain, as there is no target population and, thereby, no a priori base (cf. Section 3.1). Thus, any ingenuity in the formulation of the distribution matrix is an aspect of the very *definition* of the base, not its sampling. For example, if the investigator loses part of the nonexposed experience in the original base (e.g., through destruction of the records), this accidental modification of the distribution matrix and study size means that the base will be redefined—and not that the residual experience will be viewed as a sample of the original base. It may be well to recall here that although there is no target population for a scientific study in any substantive sense, the base of such a study commonly derives from—or is nested in—a *source poulation*, which is an entity totally unrelated to target populations (cf. Section 3.2.2).

4.2. STRATIFIED SAMPLING OF CASES

Within the domain of admissibility, the cases may be very unevenly distributed over the relevant categories of a determinant of interest. In experimental studies this should not tend to happen, because there is full control over the distribution matrix. Nor should it tend to happen in nonexperimental cohort studies, whenever selectivity by the determinant in the formation of the cohort is readily implementable (see Section 3.2.2.1). However, attention to the distribution matrix in nonexperimental cohort studies is often casual or nonexistent, for practical reasons or because of an oversight. In dynamic-population follow-up the distribution of the determinant can sometimes be influenced by the choice of the base in place and/or time (cf. Section 3.2.1.5); but often there is little that can be done.

In the face of such skewness of the distribution of the determinant in the base it may be well to consider a second-stage employment of the principle underlying the case-referent approach itself—the use of a *census of the cases from the rarest category of the determinant and only a sample of those from the most abundantly represented one(s)*. Such selectivity is indicated when costly verification of, or detail on, the information on the determinant in the abundant category is needed; when expensive data acquisition on modifiers and/or confounders remains to be carried out after the determinant status/ history is known; and when data processing involves appreciable cost (cf. Miettinen, 1982b; Walker, 1982).

EXAMPLE 4.5.   Consider a retrospective study base for studying the occurrence of cancer as a possible complication of chronic coumadin medication in patients who have been treated for myocardial infarction in a particular set of hospitals. Suppose such a treatment in the hospitals at issue has been more the rule than the exception (as has been the case in the Netherlands). Then the majority of the cases of cancer in the study base have a history of coumadin medication, even if the "null hypothesis" is correct. The basic information as to whether such treatment took place could be obtained readily (e.g., from the roster of the Thrombosis Service), but for the details, possibly extensive medical records would have to be abstracted for the treated cases. This could entail considerable expense for travel and the like. If this is the case, it is reasonable to enroll only a sample of the cases that have a history of coumadin use with all the cases that do not have such a history.

The same principle applies to *modifiers* under express study. If the distribution matrix of the base is far from ideal as to the distribution of a modifier under study, the ascertainment of cases should be complete in the most sparsely represented category, but could be based on sampling in those cases that derive from modifier categories represented with relative overabundance in the base.

EXAMPLE **4.6.**   In any study of causal determinants for lung cancer other than smoking, the effect of interest is likely to be modified by smoking habit; and if the distribution of this factor were left uncontrolled in setting the design matrix, the vast majority of cases would tend to be smokers. In such a situation one would be keen on enrolling all cases who have *not* smoked, whereas among cases who *have* smoked, a sample would do.

It should be understood that with stratified sampling of the cases from the base, the pay-off is not simply the reduced effort and cost of studying the cases. The principal savings may derive from the consequent curtailment of the necessary sampling of the base itself.

4.3.   STRATIFIED SAMPLING OF THE BASE

In the preceding section we saw that the cases may sometimes be studied advantageously by the use of determinant- and/or modifier-stratified sampling of the total set of cases. In the sampling of the base, stratification is used very commonly—and to considerable advantage in study efficiency.

In the sampling of the base the concern is to learn about the *distribution of the determinant conditional on modifiers and confounders* (cf. Section 4.1). In a way, elementary case-referent inquiries are carried out within categories based on modifiers and/or confounders. Thus, the principles that guide the size of the base sample relative to the size of the case series in the context of no concern for modifiers or confounders (Section 4.1 and Appendix 5) guide the selection of sizes for the base samples within such strata of the base as well. A suitable "rule of thumb" is that, within each stratum, a base sample that is a few times as large as the set of cases provides for harvesting essentially all of the information within the stratum.

This principle suggests that efficient sampling of the base involves *matching* to the case distribution according to the modifiers and confounders by which the occurrence relation is conditioned in the study. Specifically, such matching would seem to be of interest whenever the stratum-specific base samples would not otherwise tend to be reasonably proportional to the respective numbers of cases. Moreover, where skewness of the distribution of the determinant justifies determinant-stratified sampling of cases, this same selectivity suggests itself in the base sampling as well.

The alternative to the use of a matched reference series is, generally, the use of a *larger unmatched* sample of the base. It needs to be larger when the occurrence of cases varies according to either the modifiers to be studied or the confounders to be controlled. Otherwise, in such a situation the base sample would tend to be relatively insufficient for harvesting the information from the strata that show proportionately more cases. In other words, an unmatched reference series would need to be larger because its relative insufficiency, resulting from variability among the strata in the ratio of the number of base representatives to the number of cases; for some strata it would be insufficient and for others more than sufficient.

EXAMPLE **4.7.** Suppose that the relation between an illness and a determinant needs to be examined conditionally on gender (either because of concern for modification by gender or so as to control confounding by gender). A matched sample of the base that is, for example, fourfold relative to the number of cases assures this same ratio for both strata, regardless of the relation of the occurrence of the illness to gender. As for an unmatched sample of the base, suppose that the illness is five times as common in males as in females, and both genders are equally represented in the study base. In this situation, the ratio of base representatives to cases would be 2.4:1 in the male stratum and 12:1 in the female stratum. This means incomplete harvesting of the information from the male domain, whereas for the female stratum the base sample is unnecessarily large.

EXAMPLE **4.8.** If, in Example 4.7, gender is not a determinant of the occurrence of the illness (unconditionally), the expected gender distribution of an unmatched sample of the base is the same as that of the case series. Thus, if both series are large, there tends to be no appreciable difference in the size efficiencies of the two approaches, that is, no reason for matching, despite conditional analysis. (Even if gender bears no relation to the occurrence of the illness unconditionally, it may be a confounder and/or modifier of the relation of the illness to the determinant under study.)

EXAMPLE **4.9.** Suppose that the control of confounding requires that the occurrence relation be examined conditionally on sibship. With matching it is realistic to pursue a reasonably constant ratio of the number of reference subjects to cases over the sibships. By contrast, a simple random sample of the base would tend to mean that the case series and the base sample come from totally nonoverlapping sets of sibships. This would mean that the ratios take on the values of zero and infinity only, with no comparative information deriving from any of the strata. (cf. Example 4.4.)

These examples illustrate the *efficiency implications of matching of the reference series (base sample) according to a factor (modifier or confounder) by which the analysis is to be conditioned*:

1. The gain in efficiency tends to be *minimal* if the matching factor is essentially unrelated to the outcome and is measured on a simple scale (ordinal or quantitative, or nominal with only a few categories), particularly if the number of subjects is large.

2. The gain in efficiency tends to be *substantial* if the matching factor is strongly related to the outcome and is measured on a simple scale, with the efficiency effect accentuated in the context of a small number of subjects.

3. The gain in efficiency is *critical* if the matching factor—a confounder—is measured on a nominal scale whose categories have very sparse representations in the study base.

Till now we have taken it as given that the analysis is to involve conditioning by the matching factor, that is, that the latter is to be treated as a potential modifier and/or confounder in the analysis. This is not always known in the design stage of a study, particularly in the context of potential confounders. It is therefore necessary to appreciate the effects of matching on size efficiency *in situations in which there is no inherent need for conditional analysis*, that is, where the matching would be motivated by a concern for confounding but the potential matching factor is *not a confounder*. The effect depends on the matching factor's relation to the determinant in the study base:

1. If the potential matching factor is *unrelated* to the determinant in the base, matching would be of no consequence; a matched sample of the base is interchangeable with an unmatched one.

2. If the potential matching factor is *related* to the determinant (but not the outcome) in the base, a matched reference series would be less informative than a simple random sample of the same size, that is, matching would *reduce* size efficiency (Miettinen, 1970b; Samuels, 1981). The reason is that, in such a situation, the variability of the determinant in the base is lesser conditionally on the matching factor than it is unconditionally.

EXAMPLE 4.10. Consider the occurrence of lung cancer in relation to smoking, and suppose that habitual match-carrying is entertained as a potential confounder. Suppose, too, that it is not a confounder by virtue of not being an indicator of the risk of the illness among nonsmokers. Suppose, finally, that match-carrying is perfectly correlated with smoking in the study base. If the reference series is drawn with matching on match-carrying, then the study is completely uninformative. For the rate ratio contrasting smokers to nonsmokers the estimate is $(c_1/b_1)/(c_0/b_0)$, with $c = c_1 + c_0$ and $b = b_1 + b_0$ the numbers of cases and base representatives, respectively, and the subindices 1 and 0 referring to smokers and nonsmokers, respectively.

For the stratum of match-carriers, $c_0 = b_0 = 0$, so that the estimate is indeterminate. For the other stratum, $c_1 = b_1 = 0$ and again the estimate is indeterminate. There is no information within either stratum because there is no intrastratum variability in the determinant. The problem is not resolved by ignoring the matching in the analysis, because the stratified sample of the base cannot be regarded as a simple random sample of the entire base, given the relation between the matching factor and the determinant. Such an erroneous analysis would show that $c_1/b_1 = c_0/b_0$, so that, the estimate equals unity, which is misleading.

It is important to appreciate that, as illustrated by this example, matching by a nonconfounding correlate of the determinant—"*overmatching*"—*has its price in terms of efficiency, not validity*. Insofar as there is an impression of "dilution" of the relation under study, this arises from a failure to appreciate the stratified nature of the base sample in the analysis of the data, that is, the need to condition the analysis by the matching factor.

When matching the base sample to the case series would enhance the size efficiency of the study, a countervailing consideration is its commonly high cost, that is, it may not be justified in the more relevant sense of *cost* efficiency. In addition, in situations where the relative sizes of the base strata are not known a priori, matching by the stratification factor makes it impossible to study its role as a determinant of the occurrence of the illness.

In the context of a secondary base (Section 4.4.2) the source of reference subjects (base representatives), when the same as that of cases, often implies nonrepresentativeness as to the distribution of confounders and/or modifiers in the study base, inadvertent near-matching perhaps. In these instances the question is whether *additional* matching is called for.

When all these considerations do lead to the decision to match, there arises the need to decide how large the base sample should be relative to the case series, that is, what the *matching ratio* should be. The choice depends on whether the base itself is fixed or expandable.

In the context of a *fixed base*, the key principle is that the informativeness of the study is proportional to $1/(1/c + 1/b)$, where c is the number of cases and b represents the size of the base series. Thus, when $b = c$, half of the information in the base is captured; and in the general case of $b/c = R$—a general matching ratio—this proportion is $R/(1 + R)$. This argument applies to studies with a dynamic-population base in general, and to studies with a cross-sectional or cohort base whenever the illness occurs in only a small proportion of the base population. Otherwise the information return for the sample exceeds the fraction of $R/(1 + R)$. Either way, the return is rapidly diminishing as R becomes larger, and ratios larger than $R = 5$ have little justification, even in the context of no cost for the expansion of the reference series (cf. Section 4.1).

If the base is *expandable* at will, as when following a particular dynamic base over calendar time or when such a base can be expanded geographically, the optimal ratio depends on the relative unit costs of the cases and base representatives. The optimal ratio is the inverse of the square root of the unit cost ratio (Miettinen, 1969; Appendix 7). Thus, if the finding and work-up of 10 reference subjects is the equivalent of adding one case in terms of cost, it is optimal to take $R = b/c = [(1/10)/1]^{-1/2} = 10^{1/2} = 3$.

4.4. VALID SAMPLING

Ascertainment and possible sampling of the cases in a particular base, or sampling of the base itself, is invalid (biased) if some feature of the subject enrollment scheme is conducive to a distorted result. The essence of valid sampling is that the probability of inclusion in the sample not have any inadvertent dependence on the determinant (and/or modifiers) under study. Such dependence of selection on the determinant can invalidate even qualitative inference.

4.4.1. Valid Sampling in the Context of a Primary Base

When the study base has been defined independently of the cases, the possibility of incomplete identification of the *cases*, with the degree of incompleteness dependent on the determinant, is the main problem. It results from one or more of the following mechanisms:

1. Diagnostic activity is influenced by the determinant, as in the case of suspected undesirable effects of treatments, occupational exposures, and the like.
2. The feasibility of the diagnosis is influenced by the determinant, as in the study of the occurrence of angina pectoris in relation to physical activity.
3. The recording of the diagnosis is influenced by the determinant, as in the context of legal implications related to the determinant.
4. The determinant, by virtue of a known and appreciable etiologic role, serves as a criterion for the diagnosis of an otherwise difficult-to-diagnose illness, as is the case of oral contraceptive use and suspected thromboembolism.

In all of these mechanisms, the *determinant itself* has bearing on the cases' coming to attention, as opposed to the determinant being associated with other factors bearing on case identification. The latter problem, involving an extraneous factor, is analogous to confounding and is thereby subject to control in the analysis stage of the study, given that the information on the confounder is recorded (cf. Sections 1.5 and 2.3.3). For biased ascertainment of the cases there is no such *post hoc* remedy, even in principle. The only potential remaining avenue, after biased ascertainment of cases, is to restrict the analysis to the subset that would have come to attention regardless of the determinant, by virtue of severity or some other factor.

Valid sampling of the primary base itself is a matter of general principles of probability sampling.

4.4.2. Valid Sampling in the Context of a Base Secondary to Cases

When the definition of the base is secondary to available cases (Section 3.2.1.4) the case series is a valid sample (a census) by definition, but unbiased sampling of the *base* poses challenges, considering that there is no roster of the base—no "sampling frame." The key to successful sampling of such a base is keen appreciation of its definition—namely, the entire population experience from which all potential cases would have been captured in the case series of the study (cf. Section 3.2.1.4). The reference series is to be representative of that population experience, or its matching categories, as to the distribution of the determinant. The challenge is to probe that base when case detection may possibly be dependent on the determinant under study, but more commonly on other relevant and uncontrollable factors.

4.4.2.1. The Ideal Reference Entity and Its Source

An idealized reference series, as a sample of that base would consist of a phenocopy of the illness under study, occurring independently of the determinant. Cases of that condition or event would come to attention by the very same mechanism that leads to the enrollment of the index series of the study if only a last-minute differential diagnosis separated them from the cases of interest. They would serve as a totally representative reference series. Sharing all the selectivity in the actual cases, they would indicate what the case series would have been like if the illness under study had occurred independently of the determinant: they would represent the distribution of the case series under the "null hypothesis," on which the occurrence of the illness under study has no relation to the determinant (conditionally on the confounders).

That ideal may be approximated by the use of a reference series consisting of *cases of another illness* under the following constraints:

1. Cases of the reference illness derive from the same "registry" (e.g., a hospital) as the index cases.
2. The reference illness itself satisfies the following criteria:
    a. It is unrelated to the determinant in its occurrence.
    b. It is similar to the illness under study as to relevant selection factors bearing on ultimate appearance in the "registry."

This approach can be much better than the use of neighbors or siblings, in Examples 3.8–3.10 for instance.

EXAMPLE **4.11.**   Recall Example 3.5, concerning a case-referent study on the etiology of acute myeloid leukemia, with the cases identified from the registry of deaths in the Linköping University Hospital in 1972–1978 and confined to residents of the Östergötland county. The base implicit in these admissibility criteria for the cases (and defined in Example 3.5) was sampled with stratification (matching) by age, gender, parish, and calendar time, by the use of cases of other deaths, as follows:

> . . . these cases were identified in the parish registers of deaths and burials, from which the referents were then chosen (all deaths are registered in the home parishes, irrespectively of where the individual has died . . .)
>
> Six referents for each case were chosen from the parish registers; they were those in the nearest three register positions before and after each case if they fulfilled certain requirements. They should be of the same gender as the case and similar in age (± 7 a) and without a cancer diagnosis . . .

To regard these reference subjects as having been *members* of the study base (at the time of death), it is necessary to assume that they satisfied (at the time of death) the membership criteria presented in Example 3.5. In particular, it is necessary to assume that if, instead of their actual terminal illnesses, these people would have come down with acute myeloid leukemia, they would have presented themselves in the Linköping University Hospital; and that, in the event of death there, that death would have been listed in the hospital's registry of deaths (in addition to the home parish), with the leukemia recorded as the cause of death. This assumption might have been more readily tenable had the reference subjects also been required to be registered in the hospital's registry of deaths in addition to the parish registries of the cases. To regard them as *representative* of the base (conditionally on age and gender, as to background radiation, etc.), it is necessary to assume, in addition, that the occurrence (and case fatality) rates of their causes of death were unrelated to background radiation, solvent use, and so on, and that the illnesses involved were similar to myeloid leukemia as reason for referral to, and admittance into, the hospital. The former concern about representativeness was the basis for excluding deaths due to cancer:

> . . . there might have been a relationship between cancer and the various risk factors for leukemia and the inclusion of cancer diagnoses among the referents would then result in a distortion of the exposure frequency among the referents as compared to the source population of the cases.

EXAMPLE **4.12.**   MacMahon et al. (1981) studied the role of coffee consumption in the etiology of pancreatic cancer. The selection of the cases implies that the base was the dynamic population experience of all Caucasian residents of the United States, 79 years of age or younger, who, had they come down with pancreatic cancer, would have presented themselves "in any of 11 large hospitals in the Boston metropolitan area and Rhode Island between October 1974 and August 1979." As a sample of this base,

> . . . the interviewers also attempted to question all other patients who were under the care of the same physician in the same hospital at the time of an interview with a patient with pancreatic cancer . . . patients with diseases of the pancreas or hepato-biliary tract or diseases known to be associated with smoking or alcohol consumption were excluded.

Moreover, the reference series, just as the cases, was restricted to Caucasian residents of the United States, 79 years of age or younger. It is apparent that the reference series did consist of *members* of the base. In particular, since they were treated by the same physicians as the cases were, it is reasonable to assume that they would have appeared in the case series had they had pancreatic cancer. The question of their *representativeness* of the base involves some subtle issues:

1. The study base (defined above) was not inherently free of "diseases of the pancreas or hepato-biliary tract or diseases known to be associated with smoking or alcohol consumption," since such conditions did not constitute exclusion criteria for the cases. Thus, whereas for the reference subjects the reasons for hospitalization, or *primary diagnoses*, had to be in their occurrence unrelated to *coffee* habits, exclusions according to *secondary* diagnoses of that, or any other, type were unjustified. (The report does not specify whether the exclusions were based on primary diagnoses alone or on secondary diagnoses as well.)

2. Representativeness also required the use of reference diagnoses (primary) such that the patients with those conditions *traveled*, or "gravitated," to the study hospitals in a manner similar to that of cases of pancreatic cancer. In point of fact, though, it seems that patients hospitalized for conditions such as breast cancer and cervical cancer, and particularly those with hernia, bowel obstruction, and the like, were more local in their geographic distribution than were the cases of pancreatic cancer. For a more judicious choice of the reference conditions in this regard, an alternative is the confinement of the base itself (cases as well as reference subjects) to geograhic proximity of the study hospitals (cf. Example 3.9).

EXAMPLE **4.13.** Consider the study of an analgesic in the etiology of an acute, rare, and serious disease such as agranulocytosis. With the cases identified in various specialty wards, one might entertain cases of trauma from the same hospital(s) as the reference series. However, the occurrence of trauma may well not be independent of the use of analgesics, since their indications may be related to risk-taking or -exposure, and their effects may include change in the ability to cope with risk situations (cf. International Agranulocytosis and Aplastic Anemia Study, 1983).

4.4.2.2. Inclusions vs. Exclusions

When employing a reference series constituted under the principles outlined above, uncertainties about the assumptions suggest the use of *more than one diagnostic entity* in the reference series; if they yield similar results, this provides assurance about the correctness of the assumptions.

However, *there is no virtue in using a wide variety of diagnoses.* Each diagnosis needs to be justified as to the assumptions, and insofar as they are untenable, the errors have no tendency to cancel out on the basis of the variety. In fact, the variety has the drawbacks of conceptual complexity together with insufficient representations of individual diagnoses for comparisons designed to verify, in part, the assumption of representativeness of the base, by their interchangeability as to the distribution of the determinant.

When considering inclusions and exclusions, one should be free of the occasional misapprehension that there is a need for the diagnostic distribution of the reference series to be representative of that of the noncases in the "registry." The reference series is to serve as a sample of the base (experience of the catchment population of the "registry"), rather than of entries in the "registry" itself. For this reason, the need is to have *defensible inclusions*, and there is *no need to defend exclusions.*

4.4.2.3. The Validity of Siblings and Neighbors

The complexities involved in achieving representativeness of the base by the use of a reference series from the "registry" through which the cases are identified does not mean that siblings or neighbors, for example, are preferable as reference subjects. The relevant covariates may not be constant within such strata (cf. Section 2.7), and reference subjects obtained on such a basis need not be members of the base (cf. Section 3.2.1.4 and Miettinen, 1985).

4.4.2.4. Reference Series from Outside the Base

Membership of the base itself is not, actually, a prerequisite for the reference series to serve as a source of valid information about the base; *the reference series can be drawn validly from outside the base* as long as the source population of the reference series is interchangeable with the actual base (as to the distribution of the determinant, conditionally on the modifiers and confounders accounted for in the analysis). The use of such a proxy for the base does not mean redefinition (expansion) of the base, but simply an indirect way of probing into it.

EXAMPLE **4.14.** Jick and Slone (1969) studied the relation of the incidence of thromboembolism to ABO blood type among women using oral contraceptives. The reference series was not restricted to this domain, because the data were readily available only without this constraint, and since blood type may be presumed to be unrelated to gender, age, and the use of oral contraceptives. (cf. Example 2.22.)

5

Design of Information
on the Samples

The preceding chapter dealt with sampling—the identification of a series of cases and representatives of the base itself. Upon the enrollment of a case or a representative of the base, information is secured on the individual. If the case-referent strategy of rate assessment is a feature of the study design, it may be necessary to use presampling arrangements to make such information available.

5.1. PRESAMPLING PROVISION FOR INFORMATION

The exploitation of the efficiency implications of the case-referent strategy for rate assessment presupposes that the information on the determinant, the modifiers, and the confounders can be secured retrospectively, by the procurement of antecedent facts when the outcome manifests itself. This prerequisite for the case-referent strategy may preclude the employment of a retrospective base for the study. Moreover, the use of a prospective base tends not to provide for such information in and of itself. Instead, the use of a prospective base tends to be the solution only insofar as express arrangements are made for securing the *post hoc* availability of the requisite information (cf. Section 3.3.3).

The need for such prospective provisions for information does not mean that the case-referent approach is out of the question (cf. Example 3.19). It is necessary only to make advance arrangements such that the required information is accessible for any case that develops and for anyone who becomes a member of the base sample. To this end, in a prospective study base, whether experimental or nonexperimental, the need might be to secure and set aside records (e.g., of an interview), tracings (e.g., of electrocardiography), films (e.g., from radiography), biologic samples (e.g., of blood), and so on. Since the entire base is at risk of developing the illness, these contingency provisions must be made for the entire base, rather than for a mere sample of it.

5.2. TIME REFERENT OF INFORMATION

In the study of incidence by the use of a cohort base it may be appropriate to characterize the study subjects—the cases and a sample of the base or of the noncases—only as of the defining, *zero time* (Section 3.2.1.1) of the cohort. This is quite routine and appropriate in experimental studies, because the status of the determinant is kept constant over the follow-up period and losses to follow-up are kept to a minimum.

Those features of experimental cohorts, permitting the consideration of directly observable incidence proportions in relation to the determinant characterized as of the cohort's zero time, tend not to be shared by nonexperimental cohorts followed for long periods of time, particularly when the determinant is quite unstable over time. In these situations the cases of the illness at issue are not usefully characterized as of the cohort's zero-time. Instead, they are characterized in a manner analogous to that of a dynamic-population base—by taking their histories with respect to the determinant and other factors for the etiologically (or descriptively) *relevant time period prior to the onset* of the illness. In the end, the concern usually is to characterize each case for a series of *subintervals* of that historical period of interest. Thus, in the study of cancer etiology one might wish to characterize the periods of less than 1 year, 1–5 years, 5–10 years, and so on, prior to the diagnosis of the cancer. In the context of a potential acute adverse reaction to medications, the historical intervals would be defined in terms of hours and days immediately preceding the first manifestations of the adverse event.

The time referents of the information on the *reference series* are set in a manner completely analogous to that for the case series, as long as the reference series consists of cases of *another illness* with the duration of presampling manifestations generally similar to that in the illness under study. If the reference condition is more acute than the illness under study, comparability with the index series in terms of accuracy of information tends to require that the timings of the historical time intervals be matched. For example, if an index subject's illness first manifested itself 8 months ago, his/her reference subjects are also approached as if their illness started 8 months ago—defining the historical intervals from that point backward in time. Reference conditions with presampling duration generally longer than that in the illness under study should not be used.

When the reference series is based on anything but cases of a reference illness from the "registry" that supplies the cases of the illness under study, the timing aspects of its information are more complicated. The *basic reference point* in time is the time at which the person was first approached as a potential representative of the study base. The first concern is to determine whether this person, had he/she been an admissible case at that time, would have entered the "registry" from which the cases are drawn. If this criterion is satisfied, the subject is indeed a representative of the base from which the cases derive. More specifically, the person is a representative of the base in terms of the historical time periods considered for the actual cases. For such periods, the usual reference point is the time of the first manifestations of the illness (see example given above), and there is no counterpart among reference subjects that are not cases of another illness. However, with the reference subjects matched for cases, one can use the time lag since first manifestations in the index subject. Otherwise, a typical lag time among the cases could be employed for each reference subject.

When the cases represent an acute illness with short-term etiology, the implementation of this scheme can involve a problem of recall among the reference subjects. For practical reasons, there tends to be an appreciable time lag between the first approach to a potential reference subject and the actual interview. Thus, at the time of the interview, the subject may not remember the events immediately preceding the basic reference point in time, such as the use of particular drugs. This contrasts with the interviews of the cases at the very time of the acute event under study, and the result is a potential for serious lack of comparability of information (Section 5.6).

The problem has two major *pseudo-solutions*. One is to use only those potential reference subjects who are available for interview immediately, at the time when they are first approached. This admissibility condition of ready availability for something of no emergency in the reference subjects is not shared by the case series; and insofar as it is related to the determinant under study, it implies a bias in the sampling of the base (cf. Section 4.4). The other major pseudo-solution is to use the time of the interview as a surrogate point of reference in time, as the counterpart of the time of the cases' interviews in the hospital. Again, the arrangement implies asymmetry between the index and reference series: the cases came to the hospital as a matter of emergency, regardless of whether it would have been convenient for them to receive an interviewer at their homes in the absence of the health emergency. This difference in circumstances is readily associated with the most recent history regarding the determinant under study, and this tends to invalidate the use of the surrogate point of reference in time (cf. Miettinen, 1985).

One potentially appropriate solution is the use of a "random" surrogate for the reference point. In the first stage the reference subject agrees to provide the desired information, unspecified, as of a future point in time, also unspecified, regardless of the circumstances at that time—just as a case is hospitalized regardless of the circumstances other than being within the catchment area of the hospital. In addition, arrangements for making contact at that future time are made in the first stage, such as identifying persons who would know the subject's whereabouts at any time. The reference subjects are to be members of the study base at the surrogate time of information acquisition. Since they are also available for making these arrangements as of a particular time in advance, the imperative of comparability means that cases who would not have been available for such advance arrangements must be excluded.

It is evident that it may be very difficult to cope with the unavailability of the ideal approach to the reference information—namely, the use of a phenocopy of the illness under study, characterized by unrelatedness to the determinant under study, and distinguished from the illness of interest only within the "registry" for the latter (cf. Section 4.4.2.1).

5.3. CONDITIONAL SUFFICIENCY OF INFORMATION

Sometimes major economy of design in the context of prospective cohorts is achieved by recognizing points at which particular subjects enrolled into the study base have contributed all the information that they will contribute, so that further data acquisition may be terminated.

EXAMPLE 5.1.   Consider the evaluation of electroencephalographic monitoring during open-heart surgery as to its efficacy in the prevention of neurologic complications of the operation. A perfunctory design might have the following broad features. Patients scheduled for the operation are randomized to monitoring and nonmonitoring, respectively, and both cohorts are subjected to a thorough neurologic examination preoperatively, in the early postoperative period (during the hospitalization), and again after the condition has stabilized (within a few months). An alternative plan is based on the realization that *monitoring can be efficacious only insofar as it leads to feedback*. In other words, it is the feedback that eventually has the effect, insofar as there is any. Thus, one might as well monitor every patient and look for the signals for feedback on everyone (signs of ischemia, etc.). One would then withhold actual feedback (advice to the anesthesiologist and/or the surgeon) in a random subset of the patients on whom the signals appear. Subsequent observations would then be confined to this subdomain of patients on whom the signals occur, which would eliminate the vast majority of the patients (some 90%) from follow-up. Finally, since only a small subset of the patients would be followed, the wisdom of the across-the-board pre-operative examination is doubtful. It might be more cost-effective to forfeit the consideration of intrapatient changes and simply compare the postoperative findings between the feedback and no-feedback groups. In this example, appreciating the sufficiency of the information on those with no feedback from the monitoring means cutting a high cost down to a small fraction.

In addition to *monitoring*, opportunities for truncated data acquisition arise in the contexts of evaluating *screening, contingency provisions* for intevention, and other *processes involving identifiable stages in, or conditions for, the development of the effect.* Where such an opportunity does exist, it deserves early consideration in study design, since, as was illustrated, it can have profound implications for the entire design of the study—with great dividends in economy.

5.4. CONTENT OF INFORMATION

Planning for the content of the information to be secured on each subject in the base that is actually enrolled into the sample(s) does not, ideally, proceed according to the procedural phases of data acquisition. Instead, best results are generally achieved by planning according to the *conceptual categories* of essential information. These may be taken as:

1. Administrative information, including subject identity, avenues for tracing the subject, informed consent, and identification of the person(s) recording and checking the information.
2. Substantive information, according to the following subcategories:
    a. Admissibility.
    b. Determinant(s).
    c. Modifiers.
    d. Confounders.
    e. Other characteristics that may bear on the generalizability of the results.

Within each of the substantive categories, the design of the particulars of content is guided by principles that include the following:

1. *Primary* rather than inferential information is recorded. For example, electrocardiographic voltages are recorded rather than whether criteria for hypertrophy are met.
2. *Detailed* rather than unduly categorized information is recorded. For example, one records the actual reported number of cigarettes smoked

per day, such as 5, rather than 5–14 per day. Similarly, if admissibility involves the criterion that a particular characteristic takes on a value within a particular range, the actual value is recorded rather than simply that the condition is met.

3. *Objectivity* has no inherent dominance over *judgment*. For example, clinical judgment of heart size on the basis of a chest radiogram ("normal," "slightly enlarged," etc.) can be preferable to the measured cardiothoracic ratio. Similarly, the judgment of a trained interviewer as to whether a person has a history of heart attack can be preferable to objective recording of the subject's response(s) to a direct question or to a set of component questions.

4. That a piece or category of information is conceivably useful is insufficient *justification* for its inclusion in the data set. Particularly in collaborative studies, violation of this aspect of the broad principle of parsimony is conducive to complexity, which takes away from validity, to say nothing about adding cost and aggravation.

Overall, the content of the data should be guided by a clear vision of the *occurrence relation in empirical terms*—the outcome entity in terms of its criteria or index (Section 2.1), the determinant scale (Section 2.3), how modifiers are to be dealt with (Section 2.5), how confounders are to be expressed in operational terms (Section 2.7), and what general characteristics may bear on the generalizability of the results (Sections 1.7.2 and 9.1).

5.5. STRUCTURE OF INFORMATION

Given a detailed vision of the data to be obtained on the study subjects, and also on *how* they are to be obtained (as to record abstractions, interviews, and observations), the task that follows is the design of the forms on which the data are to be recorded.

With the content set, the essence of the data forms is their *structure*. Its design is guided by a multitude of principles. These include the following:

1. Procedurally separate aspects of data acquisition are to be served by *separate forms*. Thus, in prospective cohort studies there tend to be distinct forms, suitably labeled, for subject admission (used for administrative and admissibility data), routine follow-up visits, reporting of deaths, and so on.

2. In the data form for a particular aspect of data acquisition, the *sequencing* of the items of information is not governed by the conceptual categories of the research problem (as outlined above). Instead, the sequence is to correspond to the *natural flow of the process* of data acquisition.

3. In every other respect as well, the structure should be designed with a view to *ease of filling in* the data, not for convenience of data processing. For example, it should be feasible to record quantities in terms of different systems of measurement and different units within them, according to existing variations of custom. Similarly, when the source of data involves variation in individual adjustment of quantities (e.g., by body weight or surface area), the form should not force uniformity, but should provide for recording in terms that are inherent in the source. Finally, this principle calls to question any scheme for *self-coding* or *automatic processing* whenever this entails any added challenge or burden for the pivotal and subsequently irremediable process of data recording.

4. Within these constraints, each form should consist of sequentially numbered items of information, each calling for a single response (except in the context of inapplicable branches), on a scale with maximal a priori structure. The response may be to write down a number (with or without separate designation of unit), to check off a category on a nominal or ordinal scale, or even a verbal entry. There should commonly also be provision for indicating "unknown."

When the study has a primary focus on a particular hypothesis or quantification problem, it may also address a number of other relations as *secondary objectives*. When the base is a prospective cohort structured according to a single determinant and approached in terms of a census rather than the case-referent scheme, a variety of secondary outcome entities may be observable with relatively small added cost. Analogously, a study employing the case-referent approach can provide for ready history taking with respect to a multitude of potential determinants of secondary interest. Where such exploration is indeed considered consistent with the general outlook of parsimony in deciding upon the extent of information (Section 5.4), a keen sense of *priority* should be maintained, nevertheless. This imperative is of particular force in the context of questionnaire-based information, regardless of whether the form is filled in by an interviewer. Thus, the information bearing on the primary objective should not, in general, appear on the forms as just another item amongst a multitude. Rather, that information should be obtained first, while the respondent is still alert and well disposed.

The broad spectrum of outcome phenomena or determinants that correspond to the secondary objectives may be best approached, in the context of interview, in two stages. The first is open-ended; for example, "Have you ever had any problems with your health?" or "Have you ever used a medication of any kind on a regular basis?" The second stage is a systematic interview; for example, histories of drug use may be structured according to indication (anxiety, pain, contraception, etc.), type of drug (sedatives, analgesics, hormones, etc.), or perhaps both.

5.6. COMPARABILITY OF INFORMATION

Once it is known what information is desired, the study designer's concern turns to the *quality* aspects of that information.

As background for this topic, it may be helpful to recall two principles of representativeness: given primary commitment to a particular base, the case series and the base sample should be representative of the cases and the base, respectively (conditionally on stratification factors); and given an initial commitment to a series of cases, this series should be coupled with a reference series representative of the base for which those cases are the totality of cases (by definition). Either way, the core principle is that the case series and the base sample (or census) should be *coherent* as to what they represent: they should represent the *same* base experience—the distribution of the cases ("numerator" experience) in that base, and the distribution of that base itself ("denominator" experience), respectively. This imperative of coherence of referent for the distributions of the cases and the base sample (or census)—according to the determinant—is so strong that even the choice of the base is subordinated to it (cf. Section 4.1).

Attainment of this coherence between the case series and the base sample (or census) rests on *comparability of case detection* among the compared categories of the determinant; that is, certain parameters characterizing the inaccuracies of case detection must be unrelated to the determinant at issue:

1. If the commitment is to a particular *cohort* base, and if the experience of this base is approached in the spirit of a *census*, the identification of the cases is a matter of the quality of the data on the subjects actually enrolled. For the putative cases to be actual cases, *specificity* of diagnosis must be perfect (no "false positives"). For them to be also representative of all the cases occurring in the base, the *sensitivity* of case detection must not be associated with the determinant (nor with the modifiers under study). On these conditions of comparable outcome information on the members of the base, *relative* rates (rate ratios) will be valid. For absolute rates to be valid, the sensitivity must be not only comparable but perfect as well.

2. If the primary commitment is to a base, a cohort or dynamic-population experience, and if the experience of the base is harvested by means of the *case-referent* strategy, representativeness of the case series (of all cases in the base) is *not* singularly a matter of the quality of the information on the subjects actually enrolled (a case series and a base sample). It is possible, in principle, to exclude "false positives," but invariant sensitivity in the cases' coming to attention is a matter of *a priori presumption*, since the subjects actually enrolled do not cover the entire base of the study. Insofar as there is interest in the noncase subset of the base sample (see Appendix 6), diagnostic criteria with high spec-

ificity may constitute an aspect of quality of information on the reference subjects as well.

3. With the study built around a series of accessible cases, with "false positives" excluded, the theoretical definition of their associated base (Section 4.1) is valid even if the case detection is dependent on the determinant. Such dependence, however, greatly accentuates the inherently considerable challenge of finding a means for valid sampling of the base. A practical solution is unlikely, except by confining, where possible, the index series to cases so severe that coming to attention cannot depend on the determinant (cf. Section 4.4.1).

When the specificity of case detection is incomplete, that is, when "false positives" occur among the putative cases, even rate ratios are quantitatively invalid. Nevertheless, if specificity, as well as sensitivity, is comparable among the compared categories of the determinant, that is, if the errors (both rates of error) of outcome information are *nondifferential* over the determinant, *qualitative* inference (Section 1.7) remains valid: with only nondifferential errors in the outcome information, the empirical measure of relation tends to deviate from the null value of the parameter in the same direction as a totally valid empirical measure would tend to. More specifically, the distribution of the empirical measure is intermediate between the null and the nonnull distributions of a perfectly valid measure. (This involves the assumption that the outcome information is unbiased in the sense of nonnegative correlation between the empirical classifications of outcome and the true outcome.)

When the outcome parameter of interest is not a rate but the mean of a quantitative characteristic, errors are thought of in terms of their mean, or *bias*, and their scatter around this mean, or *imprecision*—rather than as error rates such as the false positive rate (complement of specificity) and the false negative rate (complement of sensitivity). Valid inference about the relation of the mean of a quantitative outcome to a determinant (potential) requires only that the bias be nondifferential (unrelated to the determinant); constancy of precision is not a requirement under a tenable regression model, nor is constancy of the scatter of the empirical outcomes themselves (reflecting both imprecision of the information and variability of the true outcomes).

Where the case-referent strategy is employed in the absence of preexisting and accessible records on the relevant background (retrospective) information, *it is of critical importance, insofar as the obtainable histories are inaccurate, that such inaccuracies of information about the determinant (and modifiers) be comparable between the index (case) and reference (base) series—even at the expense of accuracy.*

EXAMPLE 5.2.   Consider a case-referent study by Matroos et al. (1979) concerning the etiology of coronary heart disease. Both fatal and nonfatal cases were included, and the background information was secured by interview of the nonfatal cases themselves and, in the instances of a fatal event, of the next of kin. In the reference series, which consisted of living subjects, direct interview could have been used throughout, but it was not. Presumably the indirect information on deceased cases was less accurate, and the same inaccuracy was built into the reference series by interviewing the next of kin when the corresponding index subject was deceased. (In some instances the scheme can be improved by the use of deceased reference subjects for fatal cases.)

EXAMPLE 5.3.   Consider an occupational mortality study concerning a particular cause of death, lung cancer, for example. Suppose the case series is identified on the basis of death certificates, and that for this series the occupational information—quite inaccurate—is drawn from the death certificates themselves. The use of a living reference series (e.g., based on the population registry for the region for which the death certificates were reviewed) would provide more accurate occupational histories for the base sample than that used for the case series, given direct interviews of the subjects. Such incomparability of accuracy would be inadmissible, however. A preferable reference series is a series of cases of death from another cause, suitably chosen (see Section 4.4.2.1 and Wang and Miettinen, 1982), with the occupational history obtained from the death certificates, just as in the index series.

EXAMPLE 5.4.   Consider a study of the etiology of a congenital malformation anchored on a series of newborn cases, and suppose their exposure to drugs in the embryonic period is obtained by interviewing the mothers. A series of normal newborns, with similar interviews of the mothers, would be inappropriate in terms of comparability of histories. A satisfactory approach to the sampling of the base might be the use of a few other malformations [whose occurrence is presumed to be unrelated to the determinant(s) under study; cf. Section 4.4.2.1]. Such a reference series would have the advantage, relative to normal babies, that the mothers' preoccupation with the events of early pregnancy is likely to be more comparable to that in the index series.

EXAMPLE 5.5.   When the case series, identified and interviewed in hospitals, can be thought of as representative of all cases in a technically identifiable population in a particular span of time (e.g., a metropolitan area), a representative reference series may be drawn as a sample of that population (cf. Section 4.1 and Cole et al., 1971). Yet the added imperative of comparability of information may well suggest the use of cases of a few other illnesses identified in the same hospitals and also interviewed in circumstances similar to those with the case series.

As these examples suggest, the need for comparable information between the index and reference series—a sine qua non for even qualitatively valid

inference—is not simply a question of *how* the information is obtained on
the actual study subjects. An added issue is *who* should be used as reference
subjects. Thus, the adequacy of the reference series is not simply a matter
of *representativeness* of the base from which the cases derive as to the *actual*
distribution of the determinant (and modifiers) in the base. An added question is whether they provide *comparably inaccurate* information on the determinant (and modifiers).

As for *confounders*, comparability in the face of inaccuracy does *not*
provide for even qualitatively valid inference (cf. Section 2.7).

5.7. ACCURACY OF INFORMATION

As has been seen, inaccuracies of information on the health outcome and
the determinant [as well as the modifier(s)] are consistent with valid qualitative inference as long as the errors in outcome information are invariant
over the categories or levels of the determinant and vice versa, that is, as
long as comparability of information obtains in both of these regards.

In the context of *qualitative* research problems (Section 1.7.1), the pursuit
of accuracy beyond mere comparability thus has its motive in the quest for
more information from a study base of a given size, that is, for greater *size
efficiency* of research. Thus, in the common context of low empirical incidence (proportion) and/or rare exposure, the size of the study base may be
reduced by half if the sensitivity of case detection (in a census-type study)
or of exposure identification (in a case-referent study) can be doubled without compromising specificity.

Validity of *quantitative* research (Section 1.7.2), similarly, does *not* entail
any universal requirement of total accuracy of information on the study
subjects. Exceptions include the following:

1. When the empirical outcome phenomenon is quantitative, the compar-
    ability requirement means that bias (average error) be invariant over the
    determinant. Imprecision (variability of error)—the remaining aspect of
    accuracy—is again a determinant of size efficiency, but it has no bearing
    on the validity of studying the mean as a function of the determinant at
    issue. It is not even necessary to know the degree of imprecision in the
    measurement of a quantitative outcome criterion (cf. Section 5.6).

2. In the case of a nominal- or ordinal-scale outcome criterion, valid quan-
    titative inference is possible given a priori knowledge of the rates of
    misclassification, such as sensitivity (the complement of "false negative
    rate") in the detection of an all-or-none state or event. Thus, the pivotal
    design concern is to employ criteria for which the error rates are known,
    that is, well-characterized standard criteria (cf. Section 2.1). Ad hoc
    efforts to reduce the error rates are of little value for validity as long as

they remain unknown. The question of size efficiency is rather moot in the face of unknown validity.

3. As for inaccuracy with a determinant, valid quantitative inference is possible given a priori knowledge of the degree of imprecision or rates of misclassification, according as the determinant is measured on a quantitative or nominal/ordinal scale. The implications are the same as in the case of a nominal/ordinal outcome criterion.

Insofar as there is interest in the enhancement of the precision of some quantitative item of data per se, a major alternative to attempts at improving the technique itself is to *replicate* its application, blood-pressure reading, for example.

When a *local method* of measurement differs from what is regarded as the standard, their relative precisions (which are irrelevant for validity in the context of the outcome measure) raise a problem when the measurement concerns a determinant. The solution is *not* that of replacing each local reading by its corresponding expected value by the standard method, as read from a regression line relating the two types of reading (the relation of the mean value from the standard to the reading by the local method). The proper approach depends on the relative imprecisions of the two methods. For example, if the two methods are of equal imprecision, no translation from the local to the standard method is needed, even though the regression slope is less than unity. This equivalence corresponds, in the context of uncorrelated errors between the two methods, to lack of correlation between the sum and the difference of the two types of measurement result in a series (large) of paired readings on variable (and generally unknown) true values. [More generally, given uncorrelated errors, the error standard deviation of a given one of the two methods is the covariance (theoretical) between reading by that method and the difference between the two.]

6

Design of Analysis

In the design stage of a study, a detailed plan for the eventual analysis of the data is commonly both infeasible and unnecessary. It may be infeasible because the particulars depend on the data themselves, and it may be unnecessary because the design concerns for analysis are rather limited. The essential reasons for considering data analysis in the design stage are these:

1. It constitutes a check on whether the core objective(s) really has (have) been identified. When that task has escaped attention up to this point in the planning, a sketch of the essential analysis (analyses) stimulates the formulation of the central objective(s), even if somewhat belatedly.

2. It brings to the fore the essential entities inherent in the conceptualization of the outcome, the determinant(s), the modifiers, and the confounders. Again, this may reveal omissions in the planning, perhaps all the way back to the core objective(s), but more likely as to the elements in the actual occurrence relation (Chapter 2). Also, the appropriateness of the planned data collection gets to be checked as to whether the essential elements are addressed. An alert and critical planner will also recognize the futility of a good part of the planned data collection—and the rare decisive one will even act on this realization.

3. It has the effect of assuring that the data analyst(s) is (are) brought into the research team in the planning stage. This provides for critical examination of the entire study plan from the statistical point of view. It also assures consideration of the technical provisions for data manage-

ment and analysis. Related to all this is the assurance of informed consideration regarding the budgetary aspects of data processing and analysis.

4. Insofar as the plan involves projected data displays—expected numerical results—it can have bearing on the judgment as to whether the planned study size is adequate (often relative to the alternative of zero; cf. Section 3.2.3). However, any attempt at such a projection may be without foundation in anything but fiction, particularly in studies designed for exploration of the unknown (which is somewhat of an exception in "normal science").

The projection of the amount of information in the eventual data takes on a variety of forms. Commonly involved is an all-or-none outcome and a dichotomous determinant. Moreover, cases of the outcome phenomenon and representatives of the index category of the determinant are relatively rare among the study subjects. In such an instance the total amount of information is characterized quite well by the projected *number of exposed cases,* particularly the expected null number. For any projected observed number, the precision is conveniently approximated in terms of its coefficient of variation, which is the inverse of its square root.

The information is appreciably less than this if the reference series is not severalfold relative to the index series; if it is necessary to control a confounder whose expected distributions between the index and reference series are very different, or a confounder measured on a highly polytomous nominal scale; and if the intent is to explore modification, particularly by a nominal-scale factor with rare categories. When any one of these conditions obtains, it is good to consider hypothetical data, as realistic as possible (including chance irregularities), and to compute the corresponding interval estimate(s) of the comparative parameter(s) of primary interest. Such sketches would generally be based on tabular presentations. In the interpretation of the resulting indications of precision, it may be appropriate to anticipate more efficient analyses based on regression models.

This sketching of possible data and their informativeness can be applied to other scales as well without any appreciable distortion of a vision that is hazy at best. Different levels of exposure may be pooled into one; a continuous characteristic may be reduced to estimates (surmises) of the lowest and highest intertertile categories of its overall (unconditional) distribution, omitting the middle one; and so on. The consequence tends to be only modest underestimation of the information.

When the study is to address several outcome phenomena and/or several determinants (e.g., all congenital malformations and exposures to all drugs on which an adequate amount of information will be available), it is desirable to carry out the sketchings for the extremes of the anticipated frequencies over the various outcome entities and determinant categories. This can have helpful implications for refining the realistic range of study concerns. For example, it may reveal that, given the projected sizes of the individual index groups, the contemplated size of the common reference group is excessive.

The development of the plans for data analysis is not simply a catalyst for refining the study plan and understanding its implications. Their presentation is most helpful also to those who review the proposed study for acceptance or funding—usually a body of pundits not intimately familiar with the intricacies of the mission, particularly as to what the numerical results are likely to be. Their judgment may also be facilitated by the proposer's innocent commitment to a "t test" as opposed to a "chi square test," or conversely, or to something else, maybe as erudite-sounding as "analysis of variance."

7

Interdependencies
in Design

The presentation of epidemiologic study design in the preceding chapters has a strong implication of *sequentiality* in the process. It conveys the idea that, with the usual, amorphous research question or idea as the point of departure, a good epidemiologist first designs the occurrence relation in detail, then chooses the study base, and so on.

On the other hand, the text makes many allusions to *interdependencies* among the design decisions:

1. With fundamental interest in incidence, one may have to study prevalence for reasons of research practicability.
2. With interest in a longitudinal relation, only a cross-sectional one may be subject to study.
3. Modification of a parameter of relation by a particular factor may be of express interest, but information on it may not be accessible, or an informative distribution of it may not be attainable in an otherwise appropriate study base.
4. A retrospective base might be preferred, except that unbiased sampling of it may be infeasible or the information obtainable on the sampled subjects may be inadequate.

5. A case-referent strategy for rate assessment might be preferred for efficiency in principle, but a need for extensive presampling provisions may make a census approach just as attractive.

6. Realization of the risk of bias in case detection may lead to the abandonment of a contemplated primary base in preference to one whose definition is secondary to an accessible series of cases.

7. The risk of bias in case detection may lead to a redefinition of the very phenomenon being studied (restriction to a subtype that would come to attention regardless of the determinant).

8. Consideration of comparability or accuracy of information on study subjects may lead to a reformulation of the empirical occurrence relation to be studied.

9. Examination of the analysis of projected data may lead to modification of not only the size of the study base but even the study objectives themselves.

Overall, then, even with an express, a priori problem to be investigated, the process of study design is highly *iterative*. In the end, the question of adequacy of the design is not a matter of its component decisions but, rather, the plan *as a whole* should represent a reasonable balance among various, often conflicting considerations. These include the following desiderata:

1. Capturing and addressing the *essence of the research problem,* with a view not only to how it may have been initially expressed but also to its underlying motives, scientific and other.

2. Using a base whose character, as the direct referent of the results, provides for *generalization* beyond itself, consonant with the motivation for the study, and which represents an *efficient distribution matrix*.

3. Having representation of the base and information on the study subjects consonant with reasonable *validity* of the results with respect to the base itself (internal validity)—a prerequisite for any meaningful generalization.

4. Representing a reasonable degree of *efficiency* in the procurement of the ultimate information with respect to the research objective(s). By contrast, informativeness as it is determined by the mere size of the study base is not, in the author's view, a critical matter in study design and is not generally a point for objective criticism of a study plan.

8

Study Protocol

The end-result of study design—a study plan—is documented in writing as the *study protocol*. The purposes of this documentation are:

1. To *crystallize* the plan for the planners themselves, as its writing calls for explicitness that might not develop without the documentation.
2. To provide a basis for outside *review* of the plan for advice, acceptance, and/or funding.
3. To help orient and *train* study personnel.
4. To safeguard against the consequences of the planner's loss of *memory* (or indeed of life itself) before the completion of the study.
5. To document the study procedures for *posterity*.

The protocol documents, in all relevant detail, the *procedures* employed in the study. Indeed, it is often referred to as the "manual of operations." Thus, its essence is stipulation of the procedures. To be effective, the protocol also provides for an understanding of the nature of the intended procedures; but justification of the procedures is not within the realm of the study protocol.

For a study protocol to be intelligible it must start by stating the "objective" of the study. As all studies have the objective of learning, the issue really is the subject of learning or the *object* of the study.

In *descriptive* research, a bare minimum statement of the study object identifies the phenomenon whose occurrence is at issue, together with either a restricted type of subject or, in the context of a relatively heterogeneous referent, the major determinants that the occurrence will be related to. In these terms, the object of a study might be "the occurrence of ventricular fibrillation during ambulance transport of patients with suspected acute coronary event," with no reference to the determinants that might be considered within the referent. On the other hand, the object might be "the occurrence of ventricular fibrillation in (patients with preexisting) coronary heart disease in relation to age, time since last acute event, severity of angina, ..."

When the object is a relation that is viewed in *causal* terms, the object statement necessarily identifies the determinant in addition to the health outcome, and it reveals the concern with causality. It may be essential to specify the type of subject as well. Thus, the object might be "the effect of physical exercise habits on the risk of ventricular fibrillation" or, alternatively, "physical exercise habits in the etiology of . . . ," but it is not "the relation of . . . ." Moreover, with this objective one specifies either the domain of patients with coronary heart disease or some other limited range of a major risk indicator (e.g., age) or, alternatively, the intent to consider modification of the effect by such characteristics (cf. Section 2.5).

With the object of the study understood, the protocol proceeds to a specification, in particularistic terms, of either the *base* to which the study is directly committed or the series of *cases* on which the base depends (Section 3.2.1.4). With a direct commitment to a base, its minimum specification is of the form "cardiac transports in town T (or by company C) in the time period from T_1 to T_2"; or "patients discharged alive with the diagnosis of acute myocardial infarction from hospitals H_1, . . . and followed from the discharge for a period P of time (or "up to time T" in calendar time); or "the population of city C in the time period from T_1 to T_2." If the base is defined indirectly through a series of cases (Section 3.2.1.4), the minimum specification is of the form "the catchment population of all cases of sudden cardiac death diagnosed at institutions I_1, . . . in the time period from T_1 to T_2."

If the base is an *experimental* one, the protocol expands on its definition by stipulating the interventions applied, their subject selection, and their timing.

From the definition of the base, direct or implicit, the protocol naturally turns to the terms in which the base is to be *represented* [in the sense of sampling (Chapter 4)] together with, where relevant, any (prospective) arrangements for the availability of needed information on those representatives (Section 5.1). Thus, in the case of the cardiac transport base mentioned above, the subjects actually enrolled in the study would presumably consist of all cases in the base together with a sample of the base itself. This same strategy would be specified for the cohort of patients discharged from the hospitals; but an essential associated feature might be the (prospective) arrangements needed to procure and store, for example, 24-hour Holter tapes and the like for the availability of information on cardiac arrhythmia status and other risk indicators at the time of hospital discharge. If the base is the population of a city in a particular time period, the protocol indicates how its representation in terms of a series of cases (unbiased) and a sample of the population is to be achieved. For example, the cases might be identified by a review of the records of all coroner's offices, ambulance companies, and so on, serving the city at the time. The corresponding base sample could be drawn from the town books of all the townships within the city, with all town-specific subsamples proportional in size to the respective town populations within categories of age and gender. If the commitment is to a case series characterized more by ready accessibility than by representativeness of all the cases in a particular regional or other a priori population, a critical protocol element is the stipulation of how the ill-defined base from which the cases derive(d) is to be sampled—through neighbors, cases of another illness from the "registries" through which the cases are identified, or whatever (cf. Section 4.4.2).

At this point the reader of the protocol is poised to consider the *information* to be secured on each representative of the base (actual study subjects). For intelligibility, it should be organized in terms of the conceptual categories outlined in Section 5.4. For the same reason, it is essential to distinguish between conceptual entities on one hand and their operational criteria, measurements, or indices on the other. For example, if there is interest in "exercise tolerance," this entity must be translated into an operational scale from "excellent" to "crippled," for example, with all categories characterized in terms of their respective conceptual meaning and criteria. Thus, "excellent" tolerance might mean absence of any limitations other than lack of training, and the criterion might be a history of recent episodes of exertion up to exhaustion (which may be infeasible to meet in the context of unrelated handicaps).

A closely associated but totally distinct element in the protocol is the *data forms* (Section 5.5), conveniently presented as appendices.

With the information content understood, the reader is ready to consider the stipulated *procedures* of data acquisition: who, what, how, and on what prompting, in a sequence that is most appropriate for each component in the overall process.

The *flow* and *processing* of the information come next, including any arrangements for quality control in the sense of detection of omissions, other departures from protocol, and errors, together with the nature and particulars of remedial actions.

In large, particularly multicenter, studies the protocol also specifies the *administrative organization* of the study personnel. Best understood at the end of the protocol, this specification stipulates, by areas of responsibility, the types and numbers of people involved, their fractional time commitments, and, where known, their identities. It also delineates the intended lines of communication and authority relations.

Closely related to staffing and organization, in large-scale and long-term studies in particular, is the visualization of the *time course* of the study, and this, too, is an important aspect of the protocol. At the time as of which the project is funded, the study plan is often tentative in terms of various aspects of the procedures outlined in the then protocol. It needs to be tested for feasibility and other operational appropriateness in the first, pilot, phase of the project. A time period needs to be scheduled for this testing and finalization of the protocol. If, in a prospective cohort study, "baseline" observations are to be made on the entire base, the period of identifying the members and making these observations needs to be stipulated. In any case, the protocol stipulates the period of actual subject enrollment, whether that of the formation of a cohort for census-type follow-up or that of cases and reference subjects. In the context of a prospective cohort follow-up, the spread of follow-up examinations over time needs to be carefully delineated in order that the work load at different times during the project be understood. Beyond the data-acquisition phase, appropriate time is to be scheduled for data analysis and the preparation of the final report(s).

The study budget, though essential in an application for funding or response to a contract offer, falls outside the realm of the protocol which, it must be recalled, is the documentation of procedures, the manual of operations.

PART 2

Data Analysis

.

9

Elements of
Data Analysis
and Inference

9.1. INTRODUCTION

In science, data are not viewed in terms of documentation of the experience of interest. Thus, even when census representation of the study base provides for characterization of the empirical occurrence relation without any sampling-related or other uncertainty, the documented experience does not represent the ultimate *result* of the study. As the objective is to learn about *abstract* quantities and relations (Section 1.6), the actual result of the study could be taken as the *view* about the abstract object of the study that the study leads to, or as the change in the view brought about by the study.

The view that results from a particular study is generally *subjective* only. Thus, despite all the studies on, for example, the effects of smoking, physical exercise, or diet on the risk of myocardial infarction, or on the efficacy of anticoagulant medication in the prevention of its recurrence, the opinions of even experts on these topics remain quite diverse and, hence, subjective. The reasons for this fall into two broad categories. First, because views formulated in the absence of the information from a particular study are subjective, even objective but limited information from a particular study leaves the views, updated in the light of the study, variable among experts.

Second, the evidence itself from empirical studies commonly falls short of objectivity, even with reference to the study base itself, to say nothing about the realm of its generalization. The problem is not peculiar to nonexperimental research on causality; randomized clinical and prevention trials, too, are continually subjects of controversy as to the evidence they provide.

It is thus evident that the purpose of data analysis cannot realistically be taken as that of reaching a *conclusion* about the object of the study. Instead, the purpose, in proper terms, is to *summarize the evidence* in the data with respect to that object.

Such a summarization must *quantify the imprecision* that results from the quantitative limitations of the study base (perhaps compounded by its sampling), since it is viewed as only a sample of the larger, abstract reality of its kind (cf. Sections 1.6 and 3.1).

The quantification of the imprecision presupposes the invocation of a *statistical model*, which not only embodies the object of the study—a parameter of the theoretical occurrence relation (Section 1.3)—but also describes how the study base came about as an empirical representation of the larger reality that the relation characterizes. It is customary to construct the statistical model on the presumption that the study base came about as a *simple random sample* of the entirety of potential experience of its kind, that is, of the corresponding "*superpopulation*" experience.

EXAMPLE 9.1.   Suppose that in a series of 10 diabetics studied for a potential genetic marker, five showed the trait at issue, that is, that in the study base the prevalence *was* 50%. This gives some information as to how prevalent that trait *is* in general (in the abstract) among patients of the kind that the 10 patients represent (in the light of their source and admissibility criteria, together with descriptive information about them). One would generally adopt the view (model) that the 10 case enrollments represented "trials" with independent and equal probabilities for "success" in the sense of presence of the trait at issue—that probability being the prevalence of the trait, the object of the study. In this sense the empirical number of patients with the trait, five (out of the total number of patients, 10), is viewed as a realization for a binominal random variate (see Appendix 10) with the object of study as its parameter—unknown but subject to statistical inference under the model.

EXAMPLE 9.2.   Suppose that 10 patients with a particular type of congenital heart defect were operated on using a novel operative approach, and that five of them died during the operation. The magnitude of the corresponding theoretical intraoperative mortality rate, in clinical situations of the type represented by the 10 patients in the study base, is approached in a manner completely analogous to that outlined in Example 9.1.

This outlook in data analysis, as a foundation for inference, seems to be adequate as long as there is a keen sense of the kind of potential experience that the study base represents (is drawn from). Thus, in Example 9.1 there is probably reason to consider the ethnic composition of the source population, age of onset among the cases, and so on. In Example 9.2, a whole range of particulars about the type of patient and about the intervention itself (surgeons' skill, operative procedure, etc.) need to be specified for the direct referent in order that the abstract referent addressed by the model can be understood.

In the context of qualitative problems of research (Section 1.7.1), the data are summarized (under an adopted statistical model) for *hypothesis testing*—in contrast to quantitative research in which the summary is to serve *estimation* of the parameter(s) of the relation of interest. Somewhat different types of summary are used—without good justification (Section 9.8)—for these two purposes, respectively.

Such summaries of the data must be supplemented by whatever descriptive information on the study may have bearing on the validity (internal) of the evidence and its generalizability (external validity). This information, together with the summarized evidence, constitutes the basis for *inference* about the object of study. As noted, this use of the products of data analysis is inherently subjective.

9.2. HYPOTHESIS VS. ITS DENIAL

The development of a reasonable summary of the data for hypothesis testing presupposes the adoption of some particular strategy for inference in the face of evidence.

The strategy that suggests itself most immediately is based on the degree of consistency (compatibility) between the hypothesis and the data, with consistency enhancing the credibility of the hypothesis and inconsistency detracting from it.

This outlook is quite unsatisfactory. A study of size zero, even, would support the hypothesis, while a substantial amount of evidence would be needed to detract from it. Idle hypotheses of investigatively lazy scientists would have longevity, in conflict with the general principle of parsimony in science.

This problem is avoided by *testing not only the hypothesis itself but also its counterpoint, its denial, its corresponding "null hypothesis."* With this orientation, inference is guided, qualitatively, by the following rules:

1. If the evidence is inconsistent with the denial ("null hypothesis") but consistent with the hypothesis itself, the credibility of the hypothesis is enhanced by the evidence.
2. If the evidence is consistent with the denial but inconsistent with the hypothesis itself, the evidence detracts from the hypothesis.

3. If the evidence is consistent with both the hypothesis and its denial, the data have little or no inferential implication; the study was essentially unhelpful for modifying the credibility of the hypothesis.
4. If the evidence is inconsistent with both the hypothesis and its denial, the evidence points to another, alternative hypothesis.

This comparative outlook guides proper summarization of evidence, that is, data analysis, for hypothesis testing. For it to have full impact, the meanings of "hypothesis" and its denial (the "null hypothesis") need to be understood expressly and properly.

A *hypothesis* is a tentative piece of scientific knowledge, an *idea*, a proposition, based on insight and/or evidence, that contrasts with the a priori commitment to the simplest possible view of reality—the view in terms of which, in particular, all differences are taken to be zero unless there is express reason to think otherwise. The denial of a hypothesis thus is not really another hypothesis (*"null hypothesis"*) but, rather, a derivative of the general principle of parsimony in science. It implies specific *"null" values* for various parameters characterizing the occurrence relation (Appendix 2): rate difference (RD) = 0, rate ratio (RR) = 1, regression slope (B) = 0, etiologic fraction (EF) = 0, and so on.

An actual hypothesis corresponds to a departure from the null value—in a *particular direction* inherent in the hypothesis. Thus, a causal hypothesis implies that, conditionally on all confounders, $RD > 0$ (not $RD < 0$), whereas a preventive hypothesis has the opposite implication. There are no "two-sided" hypotheses (implying $RD \neq 0$), for ideas are more substantive than mere rebellion against the principle of parsimony, and thus, they have more specific quantitative implications than the entire complement of the null point.

9.3. THE *P*-VALUE

9.3.1. Sampling Behavior of the *P*-Value

The usual summary of evidence for hypothesis testing in epidemiology still is, alas, the so-called *P*-value. It is a function of the data—a statistic— computed under the statistical model that underlies the analysis. It is constructed in such a way that the following properties for its sampling distribution (distribution over hypothetical replications of the study) are achieved (as nearly as is possible within reason):

1. On the denial of the hypothesis (H_0) the statistic (P) has a uniform distribution in the range from zero to one, so that

$$\Pr(P < \alpha \mid H_0) = \alpha \qquad\qquad (9.1)$$

for any α in that range.

2. On the hypothesis itself (H) the distribution is still bounded by zero and one, but it is shifted to the left, so that

$$\Pr(P < \alpha \mid H) > \alpha. \qquad\qquad (9.2)$$

In any given test situation, several statistics satisfying these desiderata can be constructed. Evidently, for maximal discrimination between the hypothesis and its denial, the preference is for a statistic that has the greatest possible leftward shift in distribution when the hypothesis indeed is correct, that is, the statistic with the greatest possible "power" in the situation at hand.

9.3.2. Basic Interpretation of P-Values

A scientist sending a body of data—a sample of reality—to a statistical laboratory when testing a hypothesis is in a situation analogous to a clinician sending a stool sample to a clinical laboratory when preoccupied with the possibility of a particular gastrointestinal illness. Neither expects the laboratory to settle the issue. Instead, the scientist simply wants the P-value and other factual information, just as the clinician needs particular test results. Interpretation remains the responsibility of the scientist, just as it is the clinician's responsibility.

If the interpretation of the P-value is to parallel that of clinical laboratory results, the definitional characterization of its distributions must be refined. For actual inference it is not enough to know that, on the hypothesis itself, the distribution is shifted to the left (Section 9.3.1). One needs to know the distribution of the P-value on the hypothesis itself in much greater detail, just as the clinician needs to refer to the actual distribution of the laboratory reading in the presence of the illness, instead of simply noting that the distribution corresponding to normalcy is shifted, by an unknown amount, in a particular direction. This need is even greater in the research context, because the range of the P-value is the same regardless of whether the hypothesis obtains, and because the *degree of shift is not inherent in the scientific hypothesis, even when quantitatively specific, but depends on the amount of information in the data* as well. (Whereas for some clinical tests on a stool sample, such as the guaiac test, the range is the same regardless of the truth about the clinical question, the distribution of the test result in the presence of the illness does not depend on the size of the sample.) Moreover, computing the nonnull distribution of the P-value for any given degree of departure from the null state is generally almost as feasible as computing the P-value itself, as illustrated in Appendix 9.

Despite the need for, and feasibility of, computing the nonnull distribution of the *P*-value as an auxiliary statistic for the interpretation of the *P*-value itself, such computation has remained outside the "normal science" practice of epidemiology. Too commonly even judgment is set aside, so that the inference is drawn in a completely mechanistic manner. A value of "α" (see Section 9.2.1) is chosen in a more or less perfunctory, arbitrary way (almost always as either 0.05 or 0.01; cf. Section 3.2.3), and the *P*-value is compared with α, the "level" of the test. If $P < \alpha$, the "null hypothesis" is "rejected" and the hypothesis itself is "accepted;" if $P > \alpha$, the "null hypothesis" is "accepted" and the hypothesis itself is "rejected."

An intermediate, and rather reasonable, stance is to consider the *P*-value in conjunction with the *amount of information* in the data—an informal auxiliary statistic. Suitable guidelines for interpretation in this manner are the following:

1. If the information is *very sparse*, the nonnull distribution of the *P*-value is almost identical to the null distribution (except if a very large departure from the null state is hypothesized). In such a situation, the *P*-value *does not discriminate* between the hypothesis and its denial. Thus, whatever the value, it is devoid of information, so that it—and indeed the whole body of data—is to be *ignored*.

2. If the information is *very ample*, even very small deviations from the null state in the hypothesized direction can assure a very small *P*-value. By the same token, a minor lack of validity in the data can cause very small *P*-values. Thus, in this situation the "*P*-value test" is much *too sensitive to be useful* when "positive" (*P*-value small), which is analogous with, for example, a test for cardiac arrythmia based on the information recorded in a 24-hour Holter tape and viewed as positive as soon as a single extrasystole is found. The information base is too rich to be viewed in the qualitative spirit of hypothesis testing. Such data deserve to be analyzed quantitatively, that is, with a view to *estimation*, and this makes the misplaced testing redundant as well.

3. If the amount of information is *intermediate*, the nonnull distributions of the *P*-value, corresponding to reasonable departures from the null state, are such that large and even intermediate values are quite rare, while values close to zero are common. At the same time, trivial departures from the null state—and trivial invalidity—do not cause major shifts in the distribution relative to the uniform distribution on the denial of the hypothesis. This is the behavior characteristic of a desirable test statistic, and in this situation, therefore, the *P*-value can be used in inference. Nevertheless, as long as the nonnull distributions are not worked out expressly, only informal guidelines are feasible:

   a. A *very small P*-value is relatively more compatible with the hypothesis than its denial; it *supports* the hypothesis.

b. A *small* P-value does *not discriminate* between the hypothesis and its denial.

c. An intermediate and particularly a *large* P-value is relatively less compatible with the hypothesis than with its denial; it *detracts* from the hypothesis.

These guidelines are justified and expanded upon in Appendix 9.

If one works out the actual nonnull distributions of the P-value corresponding to different degrees of departure from the null state in the context of the actual degree of informativeness of the data (as in Appendix 9), this would obviously enhance the basis for any informal translation of the actual P-value to a modification of any given credibility (subjective) that a particular scientist attached to the hypothesis before the data. For formal inference, however, the entire P-value concept is irrelevant; the information is summarized in terms of the likelihood ratio function (Section 9.7).

It is a common belief that the P-value expresses the probability that "the data are due to chance" or the probability that the "null hypothesis" is correct. In point of fact it expresses nothing of the sort. It is, as has been described, only a statistic, a *partial summary of the evidence* for or against the denial of the hypothesis in a particular body of data. The probability that the "null hypothesis" is correct is a quantitative expression of the extent to which someone believes in the denial proposition. This depends only partly on the evidence in the data—expressed not as the P-value but as the likelihood ratio function. An additional determinant is the person's view of the hypothesis apart from the data (cf. Section 9.7.2).

EXAMPLE 9.3.   Consider testing the hypothesis that, for a normal-looking coin, the probability, when tossing the coin, of the head side landing up is greater than $\frac{1}{2}$. Suppose that the coin is tossed five times and that a head comes up each time. For this evidence the associated P-value (see Section 10.1.3) is $0 \leq P \leq (\frac{1}{2})^5$, that is, $0.00 \leq P \leq 0.03$. Yet, the probability (subjective) that the denial proposition (probability of heads equaling $\frac{1}{2}$) is correct would likely remain 100% in the minds of many people.

For further discussions on the misuse and deficiencies of the null P-value the reader is referred to Morrison and Henkel (1970) and Diamond and Forrester (1983).

9.3.3. P-Values for Data-Suggested Hypotheses

The interpretation of P-values is commonly considered to involve certain subtleties beyond the basic issues discussed above—distinctions and constraints that have to do with particular types of inferential setting.

One of these notions is that a P-value is interpretable at its "face value" only insofar as the investigator(s) had the hypothesis "in mind" a priori, before the data were at hand. Only in such instances of prior or "advance hypotheses," so goes the thinking, can one speak and think of actual hypothesis testing. These are taken to contrast with situations in which the *hypothesis is suggested by the data*. In these latter types of instance one speaks of "hypothesis generation," and P-values are said to be "nominal" only and to be devoid of the null property of $\Pr(P < \alpha \mid H_0) = \alpha$ (cf. Section 9.3.1). The notion is that if the investigator(s) did not have the hypothesis in mind before the data were collected, $\Pr(P < \alpha \mid H_0) > \alpha$. It is taken as a corollary of this that a "hypothesis suggested by the data" cannot be properly tested by the use of those same data, but requires new data for proper (actual) testing. This notion, were it held as a principle, would be of major consequence in epidemiologic research. For even if a study is motivated by a particular hypothesis that the investigator(s) have in mind quite expressly and strongly, a large body of secondary, exploratory information is commonly obtained on the study subjects (cf. Section 5.5), with hypotheses only questionably in mind.

It is indeed clear that data may be used to test a hypothesis that existed as an idea prior to the collection of the data, and that they may also give rise to ideas that did not exist before. But it seems equally clear that in either situation the data provide *evidence* only, whether summarized in terms of a P-value, a likelihood ratio, or whatever, and that this evidence is altogether independent of the investigator's—and everyone else's—mind-set before becoming aware of that evidence. When an investigator familiar with the subject matter did not have in mind a relation for which there is evidence in the data, it tends to be that the advance credibility for that relation, or the data-suggested hypothesis, was quite low for experts in general. For this reason the credibility remains low even after the data are obtained (cf. Example 9.3). This, however, is no reflection of the P-value having been only "nominal." Indeed, even when nobody has the hypothesis in mind before the data are collected, the evidence and its consequent consideration of the relation can lead to the realization that it indeed has a strong rationale quite apart from the data, that is, that everyone concerned actually *should* have had it in mind before becoming aware of the data. In this case, the prior credibility, formulated a posteriori, is high, and with the evidence from the hypothesis-generating data it should naturally be even higher.

Finally, it is good to bear in mind that the entire stress on prior hypotheses has no actual foundation in the mathematical aspects of the P-value. It is a statistic considered in "frequentist" statistics only. None of the formulations involved address the history of the mind-set of the investigator in any way. Bayesian statistics does address subjective credibility of hypotheses, but its formulations for inference make no distinction between prior hypotheses and those suggested by the data (see Section 9.7.2).

9.3.4. *P*-Values for Multiple Hypotheses

Another prevalent belief among epidemiologists is that the interpretation of a P-value must be modified whenever *more than one hypothesis* is tested within a single study. It is said, for example, that if 20 hypotheses are tested at the level $\alpha = 0.05$, one should expect one P-value to be "significant" ($P < \alpha$), even if all 20 "null hypotheses" are correct, and that therefore such significance is only "nominal" or insignificant. The point, if tenable, is again of substantial moment in epidemiologic research, because of the commonality of multiple secondary objectives even in the context of a single core object for the study (Section 5.5).

This notion, just as the previous one, has remained alien to the author. It is unarguably true, of course, that the larger the number of hypotheses tested, the larger the number for which there is supportive evidence; and the same applies to detracting evidence as well. In no way does this seem to imply that whoever tests a multitude of hypotheses inherently has less than the "nominal" amount of evidence for or against any *particular one*, regardless of whether the evidence is provided by a single study or by a series of studies, parallel or sequential. Indeed, it is not even clear what constitutes a single study or body of data as opposed to a multitude of separate studies or bodies of data. The common-sense posture would seem to be that, when testing a particular hypothesis, the existence of data bearing on other, completely unrelated hypotheses is immaterial, regardless of whether those data were obtained as part of the same study or in another one (whatever the distinction). A clinician, too, when diagnosing a particular illness in a patient, is not burdened by any other illnesses that he/she is also diagnosing on the patient—as long as those other illnesses do not manifest themselves in the same symptoms, signs, or laboratory tests.

As the theoretical basis for the "multiple testing problem" one usually refers to the "frequentist" mathematics concerning the testing of "omnibus" hypotheses—ones that concern, simultaneously, a multitude of contrasts in terms of a single determinant. This has nothing to do with a series of tests concerned with separate and unrelated determinants/hypotheses. Indeed, "frequentist" statistics does not even admit the concepts of "related" and "unrelated" hypotheses, and it provides, therefore, no source of insights in this context. Bayesian statistics, on the other hand, does address these concepts and this distinction. One speaks of "correlated" and "uncorrelated" hypotheses, respectively, and the theory is in conformity with common sense: related hypotheses must be examined jointly, whereas unrelated ones can be tested separately; and in the latter case, it is altogether immaterial how many hypotheses are tested within a single study.

EXAMPLE **9.4.** Consider the study of the etiology of traffic accidents and, in particular, the separate hypotheses that implicate speed, alcohol, sedatives, tiredness, darkness, heavy rain, road conditions, and traffic density, respectively. To test the effect of speed, one must control potential confounding by the other factors insofar as they may be associated with speed (positively or negatively). In viewing the evidence (P-value) on the speed relation obtained in this way, one must ask whether it represents the entirety of the evidence on this relation in the data. In other words, one asks whether evidence (or a priori knowledge) about the existence of, for example, an alcohol effect has bearing on the credibility of the speed hypothesis. If alcohol effect means effect conditionally on speed (with speed controlled in the analysis), it has no relevance. The same unrelatedness characterizes all the other hypotheses relative to the speed hypotheses. However, the alcohol, sedative, and tiredness hypotheses are mutually related—meaning that insofar as one of them is known or suspected to be correct, this has bearing on the credibility of the other two. Thus, in considering any one of them, it is necessary to take cognizance of the evidence (and a priori information) on the other two.

EXAMPLE 9.5.   Consider the evidence bearing on a particular, single hypothesis, viewed according to categories of potential modifiers, age and gender, for example. By and large, if the effect exists in one category, it exists in the others as well. Therefore, the basic existence of the effect should be tested by considering the evidence from all the categories jointly, rather than category by category. Once such an effect is considered to exist, it remains to study its possible quantitative modification by age and gender.

9.3.5. *P*-Values in Repeat Testing

Another putative subtlety that occurs frequently in the analysis and interpretation of epidemiologic data relates to *repeated testing* of the same hypothesis, which is associated with periodic updatings of the data base in the course of the accrual of study experience. The common belief is that a history of such "sequential testing" again causes the *P*-values on the total data to be "nominal" only, unless particular procedures specific for such testing (Armitage, 1975) are employed. In particular, the thinking is again that for the "nominal" statistic from the total data, $\Pr(P < \alpha \mid H_0) > \alpha$, thus rendering the test invalid (cf. Section 9.3.1). It does stand to reason that consideration of only the smallest *P*-value along the way would entail this problem, but when *all* the accrued evidence is considered, it is quite inapparent to the author how the evidence in the data—whether for or against the hypothesis—is reduced by the previous examinations of the less complete data. Once again, Bayesian theory conforms with intuition: the evidence in the accrued data (summarized in a likelihood ratio) is in no way dependent on the previous testings (Cornfield, 1966).

When faced with these common guidelines to scientific inference, it is well to be aware of their origins. As noted, those tenets are not closely argued corollaries of express theory. Insofar as theory is involved at all, it is some aspect of "frequentist" statistics—theory that never addresses scientific insights and the consequent beliefs about particular propositions, the mental entities that scientific inference is to modify. Subjective Bayesian statistics does deal with beliefs; regrettably, however, it does not play much of a role in the training of epidemiologists (or biostatisticians) nor in the practice of epidemiologic data analysis and inference.

9.4. TESTING VS. ESTIMATION

In hypothesis testing, an inherently quantitative problem is viewed qualitatively. The concern is to learn *whether* there is a relation between the occurrence of the outcome phenomenon and the potential determinant. Such a viewpoint is appropriate in the context of *discovery* and its *verification* or *refutation*, which are aspects of hypothesis testing. (The use of those terms reflects a presumption as to what the proper "conclusion" is—an outlook that is readily at variance with the realities of research, as discussed in Section 9.1).

Once a hypothesis has gained substantial credibility among experts in general, interest shifts from its testing to the quantitative particulars of the relation—to estimation of parameters of the relation (Appendix 2).

The problem in the estimation phase of the evolution of knowledge is but an extension of the qualitative one. In hypothesis testing the focus of inference is the null value of the parameter of interest relative to the hypothesized range of values. More specifically, in epidemiology, hypothesis testing commonly addresses discrimination between the null value and a semi-infinite range of hypothesized values, with that range bounded by the null value (Section 9.1). In estimation, by contrast, the null value has no particular status. Either the parsimonious posture that it represents has already been "rejected," or there was no hypothesis to begin with (as is commonplace in comparative clinical trials, for example). Thus the focus of the analysis and inference is extended from the null value to other particular values of the parameter, and preoccupation with the hypothesized range as a whole is replaced by concern for more specific ranges.

9.5. INTERVAL ESTIMATES

9.5.1. One-Sided Interval Estimate

In hypothesis testing there is, as was observed, an a priori value of focal concern for the comparative parameter (the null value), and in the ordinary ("classical" or "frequentist") approach one derives its associated *P*-value.

It is a simple variation of that theme to make an a priori commitment to a particular *P*-value ($P = \alpha$) and to derive its associated value for the parameter. Thus, while in hypothesis testing one derives the *P*-value for the null proposition of no association (i.e., rate ratio equal to unity, etc.), one may take an interest in $P = 0.05$, for example, and derive that value of rate ratio (*RR*) for which, were it tested as the null value, the *P*-value would equal 0.05. Clearly, if, for the null value, $P < 0.05$, and if the hypothesis implies $RR > 1$, the value of RR corresponding to $P = 0.05$ is larger than the null value of unity. Similarly, if $P > 0.05$ for $RR = 1$, then, with a hypothesis implying $RR > 1$, $P = 0.05$ corresponds to a value of RR less than unity. If P equals 0.05 against $RR = 1$, the parameter value for which the P-value is 0.05 is the null value itself.

Such a value of the parameter—the one that corresponds to a particular, a priori P-value—is termed a "confidence limit" or "confidence bound." In particular, with the P-value set at some $P = \alpha$, the corresponding value of the parameter is referred to as a "one-sided 100 $(1 - \alpha)\%$ confidence bound." If the hypothesis implies parameter values larger than the null value, this particular value is the "lower" one-sided bound; otherwise, it is the "upper" one-sided bound, at the "confidence level" of $1 - \alpha$. A lower bound is associated with an "upper-tail" P-value; conversely, an upper bound is based on a "lower-tail" P-value. (For definitions of these P-values, see Section 10.1.1.)

The frequency behavior of a one-sided confidence bound is, of course, a derivative of that of the P-value. Thus, with the hypothesis implying exceedance of the null value of the parameter, the value corresponding to $P = \alpha$ (the lower one-sided bound at the "confidence level" of $1 - \alpha$) is such that in $100\alpha\%$ of applications it exceeds the actual (but generally unknown) value of the parameter. By the same token, in $100(1 - \alpha)\%$ of applications it falls below the actual value of the parameter. In these latter instances the corresponding *confidence interval* or *interval estimate*, which ranges from the lower bound to the highest conceivable value of the parameter, covers the actual value of the parameter, so that the coverage rate is $100(1 - \alpha)\%$. If the hypothesis implies that the parameter value is smaller than the null value, the bound corresponding to $P = \alpha$ (the upper one-sided bound at the level of $1 - \alpha$) falls below the actual parameter value in $100\alpha\%$ of applications, so that the interval (the range of values smaller than the bound) fails to cover the actual value of the parameter. In the remaining $100(1 - \alpha)\%$ of applications the bound exceeds the parameter's actual value and the interval covers it.

The frequency behavior of confidence intervals justifies the data-prognostic idea that one may be $100(1 - \alpha)\%$ confident that a $100(1 - \alpha)\%$ interval, yet to be derived, will cover the parameter's actual value. This does not mean, however, that one attaches $100(1 - \alpha)\%$ confidence for the coverage of an interval already computed and known to the person whose confidence (subjective credence) is at issue. For example, one cannot generally be 95% confident that a 95% confidence interval, already known, covers the actual value of the parameter, even if there is no uncertainty about the *validity* of the interval, that is, of the validity of the data themselves nor of the structure or computation of the interval. Such confidence is justified only when there is *no prior information* about the magnitude of the parameter.

EXAMPLE 9.6.   As an illustration of the latter condition, recall Example 9.3. With five heads out of five tosses of a coin, the lower one-sided 95% confidence bound for the rate of heads, in terms of the "exact" procedure based on mid-P (Section 10.1.3), is the solution of $\frac{1}{2}R^5 = 0.05$. That bound has the value of 0.63. From this statistic it does not follow that a reasonable person would be 95% confident that the probability of heads is at least 0.63— or even as high as 0.55. Rather, one would infer that here is one of the instances in which the interval fails to cover the parameter.

Total absence of prior information is very rare in epidemiologic research. Therefore, in general, one is not at all $100(1 - \alpha)\%$ confident that a particular $100(1 - \alpha)\%$ "confidence" interval, however valid, covers the value of the parameter of interest. Thus, the role of an interval estimate is analogous to that of a P-value: it is a statistic only, an element in the summarization of the evidence in the data. Indeed, the presentation of a multitude of confidence bounds, each corresponding to a particular level of "confidence" ($1 - \alpha$)—a particular P-value—constitutes a thorough summary of the data. Such a summary is tantamount to presenting the P-value as a function of the parameter of interest, the *P-value function* (cf. Folks, 1981).

EXAMPLE 9.7.   Recall the "data" representing five heads out of five tosses of a coin, with the null rate of heads equal to $\frac{1}{2}$ and the hypothesis (suggested by the data) that the theoretical rate exceeds $\frac{1}{2}$ (Examples 9.3 and 9.6). For any value R (unspecified) of the rate the corresponding P-value ("upper-tail mid-P"; see Section 10.1.3) is $\frac{1}{2}R^5$. Its value of $\alpha = 0.05$ corresponds to $R = 0.63$, which is thus the lower one-sided 95% the confidence bound (Example 9.6). The corresponding 90% bound corresponds to $P = 0.10$, that is, the bound is the solution of $\frac{1}{2}R^5 = 0.10$. This confidence bound is $R = 0.72$. The 80% bound is the solution of $\frac{1}{2}R^5 = 0.20$, which is 0.83; and so on. Clearly, insofar as a particular statistic, for example the 95% bound, is informative, a whole series of such statistics is even more so. Moreover, such a summary (analysis) of the evidence (five heads out of five tosses) is a trivial derivative of the P-value as a function of the parameter: the point $(P,R) = (0.05,0.63)$ implies the 95% one-sided confidence bound.

These concepts are illustrated in Figure 9.1, which deals with the example given above.

As illustrated, the extension of hypothesis testing (of P-value computation against the null value) to one-sided interval estimation leads to a whole series of statistics—confidence bounds corresponding to various confidence levels (P-values) of interest. This raises the question of what confidence levels, or what range of the P-value function, should be accented in the presentation of the results of an analysis. The answer depends on the end to which the evidence is presented. If the concern is to show evidence for a *discovery* (in the context of a new hypothesis) or presumed *verification* (of a previous hypothesis), the main interest is in small P-values and, thus, in parameter

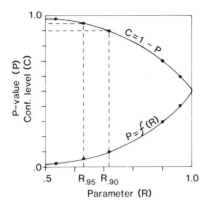

Figure 9.1. Derivation of lower one-sided confidence bounds for the theoretical rate (R), given five events out of five trials (Example 9.7). The 95% bound corresponds to $P = 0.05$, the 90% bound to $P = 0.10$, and so on.

values (confidence bounds) that correspond to high levels of confidence. Hence, if the P-value against the null point is 0.003, for example, one might wish to ascertain what parameter values correspond to the P-values of 0.01, 0.05, and 0.10; that is, one might wish to supplement the evidence in the P-value computed against the null proposition with one-sided confidence bounds corresponding to the confidence levels of 99, 95, and 90%, respectively. Alternatively, the P-value function could be shown graphically in the range from the null P-value (0.003) to $P = 0.10$.

If the evidence is summarized in the spirit of a presumed *refutation* of a previous hypothesis, in which case the null P-value is intermediate or large, the supplementary confidence bounds should correspond to large P-values (low confidence levels). For example, if the hypothesis implies a positive association and the P-value against the "null hypothesis" is 0.20, one ascertains how close to the null value of the chosen parameter (e.g., the rate ratio) are the values corresponding to the P-values of 0.90, 0.95, and 0.99; that is, one wants to supplement the null P-value with one-sided upper confidence bounds corresponding to the confidence levels of 90, 95, and 99%, respectively. (These bounds must be close to the null value for the data to detract from the hypothesis. If they are "deep" in the hypothesis-implied region of the parameter, the data are rather uninformative about the correctness of the hypothesis, and too sparse for appreciable modification of its credibility (cf. Section 9.3.2).

9.5.2. Two-Sided Interval Estimate

One-sided confidence bounds serve to supplement the P-value corresponding to the null proposition whenever the thrust of the analysis is hypothesis testing.

When the concern is not to test a hypothesis but to estimate—to quantify—a parameter, the P-value function still serves as the basic, overall summary of the evidence in the data. If the quantification addresses a com-

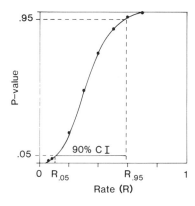

Figure 9.2. Derivation of two-sided confidence bounds (interval estimates), given three events out of 10 trials (Example 9.8). The bounds of the 90% interval, $R_{.05}$ and $R_{0.95}$, correspond to $P = 0.05$ and $P = 0.95$, respectively, and their values are 0.11 and 0.59, respectively.

parative parameter (Appendix 2), the P-values are computed analogously with that for the null value of the parameter. Thus, if the original hypothesis implies a positive relation, the "upper-tail" P-value (the increasing P-value function) is considered; and in the context of negative relation, the "lower-tail" P-value (the decreasing P-value function) is appropriate (see Sections 10.1.1 and 10.1.3).

Given a P-value function, the quantitative concern with it is to identify what range of the parameter seems reasonably consistent with the data, and, thus, what ranges seem rather inconsistent with them. In this spirit, there is equal interest in identifying the parameter values that correspond to small P-values, such as 0.05, and large ones, such as 0.95. In other words, in quantification the interest is in *two-sided confidence intervals*—ranges of parameter values bounded by those corresponding to two equally extreme P-values, one corresponding to $P = \alpha/2$ and the other to $P = 1 - \alpha/2$. Values within the interval are regarded as consistent with the data, at the chosen confidence level of $100(1 - \alpha)\%$, and those outside the interval inconsistent with the data at that level.

EXAMPLE 9.8.   Suppose that a new treatment is introduced and tried on 10 patients, and that three of them show a favorable outcome, despite uniform failures of past treatments. It is obvious that the treatment is efficacious, and it remains to quantify the success rate R. For any given value of R, the "upper-tail" mid-P (Equation 10.26) is the corresponding probability of at least four successes out of 10 trials plus half of the probability of the observed number, three. Equivalently, $P = 1 - \text{Pr}(0-2 \text{ successes}) - \frac{1}{2}\text{Pr}(3 \text{ successes})$. Based on tables of binomial probabilities (Section A.10.1), this P-value, a function of R, is presented in Figure 9.2. The figure also shows an example of two-sided confidence intervals implied by the P-value function.

Such a two-sided interval, with the "nonconfidence" (α) equally split, is designed not only to cover the actual parameter value (unknown) in $100(1 - \alpha)\%$ of applications, but also to have the two types of noncoverage occur with equal frequencies: in $100(\alpha/2)\%$ of applications the lower bound (and thus the whole interval) is above the target value, and with this same frequency the upper bound falls below the actual value of the parameter.

This frequency behavior of a $100(1 - \alpha)\%$ confidence interval does not mean that one may be $100(1 - \alpha)\%$ confident that the actual value lies within a particular interval already known, or that the probability (credibility) of its falling below (above) the interval is $100(\alpha/2)\%$ (see Section 9.5.1).

9.6. POINT ESTIMATE

From the preceding sections it is evident that a 50% one-sided bound equals both the upper and lower bounds of a 0% two-sided interval. That point of merger of two-sided limits (that point interval) is a "point estimate" of the parameter.

A fundamental *validity* criterion for the point estimate, inherent in a 0% two-sided interval, is that each of the two types of error occur $100(\alpha/2)\%$ = 50% of the time (Section 9.5.2). Hence, a point estimate is valid if the actual value of the parameter is the median of the sampling distribution of the point estimator, or the fundamental validity criterion for point estimates is *median unbiasedness*. This contrasts sharply with mean unbiasedness, meaning that the mean (rather than the median) of the sampling distribution of the point estimate equals the target value. This latter property is not a desideratum for point estimates. Thus, ordinary point estimators of rate ratio in epidemiology take on the value of infinity with nonzero probability; and even though this signifies that their means—and thereby their mean biases— are infinite, this is no detriment to their use.

Given median unbiasedness, the remaining desideratum is *efficiency*, or maximal attainable precision, that is, minimal attainable sampling variability.

Both of these properties are, in general, attained quite well by the use of the *empirical value* of the parameter, for example, the empirical rate ratio as a point estimate of the theoretical rate ratio. This can also be said about the *maximum likelihood* estimator (cf. Birnbaum, 1962), which is the value of the parameter that corresponds to the maximum of the likelihood ratio function (Section 9.7.1).

9.7. THE LIKELIHOOD RATIO

9.7.1. Essence of the Likelihood Ratio

We have seen that insofar as the essential statistics resulting from data analysis are taken to be the P-value (against the null proposition) together with interval and point estimates, it suffices to derive the P-value function, since all of these statistics can then be deduced ("read") from this function (cf.

Folks, 1981). Its "reading" might best be left to the paper's audience, in part because individual interests in the audience, in terms of what values to accent in the function, may not coincide with those of the investigator(s).

Even though the statistics that may be read directly from a P-value function are of the sort almost singularly used in epidemiology, there is an important alternative to the P-value concept, and thus to the P-value function, namely the *likelihood ratio* (*LR*) and the *LR* function.

Unlike the P-value, the *LR* is not designed to have a particular type of sampling distribution, which is conditional on any given value for the parameter at issue. Instead, it addresses the relative merits of any given value of the parameter and its null value, in "explaining" the data that were actually obtained. Specifically, in the context of discretely (as against continuously) distributed data, the *LR* may be defined as

$$LR_h = \frac{\text{Pr}(\text{Data} \mid H_h)}{\text{Pr}(\text{Data} \mid H_0)} \tag{9.3}$$

where H_h represents a particular value of the parameter at issue within the hypothesis-implied range, and H_0 is the null value.

EXAMPLE 9.9. Consider, on a single subject, the datum that a screening test shows a positive result. Its probability on the "hypothesis" (that the disease is present) equals the "sensitivity" of the test, $1 - $ false negative rate (*fnr*). On the "null hypothesis" (of no disease) it equals the false positive rate (*fpr*). Thus, for the category in which the disease is present the *LR* is $LR_d = (1 - fnr)/(fpr)$; for the other, null category it is $LR_0 = (fpr)/(fpr) = 1$.

EXAMPLE 9.10. Consider, from a single study, the datum that $P < \alpha$ (with α an a priori level for the test and the P-value computed on H_0). For this datum, the probability on a particular nonnull value (H_h) of the hypothesis equals the power of the test at that value, $1 - \beta_h$. On H_0 the probability is (designed to be) α. Thus, $LR = LR_h = (1 - \beta_h)/\alpha$ at H_h, and $LR = LR_0 = 1$ against H_0.

In the context of continuously distributed data, the probability of the observed data (which is zero, theoretically) is replaced by the corresponding *probability density, f*( ):

$$LR_h = \frac{f(\text{Data} \mid H_h)}{f(\text{Data} \mid H_0)} \tag{9.4}$$

EXAMPLE 9.11. Consider the difference in mean outcomes between two categories of a potential determinant (of the mean). Given a theoretical mean difference *MD*, the empirical one (*md*) might be taken to have a Gaussian distribution with mean *MD* and variance V_{md}, with the latter estimated from the data and presumed to be independent of *MD* itself. Under this model (see Section A.10.5), $LR_h = \exp[-(1/2)(md - MD_h)^2/V_{md}]/\exp[-(1/2)(md - 0)^2/V_{md}]$. It is seen to be a function of MD_h, *with its maximum corresponding to* $MD_h = md$, and the value of unity corresponding to $MD_h = 0$, the null value. At $MD_h = md$ the value is seen to be $\exp[(1/2)(md)^2/V_{md}]$.

In Example 9.11, and in general, the *LR* function, as defined, takes on the value of unity at the null point and reaches its maximum at the *maximum-likelihood* point estimate of the parameter. At each point, the value of the function expresses the relative probability or probability density for the data, contrasting that value of the parameter with the null value.

9.7.2. Interpretation of the Likelihood Ratio

The *LR* function, in contrast to the *P*-value function, provides for the computation of the probability that a hypothesis is correct or, more generally, the probabilities of various ranges of the parameter's values.

If the hypothesis is "simple," implying a single value for the probability of the data, and if there are no alternative hypotheses and no concerns about validity, the interpretation can be done formally by simple application of Bayes' Theorem. Specifically, if P' denotes the prior credibility of the hypothesis, its posterior credibility, or probability of correctness, is

$$P'' = \frac{1}{1 + [(1 - P')/P']/(LR)} \tag{9.5}$$

This function implies, for example, that if $P' = 0$, then $P'' = 0$ regardless of the data (cf. Example 9.1), and that if $P' = 1$, then $P'' = 1$. In other words, it implies that evidence does not change the mind of someone who is fully committed to either the a priori parsimonious view (the "null hypothesis") or to the hypothesis itself, that is, that evidence changes the views of the open-minded only. The function also shows that if $LR = 1$ (i.e., if the data are explained equally well by the hypothesis and its denial), then $P'' = P'$ and the data lead to no change in view (cf. Section 9.3.2).

EXAMPLE 9.12.   Recall Example 9.9 concerning a positive result from a screening test. The "hypothesis" (that the disease is present) implies the singular value of $1 - fnr$ for the probability of this result, and it has no alternative—only the denial, the null proposition of the absence of the disease. Thus, it is appropriate to use the formula given above, with $LR_d = (1 - fnr)/(fpr)$ for the instances of test positivity. In particular, if the prior credibility of the presence of the disease is 50%, and if, for the test, $fnr = 20\%$ and $fpr = 5\%$, the probability of the disease in the face of a positive test result is $P'' = 1/\{1 + [(1 - 0.5)/0.5]\,0.05/(1-0.20)\} = 94\%$. For a *negative* test result the probabilities conditional on the presence and absence of the disease are *fnr* and $1 - fpr$, respectively, so that $LR_d = (fnr)/(1 - fpr)$. The corresponding P'' (with $P' = 50\%$, $fnr = 20\%$, and $fpr = 5\%$) is 15%.

EXAMPLE 9.13. Recall Example 9.10, dealing with the *LR* corresponding to a "significant" result ($P < \alpha$) of a statistical test. It was found that its corresponding likelihood function is $(1 - \beta_h)/\alpha$. If the data are sparse, the power $1 - \beta_h$ remains close to the level ("null power") α of the test throughout the hypothesized range. This means that LR_h remains close to one throughout, and therefore P'' remains close to P', regardless of the "significance" of the result. In the other extreme, the case of ample data, β_h is essentially zero at minor deviations from H_0 already. Theoretically, then, $P'' = 1/\{1 + [(1 - P')/P']\alpha\}$—a value close to one. In this type of situation, however, it is unrealistic to regard α, the nominal level of the test, as the actual level α^*. Points in the immediate vicinity of the null value are regarded as essentially null (as opposed to nonnull) values, a rate ratio of 1.1, for example. This reflects a lack of theoretical interest in trivial deviations from the idealized null value, and insufficient validity of the data for their pursuit. Thus, points next to the theoretical null value are in the operative null region, and with ample information (I) the value of α^* can approach unity within this region. With $I \to \infty$, the consequence is $\alpha^* \to 1$; this means that $LR \to 1$, which implies that $P'' \to P'$ (cf. Section 9.3.2).

If the interpreter allows for alternative hypotheses as well, the prior credibility is to be divided among all the hypotheses and their shared denial. In this case,

$$P'_0 + \sum_h P'_h = 1, \tag{9.6}$$

where P'_0 and P'_h are the prior probabilities of the "null hypothesis" and the hth hypothesis, with the summation ranging over all the alternative hypotheses. For the hth hypothesis, the posterior credibility is

$$P''_h = \frac{P'_h(LR_h)}{P'_0 + \sum_h P'_h(LR_h)}, \tag{9.7}$$

where LR_h is the *LR* contrasting the hth hypothesis to the "null hypothesis." The posterior credibility of the "null hypothesis" in the context of several hypotheses is not the complement of P''_h but $1 - \sum_h P''_h$, that is,

$$P''_0 = [1 + \sum_h (P'_h/P'_0)(LR_h)]^{-1}. \tag{9.8}$$

These formulations apply also to solitary "complex" hypotheses, that is, to epidemiologic hypotheses of the ordinary, qualitative kind. The hypothesis can be viewed as consisting of multiple quantitative alternatives, or as multiple "simple" hypotheses that are alternatives to one another. Thus, given the *LR* function from the data (and the presumption of validity), any personal prior view can be translated into the corresponding posterior credibility P'' = $1 - P_0''$, using Equation 9.8. Clearly, this probability depends not only on the prior credibility of H, or of H_0, per se, but also on how the prior probability of H is distributed over various quantitative subdomains within H.

Because the distribution of prior probability within H is a subjective matter, general discourse may be aided by considering the *maximal impact of the data* on the credibility of H over all possible distributions of the prior credibility of H over the particular values within its range. This extreme corresponds to assigning the entire prior probability of H to the value at which the *LR* assumes its maximum value. Thus,

$$P''_{max} = 1 - (P_0'')_{min}$$

$$= 1 - \left\{ 1 + \left(\frac{1 - P_0'}{P_0'} \right) [max_h(LR_h)] \right\}^{-1} \qquad (9.9)$$

$$= \left[1 + \frac{P_0'/(1 - P_0')}{max_h(LR_h)} \right]^{-1}.$$

This formulation presupposes that the value of the empirical test criterion falls in the hypothesized range of the parameter values. With the details of the subjective prior distribution thus suppressed, it is possible to report the extreme posterior probabilities corresponding to various individual prior probabilities for the hypothesis.

EXAMPLE 9.14.   In the Boston Collaborative Drug Surveillance Program, a multitude of diagnostic entities were compared as to the patients' distributions by a variety of blood antigen systems. Such screenings indicated that the *ss* phenotype in the *S* antigen system may occur with relatively high frequency among breast cancer patients. Since this was a data-suggested hypothesis, another case-referent study was carried out, in accordance with the prevailing "frequentist" principles (Section 9.3.3). This new study also showed a "significant" association, with a chi square (1 degree of freedom) value of 8.9. Thus, in the "frequentist" spirit, the "null hypothesis" of no association was "rejected" and the previous, data-suggested hypothesis was "accepted" (cf. Section 9.3.2). The "discovery" was published in a major medical journal (Boston Collaborative Drug Surveillance Program, 1971), with the author of this text as a member of the research team. However, data from two subsequent studies by others strongly refuted that "discovery," a proposition that had very low inherent credibility anyway, and the consensus now is that the original "finding" was false—an example of erroneous rejection of a correct null hypothesis, a case of a "Type I error." Suppose now that the data had been summarized in terms of the maximum of the *LR* function, and that its associated maximum posterior credibility in the context of a reasonable prior credibility had been considered (Equation 9.9). For LR_{max} the value could have been taken (Equation 10.18) as exp $[(\frac{1}{2})(8.9)] = 87$. Thus, for any given prior probability P' for the hypothesis, the *maximum* posterior probability would have been $\{1 + [(1 - P')/P']/(87)\}^{-1}$. As for a reasonable value for the original prior credibility, it would scarcely have exceeded 1%, since any given blood antigen system would have been an unlikely marker for any particular cancer, and the S antigen system and breast cancer would not have been regarded as exceptions to this general view. For that 1% prior probability the corresponding *maximum* posterior probability is $[1 + (0.99/0.01)/87]^{-1} = 47\%$, when using the second set of data only. Had the prior probability after the initial data been set to 5%, the corresponding maximal posterior probability would have been 82%. With analyses of this type, the hypothesis would probably not have engaged the investigators nor impressed the editor of the journal.

9.8. REVIEW

In this chapter, data analysis is viewed as the process of *summarizing the evidence* in the data with reference to the research problem, that is, as the process of deriving, under a chosen statistical model for the origin of the data, suitable statistics as a basis for inference. Although elements of inference are also introduced, a sharp distinction between analysis and inference is maintained, and more emphasis is placed on analysis than on inference. The main reason is that *analysis is a task within each research project, something for an investigator to at least understand, if not necessarily carry out personally, whereas inference is not a concern specific to the investigator(s). In the end, inference, which is inherently subjective, will be made by readers of the study report*, independently (ideally at least) of the investigator(s)' own inference.

As for the elements in such summarization, the distinction between testing and estimation is rather immaterial. To be sure, there are problems of hypothesis testing, distinct from those of quantification, with the latter characteristic of situations in which the hypothesis has already been accepted (more or less) or in which there was no hypothesis in the first place. Yet in data analysis one should not aim at presenting one set of statistics in hypothesis testing and another in estimation—in classical terms, the P-value for the null point in the former and a point and interval estimate in the latter. For it is clear that point and interval estimates do supplement the null P-value in summarizing the evidence for hypothesis testing, even if the null P-value is somewhat superfluous for the purpose of estimation. Thus, *the distinction between testing and estimation, which is often very natural and clear in the formulation of the research problem and, thereby, central to inference as well, has no major relevance to data analysis*.

A related point of emphasis has been that *all of the elements in classical ("frequentist") summaries of evidence—the null P-value, confidence limits, and the point estimate—are derivatives of a single statistic, the P-value as a function of the parameter of interest;* they can be "read" from a graphical display of the *P*-value function. Because of this, and considering that particular readers of the research report may wish to derive statistics other than those considered sufficient by the investigator(s), it is recommended that a rather comprehensive presentation of the *P*-value function become routine in the reporting of data analyses. Such presentations could be numerical, graphical, and/or mathematical.

Whatever classical statistics are derived and presented, they are defined in terms of their frequency properties, that is, their sampling distributions conditional on the value of the parameter of interest; they are "frequentist" statistics. They permit quantification of the frequency with which, over many studies, the "rejection" of a "null hypothesis" at a given level of testing is in error (Type I error rate), conditional on the denial proposition being correct. They similarly permit quantification of the frequency with which, over many studies, the "acceptance" of the null proposition is erroneous (Type II error rate), conditional on the hypothesis itself being correct. But they do not, generally, provide a firm basis for quantitative inference about a hypothesis, as the error rates are conditional on the very object of testing— the correctness or incorrectness of the hypothesis. Moreover, in inference the concern for error is not directed to studies at large; it is an ad hoc problem, a matter of correctness in the study at hand. In classical interval estimation, similarly, one focuses on the frequency of coverage/noncoverage among studies at large, but does not deal with whether *this* interval, computed and known, covers the parameter value under study.

For actual quantitative inference, which has to do with modification of views (about the merits of a hypothesis or about the magnitude of a parameter), *the intellectual framework is found in Bayesian statistics.* Despite all its unresolved problems, the one relevant to data analysis, as defined, is well settled; the information in the data, insofar as it is valid, is summarized in the *LR* function, for testing and for estimation. If that function is reported by the investigator(s), or if it can be deduced from the "frequentist" statistics that are given, the reader of the research report has the opportunity to engage in the *inherently personal, subjective task of quantitative scientific inference*—a meta-analytic challenge.

10

Analysis of
a Single Rate

In Chapter 9 we saw that data analysis with reference to a particular parameter is a matter of deriving the *P*-value function for the "frequentist" audience and the *LR* function for the Bayesian audience. From the former, the "frequentist" reads "the" *P*-value (at the null point of the parameter)—the null *P*-value—when the viewpoint is one of hypothesis testing. Whether the problem is one of testing or estimation, one reads one or more confidence bounds: for a one-sided interval one identifies the point (parameter value) at which the "upper-tail" *P*-value equals the nonconfidence level ($P = \alpha$, lower one-sided bound) or the confidence level ($1 - \alpha$, upper one-sided confidence bound), and for a two-sided interval one identifies the points at which $P = \alpha/2$ and $P = 1 - \alpha/2$, respectively. For the Bayesian reader the *LR* function is the summary of the evidence, the statistic that the reader couples with the personal prior view (prior probability function) to derive the corresponding posterior view—the posterior probability of the hypothesis or posterior probabilities for various ranges of the parameter.

In this first chapter on the procedures of data analysis we deal with the simplest data-analytic situation in epidemiology—the problem of assessing a rate without relating it to any determinant. In the context of this simple, noncomparative, problem some basic principles are introduced expressly, whereas in later chapters the reader's familiarity with them is assumed.

10.1. SINGLE PROPORTION

When the rate at issue is a proportion (Appendix 1), the data reduce two numbers, the empirical number of cases c and the number of subjects S, the latter constituting the observation base. In these terms, the empirical rate is

$$r = \frac{c}{S}. \tag{10.1}$$

In this expression r denotes the *empirical rate*, as distinguished from the *theoretical rate R*. The latter is the object of the study, and thus the object of inference in light of the data or, more specifically, in light of the statistics resulting from the analysis of the data.

10.1.1. Chi Square Function

In the context of a single rate, direct and exact computation of P-values for various values of the rate (theoretical) is a rather simple matter, and they can also be read from readily available tables. But since the nature of most data-analytic situations in epidemiology precludes exact analysis, for theoretical or practical reasons, consideration of this exact analysis is deferred to Section 10.1.3.

The usual approach to the derivation of P-values is "*asymptotic*," meaning that it provides exact results only in the limiting situation of an infinite amount of information in the data. Despite this theoretical limitation, asymptotic statistics tend to be quite adequate in ordinary situations of data analysis, but caution and judgment should always be exercised.

Asymptotic P-values are usually derived, in epidemiologic data analysis, on the basis of a chi square statistic, with 1 degree of freedom (df). Such a statistic is the square of a statistic whose distribution is, asymptotically, Gaussian ("normal") with mean zero and variance one (Appendix 10).

In the problem at issue, the *exact statistical model* underlying both the exact and the asymptotic analysis is that the observed number of cases c is a realization for a *binomial* distribution (Section A.10.1) with S "trials" (selections of study subject) and the probability of "success" (case) equal to R. Thus, the basic model reflects the presumption, philosophically somewhat problematic, that the study population is a simple random sample of the abstract reality to which the scientific inference refers (Section 9.1).

In a basic asymptotic analysis, the expectation (E_r) and variance (V_r) of the empirical rate are derived, without modification, from the underlying binomial model:

$$E_r = R, \tag{10.2}$$

$$V_r = \frac{R(1 - R)}{S}.$$

The approximation is only that the form of the distribution is taken to be Gaussian. In other words, the asymptotic model is that the sampling distribution of r is Gaussian with mean R and variance $R(1 - R)/S$. This implies that the statistic

$$X_R = \frac{r - R}{[R(1 - R)/S]^{1/2}} \tag{10.3}$$

is taken to be Gaussian with mean zero and variance one, that is, "standard" Gaussian, in its distribution. (This distribution is tabulated in Appendix 11.) Equivalently,

$$X_R^2 = \frac{(r - R)^2}{R(1 - R)/S} \tag{10.4}$$

is taken to have a chi square (χ^2) distribution with 1 df (tabulated in Appendix 12).

The Gaussian approximation may apply better to the *stable-variance metameter of the empirical rate* than to the rate itself. This metameter for a proportion is arc $\sin(r^{1/2}) = \sin^{-1}(r^{1/2})$, and its variance (to a first-order Taylor series approximation) is $1/(4S)$ on the radian scale, independent of R (Fisher, 1925). Its expectation (also to a first-order approximation) is $\sin^{-1}(R^{1/2})$. Thus, an alternative to the statistic given above is

$$X_R^2 = \frac{[\sin^{-1}(r^{1/2}) - \sin^{-1}(R^{1/2})]^2}{1/(4S)}. \tag{10.5}$$

The asymptotic P-value may be thought of as a transformation of the X-statistic (the standard Gaussian or "chi" statistic)—and, indeed, of the asymptotic model itself. The null property of uniform distribution in the 0–1 range (Section 9.3.1) is satisfied (asymptotically) by the cumulative Gaussian probability at X, $F_g(X)$, and also by its complement, $1 - F_g(X)$. The former is the "lower-tail" P-value against the value R:

$$P_{lt} = F_g(X), \tag{10.6}$$

with the probability derived from a tabulation of the standard Gaussian model (Appendix 11). Its complement is the "upper-tail" P-value:

$$P_{ut} = 1 - F_g(X). \tag{10.7}$$

The actual P-value represents a choice between these two, with the aim of satisfying the nonnull property of P-values (Section 9.3.1) in instances in which there is a hypothesis. Specifically, if the hypothesis implies that $R > R_0$, then $P = P_{ut}$; if the hypothesis implies that $R < R_0$, then $P = P_{lt}$.

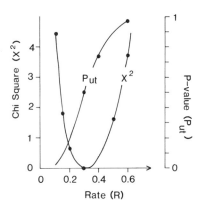

Figure 10.1. Basic X^2 function (Equation 10.4) and its associated "upper-tail" P-value function, given three events out of 10 trials (Example 10.1). For comparison with the corresponding exact P-value function, see Figure 9.2 and Table 10.1.

In terms of the cumulative probability of the chi square distribution (1 df) at X^2, $F_{\chi^2}(X^2)$, the derivation of the P-value requires cognizance of whether $R < r$ or $R > r$, because the X^2 statistic reflects only the absolute value of $(r - R)$. Where $R < r$,

$$P_{lt} = 1 - (\tfrac{1}{2})[1 - F_{\chi^2}(X^2)],$$
$$P_{ut} = (\tfrac{1}{2})[1 - F_{\chi^2}(X^2)]. \tag{10.8}$$

For the range of $R > r$,

$$P_{lt} = (\tfrac{1}{2})[1 - F_{\chi^2}(X^2)],$$
$$P_{ut} = 1 - (\tfrac{1}{2})[1 - F_{\chi^2}(X^2)]. \tag{10.9}$$

These relations define the *P-value function* on the basis of the X^2 function (Equations 10.4 and 10.5).

EXAMPLE 10.1. Recall the example of three therapeutic successes out of 10 instances of treatment (Example 9.8 and Figure 9.2). The basic X^2 function (without transformation, Equation 10.4) assumes the form $X_R^2 = (0.3 - R)^2/[R(1 - R)/10]$, depicted in Figure 10.1. Its value at $R = 0.1$, for example, is 4.44. The associated "upper-tail" P-value (Example 9.8) is derived by the use of Equation 10.8, since $0.1 < r (= 0.3)$. At 4.44, the complement of the cumulative probability is 0.035 (Appendix 12), and therefore $P_{ut} = 0.017$. At $R = 0.5$, $X^2 = 1.60$. Its associated exceedance probability is 0.21 (Appendix 12) and $P_{ut} = 0.90$ (Equation 10.9). Other points of the asymptotic P-value function may be derived in like manner, using Equation 10.8 on the left of $r = 0.3$, and Equation 10.9 to the right of this empirical value. This function is also shown in Figure 10.1. More accurate results are obtained by the use of the X^2 function based on the inverse-sine metameters of the rates. The value of $\sin^{-1}(0.3)^{1/2} = \sin^{-1}(0.548)$ is 33.2° (as obtained by the $\sin^{-1}$ function in a hand calculator). For $R = 0.1$, it is 18.4°. Thus, at $R = 0.1$, the value of the X^2 function in Equation 10.5 is $[(33.2 - 18.4)\,\pi/180]^2/$

$\{1/[4(10)]\} = 2.67$, where $\pi/180$ provides for the translation of degrees to radians. The corresponding P_{ut} is 0.05, as opposed to the value of 0.02 given above, and the exact mid-P value of 0.04. See Example 10.2 and Table 10.1.

Since the asymptotic X^2 function involves an approximation (Gaussian), P-values derived from it must always be viewed with caution and judgment, with the latter developed by combining theoretical principles and experience.

Theoretically, the question is whether the Gaussian approximation of the distribution of r (or its inverse-sine metameter, as the case may be) is tenable conditionally on R and S. When $R = 0.5$, the sampling distribution of r is symmetrical, and on this condition, very small series, such as $S < 5$ even, assure reasonable results from the asymptotic approach. On the other hand, if R is close to zero or one, the magnitude of $SR(1 - R)$—the variance of the empirical number of cases (c)—must be of sufficient magnitude. How large it is to be depends on what part of the P-value function is considered; the more extreme the theoretical value (R) under consideration—and the larger the X^2—the larger the information measure (the variance of c) needs to be.

Finally, the adequacy of the P-values, and their consequent confidence bounds (Section 9.5), depends on the use of the proper X^2 function, the basic one in Equation 10.4 or its modification in Equation 10.5. It deserves emphasis that the theoretically proper formulation in the absence of a variance-stabilizing transformation involves the *theoretical variance* of r, namely, $R(1 - R)/S$, not the empirical $r(1 - r)/S$.

Even though this principle has been known for a long time (see, for example, Wilson, 1927), its application has not become routine in epidemiology. It remains commonplace to derive two-sided $100(1 - \alpha)\%$ confidence bounds as

$$R_{\alpha/2}, R_{1-\alpha/2} = r \mp \chi_\alpha \left[\frac{r(1 - r)}{S}\right]^{1/2}. \tag{10.10}$$

These derive from

$$X_R^2 = \frac{(r - R)^2}{r(1 - r)/S}, \tag{10.11}$$

upon equating this function to the $100(1 - \alpha)$ centile, χ_α^2, of the χ^2 distribution. (Its value for 95% limits is $\chi_{0.05}^2 = 3.84$.)

The theoretically proper basic X^2 function (Equation 10.4), with $X_R^2 = \chi_\alpha^2$, yields the "quadratic" bounds of

$$R_{\alpha/2}, R_{1-\alpha/2} = \frac{-B \mp (B^2 - 4AC)^{1/2}}{2A} \tag{10.12}$$

where $A = 1 + \chi_\alpha^2/S$, $B = -(2r + \chi_\alpha^2/S)$, and $C = r^2$.

TABLE 10.1.

Comparison of the basic theoretically correct X^2 function (Equation 10.4), its variance-stabilized refinement (Equation 10.5), and the usual function (Equation 10.11) in the context of three cases in a series of 10 subjects (Examples 10.1 and 10.2); the exact mid-P (Equation 10.26) is also shown

| | Asymptotic Approach | | | | | | |
| | Equation 10.4 | | Equation 10.5 | | Equation 10.11 | | Exact |
R	X^2	P_{ut}	X^2	P_{ut}	X^2	P_{ut}	P_{ut}
0.1	4.44	0.02	2.67	0.05	1.90	0.08	0.04
0.3	0.00	0.50	0.00	0.50	0.00	0.50	0.48
0.5	1.60	0.90	1.69	0.90	1.90	0.92	0.89
0.6	3.75	0.97	3.76	0.97	4.29	0.99	0.97
0.7	7.62	0.997	6.77	0.995	7.62	0.997	0.994

The X^2 function that involves a variance-stabilizing transformation of the rates (Equation 10.5) gives

$$(R_{\alpha/2})^{1/2}, (R_{1-\alpha/2})^{1/2} = \sin\left[\sin^{-1}(r^{1/2}) \mp \frac{\chi_\alpha}{2S^{1/2}}\right]. \quad (10.13)$$

To gain a bit of experience, it may be helpful to consider a couple of numerical examples.

EXAMPLE 10.2. The X^2 function considered in Example 10.1, based on the theoretically correct formulation (Equation 10.4), and the commonly used incorrect function (Equation 10.11), are tabulated in Table 10.1. The corresponding asymptotic P-values are also shown, together with the exact mid-P (Section 10.1.3; see Example 9.8 and Figure 9.2).

EXAMPLE 10.3. Suppose that no cases appeared among 10 subjects. This makes the ordinary confidence limits (Equation 10.10) both equal to zero for any chosen confidence level. This is unappealing. The basic approach advocated here (Equation 10.12) gives, as the 95% interval, $R_{0.025}, R_{0.975} = (0.384 \mp 0.384)/[2(1.384)] = 0.00, 0.28$. For the "angular" interval (Equation 10.13), $\sin^{-1}(r^{1/2}) = 0$; $\chi_\alpha/(2S^{1/2}) = (3.84)^{1/2}/[2(10)^{1/2}] = 0.310$ on the radian scale, $0.310(180)/\pi = 17.8$ in terms of degrees; $\sin(\mp0.310\,\text{rad}) = \sin(\mp17.8°) = -0.305, 0.305$. It follows that $R_{0.025} = 0.00$ and $R_{0.975} = (0.305)^2 = 0.09$, a poor result. (In terms of the exact mid-P, $R_{0.975}$ is the solution of $(1/2)(1 - R)^{10} = 0.025$; its value is 0.26.)

10.1.2. Asymptotic LR Function

The asymptotic "likelihood" (Section 9.7.1) that corresponds to the empirical rate r reflects the Gaussian approximation of its distribution conditionally on the theoretical value of the rate. The likelihood is the Gaussian density (Section A.10.5) at r,

$$f(r \mid R) = (2\pi V_r^{1/2})^{-1} \exp \left[-\frac{1}{2} \frac{(r - R)^2}{V_r} \right], \qquad (10.14)$$

where V_r is the variance of r, that is, $V_r = R(1 - R)/S$ (Equation 10.2). This function is, evidently, specific for the data at hand (r) and it is construed as a function of the potential values of the parameter under study (R).

Insofar as there is a hypothesis about the value, and its associated null value (Section 9.2) $R = R_0$, the basic LR function, as defined in Section 9.7.1, is

$$LR_R = \frac{f(r \mid R)}{f(r \mid R_0)}. \qquad (10.15)$$

Specifically, then,

$$LR_R = \left[\frac{R_0(1 - R_0)}{R(1 - R)} \right]^{1/2} \exp \left\{ -\frac{1}{2} \left[\frac{(r - R)^2}{R(1 - R)/S} - \frac{(r - R_0)^2}{R_0(1 - R_0)/S} \right] \right\} \qquad (10.16)$$

$$= \left(\frac{V_r \mid R_0}{V_r \mid R} \right)^{1/2} \exp \left[-\tfrac{1}{2}(X_R^2 - X_{R_0}^2) \right].$$

This function reflects the inconstancy of the variance of the empirical rate (variance conditional on, or restricted by, the theoretical rate) over the possible values of the theoretical rate. If the X^2 function is based on the *variance-stabilizing transformation* (Equation 10.5),

$$LR_R = \exp \left[-\tfrac{1}{2}(X_R^2 - X_{R_0}^2) \right], \qquad (10.17)$$

a simple derivative of the X^2 function alone.

The maximum of the function, it may be recalled, is of interest when one considers the *maximal impact of the data* on the probability (credibility) of a hypothesis over various distributions of the prior probability within the hypothesized region (Section 9.7.2). It is attained at $R = r$ and equals

$$\max_R(LR_R) = \exp(\tfrac{1}{2}X_{R_0}^2) \qquad (10.18)$$

if the variance-stabilizing transformation is used in X^2 (Equation 10.5).

10.1.3. Exact P-Value Function

Exact analyses of a single rate are based on the binomial model per se, without any Gaussian approximation (Section 10.1.1). The exact counterparts of the asymptotic P-values (Equations 10.6 and 10.7) are commonly taken as

$$P_{\mathrm{lt}} = \sum_{x=0}^{c} P_{x|R,S} \qquad (10.19)$$

and

$$P_{\mathrm{ut}} = \sum_{x=c}^{S} P_{x|R,S} \qquad (10.20)$$

with c the observed number of cases and $P_{x|R,S}$ the binomial probability of x "successes" out of S "trials," given that the probability of "success" is R (Section A.10.1). Owing to the discreteness of the distribution, these P-values do not satisfy the null property of $\Pr(P < \alpha) = \alpha$ (Section 9.3.1); they do not even add up to unity (but to $1 + P_{c|R,S}$).

Theoretically, the solution to this is the use of randomized P-values (Tocher, 1950). In these terms

$$P_{\mathrm{lt}} = \sum_{x=0}^{c-1} P_{x|R,S} + UP_{c|R,S} \qquad (10.21)$$

and

$$P_{\mathrm{ut}} = (1 - U)P_{c|R,S} + \sum_{x=c+1}^{S} P_{x|R,S}, \qquad (10.22)$$

where U represents a random variate with uniform distribution in the 0–1 range. These P-values have exactly the property that $\Pr(P < \alpha) = \alpha$ (as long as R is the correct value for the parameter). However, the random element is an extraneous one and unattractive as such.

The problem with randomized P-values is resolved by appreciating that there is no imperative to arrive at a point value for the P-value statistic. The discreteness of the distribution can be taken to mean that the exact P-value can be defined only as to its range, with the bounds corresponding to $U = 0$ and $U = 1$, respectively (Miettinen, 1974c). In these terms,

$$\sum_{x=0}^{c-1} P_{x|R,S} \leq P_{\mathrm{lt}} \leq \sum_{x=0}^{c} P_{x|R,S} \qquad (10.23)$$

and

$$\sum_{x=c+1}^{S} P_{x|R,S} \leq P_{\mathrm{ut}} \leq \sum_{x=c}^{S} P_{x|R,S}. \qquad (10.24)$$

Insofar as the consideration of these ranges lacks appeal, the most reasonable solution, in the author's opinion, is not to resort to the ordinary approach of using $U = 1$ in P_{lt} and $U = 0$ in P_{ut} (Equations 10.19 and 10.20). Instead, it seems reasonable to use $U = \frac{1}{2}$ in both (Lancaster, 1952; Miettinen, 1974c). The resulting mid-P from the "lower tail" is

$$P_{\mathrm{lt}} = \sum_{x=0}^{c-1} P_{x|R,S} + \tfrac{1}{2}P_{c|R,S},\tag{10.25}$$

and the corresponding "upper-tail" value is

$$P_{\mathrm{ut}} = \tfrac{1}{2}P_{c|R,S} + \sum_{x=c+1}^{S} P_{x|R,S}.\tag{10.26}$$

(These mid-P formulations were used in various examples above.)

10.1.4. Exact *LR* Function

For the asymptotic form of the *LR* function of a proportion-type rate (Equation 10.16), the exact counterpart is quite simple, conceptually and in form. Conceptually it is

$$LR_R = \frac{P_{c|R}}{P_{c|R_0}},\tag{10.27}$$

with $P_{c|R}$ representing, as before, the exact binomial probability (Section A.10.1) of the observed number (c) of cases, given the theoretical rate R. Specifically, then

$$\begin{aligned}
LR_R &= \frac{R^c(1 - R)^{S-c}}{R_0^c(1 - R_0)^{S-c}}\\
&= \left(\frac{R}{R_0}\right)^c \left(\frac{1 - R}{1 - R_0}\right)^{S-c}.
\end{aligned}\tag{10.28}$$

10.2. SINGLE DENSITY

Thus far we have considered rates of the form of a proportion. It remains to examine what modifications of the formulations given above are needed for the situation in which the empirical rate is of the form of incidence density,

$$r = \frac{c}{T},\tag{10.29}$$

where c is the empirical number of cases, as before, and T represents the amount of population time in which the cases appeared (cf. Equation 10.1).

The counterpart of the binomial model shown above is that c is a realization of the *Poisson* distribution (Section A.10.2) with expectation (and variance) equal to TR. Thus (cf. Equation 10.2),

$$E_r = R, \qquad V_r = \frac{R}{T}. \qquad (10.30)$$

The basic asymptotic model postulates a Gaussian distribution for r, with the mean and variance given above. The Gaussian form may be attained again, to a better approximation, by the use of a suitable transformation of the rate. Both the logarithmic and the square-root tranformation provide for good results, but the latter makes the variance of the metameter ($r^{1/2}$) independent of R itself. Specifically, in terms of a first-order Taylor series approximation,

$$E_{r^{1/2}} = R^{1/2}, \qquad (10.31)$$

$$V_{r^{1/2}} = \frac{1}{4T}.$$

Thus the chi square function may be taken as (cf. Equation 10.5)

$$\begin{aligned} X_R^2 &= \frac{(r^{1/2} - R^{1/2})^2}{1/(4T)} \\ &= \frac{[c^{1/2} - (TR)^{1/2}]^2}{1/4}. \end{aligned} \qquad (10.32)$$

EXAMPLE 10.4.   Given 5 cases in the context of 20 person-years of observation, $X_R^2 = \{[5/(20y)]^{1/2} - R^{1/2}\}^2/[1/(80y)]$. Its realization at $R = 5/(10y)$, for example, is $\{[5/(20y)]^{1/2} - [5/(10y)]^{1/2}\}^2/[1/(80y)] = [(1/2)^{1/2} - 1]^2(40) = 3.4$. More simply, $X^2 = [5^{1/2} - \{20y[5/(10y)]\}^{1/2}]^2/(1/4) = 3.4$.

The asymptotic *LR* function is that in Equation 10.17, as long as the X^2 function in it is based on the variance-stabilizing transformation (Equation 10.32).

The issues with the exact *P*-value function are analogous to those discussed for proportions (Section 10.1.3), except that the Poisson probability function (Section A.10.2) is used, and for P_{ut} the summation ranges, in principle, all the way to infinity (the maximum of the range of c). In practice, the consideration of a few terms tends to suffice. Moreover, the problem is obviated by writing

$$\begin{aligned} P_{ut} &= 1 - P_{lt} \\ &= \sum_{x=0}^{c-1} P_{x|R,T} + U P_{c|R,T} \end{aligned} \qquad (10.33)$$

(cf. Equations 10.21 and 10.22), with $U = \frac{1}{2}$ for the mid-P (cf. Equations 10.25 and 10.26).

The exact LR function (Equation 10.27) takes on the form

$$LR_R = \left(\frac{R}{R_0}\right)^c \exp[-T(R - R_0)]. \tag{10.34}$$

11

Comparative Analysis of Two Rates I:

NULL CHI SQUARE

In Chapter 10, the analysis of a single rate was considered as a topic of interest per se and also as a framework for introducing general first principles of data analysis. Here we turn to comparative analysis of two rates, that is, to the analyses directed to measures of occurrence *relation* (Section A.2.2).

In the context of measures of occurrence relation, each parameter that might be considered (e.g., rate difference) has a particular null value. These null values correspond to the null proposition of no relation between the absolute parameter of occurrence (e.g., rate) and the potential determinant at issue. It follows that there is complete interchangeability among the null propositions of rate difference = 0, rate ratio = 1, and odds ratio = 1 (cf. Section 9.2).

The interchangeability of the null propositions for different measures of relation implies that, in the context of unstratified data, the chi square (X^2) functions (Section 10.1.1) specific for different parameters take on the same value in the null situation. Given this special feature of the null X^2 value, and the preoccupation with the null point in comparative analysis, it is natural to consider the null X^2 statistic first. Added reasons are its familiarity

TABLE 11.1.

Data layout and notation for comparative analysis (unstratified) of
two proportion-type rates. The compared rates represent an index
($D = 1$) and a reference ($D = 0$) category of a determinant D,
with other categories in the data extraneous for the comparison
(Section 2.3)

	Category of Determinant			
	$D = 1$	$D = 0$	Other	Total
Cases	c_1	c_0	c'	$c + c'$
Noncases	$S_1 - c_1$	$S_0 - c_0$	$S' - c'$	$S - c + S'-c'$
Subjects	S_1	S_0	S'	$S + S'$

and relative simplicity. [However, presentation of the evidence in the data,
even for hypothesis testing, covers parts of the hypothesized (nonnull) region
as well, as discussed in Section 9.5.1].

11.1. TWO PROPORTIONS

11.1.1. Unstratified Series

For rates of the form of proportions, consider first the data layout in Table
11.1, representing the situation of unconditional (unstratified) analyses. In
terms of rate difference, the test statistic analogous to that in Equation 10.4
involves the empirical rate difference

$$rd = \frac{c_1}{S_1} - \frac{c_0}{S_0} \tag{11.1}$$

in place of the single empirical rate. The corresponding theoretical value is
generally an unspecified rate difference RD, which is analogous with R in
Equation 10.4; but in the null situation, which is at issue here, $RD = 0$.

It remains to formulate the variance of the empirical value (rd) of the
measure of relation, conditional on no relation ($RD = 0$). In contrast to the
case of a single rate, here the null proposition ($RD = 0$) does not imply the
variance of rd; it must be *estimated* conditionally on $RD = 0$. On this condition, $R_1 = R_0 = R$, so that the theoretical null variance is

$$V_{rd \mid RD=0} = R(1 - R) \left(\frac{1}{S_1} + \frac{1}{S_0} \right). \tag{11.2}$$

TABLE 11.2.

Heart disease mortality among patients with adult-onset diabetes, randomized to treatment with either tolbutamide or placebo (University Group Diabetes Program, 1970)[a]

	Treatment		
	Tolbutamide	Placebo	Total
Heart disease deaths	19 (= c_1)	5 (= c_0)	24 (= c)
Patients in trial	204 (= S_1)	205 (= S_0)	409 (= S)

[a] Experiences of patients on other treatments are not shown; see Table 11.1.

In this equation, $R(1 - R)$ represents the null variance of individual outcomes when coded by 1 for a case and 0 for a noncase—the variance of an indicator, or Bernoulli, variate.

The *unbiased* estimator for the Bernoulli variance is $r(1 - r)S/(S - 1)$, where $r = c/S$, and thus the unbiased estimator of $V_{rd \mid RD = 0}$ is

$$\hat{V}_{rd \mid RD = 0} = r(1 - r) \frac{S}{S - 1} \left(\frac{1}{S_1} + \frac{1}{S_0} \right). \tag{11.3}$$

In these terms the *null chi square statistic* is (cf. Pearson, 1947; Barnard, 1947)

$$X_0^2 = \frac{(rd - 0)^2}{\hat{V}_{rd \mid RD = 0}}$$

$$= \frac{(rd)^2}{\hat{V}_{rd \mid RD = 0}} \tag{11.4}$$

$$= \frac{(rd)^2}{r(1 - r)[S/(S - 1)](1/S_1 + 1/S_0)}.$$

EXAMPLE 11.1. Consider the data in Table 11.2. The empirical rate difference rd was $19/204 - 5/205 = 0.0687$. For its null variance the unbiased estimate is $(24/409)(1 - 24/409)(409/408)(1/204 + 1/205) = 0.000542$. Thus the statistic in Equation 11.4 takes on the value $(0.0687)^2/0.000542 = 8.7$.

This statistic is securely satisfactory in situations in which either of the marginal proportions (S_1/S or c/S) is close to $\frac{1}{2}$ and in the other margin the smaller frequency is not too close to zero. With both of the marginal proportions far from $\frac{1}{2}$ it may be desirable to assure near-Gaussian distribution of rd by applying the variance-stabilizing transformation to r_1 and r_0. In these terms the null X^2 statistic (cf. Equation 10.5) is

$$X_0^2 = \frac{[\sin^{-1}(r_1^{1/2}) - \sin^{-1}(r_0^{1/2})]^2}{(1/4)(1/S_1 + 1/S_0)}. \tag{11.5}$$

EXAMPLE 11.2.   Consider, as in Example 11.1, the data in Table 11.2. For the index rate the angular (inverse sine) metameter is $\sin^{-1}(19/204)^{1/2} = 17.8° = 17.8\,(\pi/180)\text{rad} = 0.310$, and for the reference rate it is 0.157. Thus, the null X^2 value is $(0.310 - 0.157)^2/[(1/4)(1/204 + 1/205)] = 9.6$, as opposed to 8.7 in Example 11.1. The transformation makes little difference here, because one of the marginal proportions is very close to $\frac{1}{2}$ ($S_1/S = 204/409$).

11.1.2.   Stratified Series in General

11.1.2.1.   The Cochran–Mantel–Haenszel Statistic

For the purpose of conditional, or stratified, analysis, Cochran (1954) generalized the basic form for the statistic (Equation 11.4). The empirical rate differences in the individual strata ($rd_j, j = 1, \ldots$) were weighted proportionately to their respective amounts of information. In principle, the information in any given stratum-specific difference is the inverse of the respective variance of rd (Equation 11.2). Cochran assumed that $R_j(1 - R_j)$ is constant over the strata, and thus he took the weights as

$$W_j = \left(\frac{1}{S_{1j}} + \frac{1}{S_{0j}} \right)^{-1}. \tag{11.6}$$

The resulting stratified null chi square statistic, based on the ideas of Pearson (1947), Barnard (1947), and Cochran (1954), is

$$\begin{aligned} X_0^2 &= \frac{[\sum_j W_j(rd_j)]^2}{\sum_j [W_j^2 \hat{V}_{rd|RD=0}]} \\ &= \frac{[\sum_j W_j(rd_j)]^2}{\sum_j [W_j r_j(1 - r_j)S_j/(S_j - 1)]}. \end{aligned} \tag{11.7}$$

Cochran actually used the maximum likelihood estimator of the unit variance, $R(1 - R)$, instead of the unbiased estimator involved in Equations 11.4 and 11.7; that is, he used $r_j(1 - r_j)$ in place of the $r_j(1 - r_j)S_j/(S_j - 1)$ in the statistic given above. This distinction is often immaterial, but it is of critical relevance in the context of pairwise matching and in other situations in which the stratum-specific information is sparse.

EXAMPLE 11.3.   Consider the data in Table 11.3. For the male stratum ($j = 1$), the empirical rate difference (rd_1) is $5/38 - 36/681 = 7.87\%$. The

TABLE 11.3.

Incidence by gender of drug-attributed rash in relation to allopurinol exposure among recipients of ampicillin (Boston Collaborative Drug Surveillance Program, 1972)[a]

Stratum	Component of Rate	Exposure to Allopurinol +	−	Total
Male ($j = 1$)	Cases	5 (c_{11})	36 (c_{01})	41 (c_1)
	Noncases	33	645	678 (c_1)
	Subjects	38 (S_{11})	681 (S_{01})	719 (S_1)
Female ($j = 2$)	Cases	10 (c_{12})	58 (c_{02})	68 (c_2)
	Noncases	19	518	537 (c_2)
	Subjects	29 (S_{12})	576 (S_{02})	605 (S_2)

[a] See also Table 11.1.

corresponding weight is $(1/38 + 1/681)^{-1} = 36.0$, and the null estimate (unbiased) of the variance of the outcome (Bernoulli) is $(c_1/S_1)(1 - c_1/S_1)[S_1/(S_1 - 1)] = 0.0538$. Thus, from the male stratum, the numerator contribution before squaring is $36.0(0.0787) = 2.83$, whereas the denominator element becomes $36.0(0.0538) = 1.94$. From the female stratum the corresponding elements are $6.74 [= 27.6(0.244)]$ and $2.76 [= 27.6(0.0999)]$. Thus, the value of the null X^2 statistic is 19.5.

We may seek better assurance of the tenability of the Gaussian assumption by employing the angular transformation. Indeed, such a need is apparent in Example 11.3, considering that *both of the marginal proportions are far from the value $\frac{1}{2}$, which would assure symmetry of distribution (conditionally on both margins). The realizations in the index series (Table 11.3) are in the "long tail" of the null distribution, and therefore the null X^2 in Example 11.3 is, presumably, too large.* A remedy for such a problem is, again, the employment of Fisher's angular transformation of proportions. To this end we first rewrite the basic statistic (Equation 11.7) as

$$X_0^2 = \frac{(r_1^* - r_0^*)^2}{\dfrac{\sum_j W_j r_j (1 - r_j) S_j/(S_j - 1)}{(\sum_j W_j)^2}}, \qquad (11.8)$$

where r_1^* and r_0^* are the mutually standardized rates for the index and reference series, respectively, with the standard weights proportional to the comparative information within the strata:

$$r_1^* = \sum_j W_j r_{1j}/\sum_j W_j \text{ and } r_0^* = \sum_j W_j r_{0j}/\sum_j W_j.$$

(As before, $r_{ij} = c_{ij}/S_{ij}$ and $r_j = c_j/S_j$.) Then,

$$X_0^2 = \frac{\{\sin^{-1}[(r_1^*)^{1/2}] - \sin^{-1}[(r_0^*)^{1/2}]\}^2}{\frac{1}{4} \frac{\sum_j W_j r_j (1 - r_j) S_j/(S_j - 1)}{(\sum_j W_j)^2 r^*(1 - r^*)}}, \qquad (11.9)$$

where

$$r^* = \frac{\sum_j W_j r_j}{\sum_j W_j}.$$

EXAMPLE 11.4.   As in Example 11.3, consider the data in Table 11.3. The rate for the index series, based on weighting by the amount of comparative information, is $[36.0(5/38) + 27.6(10/29)]/(36.0 + 27.6) = 0.244$ (cf. Example 11.3). For the reference and overall rates the corresponding values are 0.0736 and 0.0811, respectively. The angular metameters are $\sin^{-1}$ $(0.224)^{-1} = 28.2° = 28.2(\pi/180)\text{rad} = 0.493\text{rad}$ and 0.275rad, respectively. Thus, the numerator of the statistic is $(0.493 - 0.275)^2 = 0.0475$. The denominator is $(1/4)(1.94 + 2.76)/[(36.0 + 27.6)^2(0.0811)(1 - 0.0811)] = 0.00390$. Thus, $X_0^2 = 12.2$, rather than the presumably excessive 19.5 in Example 11.3.

The null chi square statistic presented in Equations 11.7 and 11.8 was derived by the use of a rationale that does not involve *conditioning by the marginal rates* (r_j), any more than does the statistic for a single 2×2 table in Equation 11.4; but the alternative deserves note here. For a single 2×2 table, the argument that is conditional on the marginal rate ($r = c/S$) involves the *hypergeometric* model (Appendix 10) for the distribution of one of the cell frequencies, generally for the number cases from the index category of the determinant. Based on this number, the null model implies the chi square statistic

$$X_0^2 = \frac{(c_1 - E_{c_1|c})^2}{V_{c_1|c}}, \qquad (11.10)$$

where the expectation and variance (conditional on the marginal number of cases c) are

$$E_{c_1|c} = \frac{S_1 c}{S},$$

$$V_{c_1|c} = \frac{S_1 S_0 c(S - c)}{S^2(S - 1)}.$$

(In this conditional argument it is possible to use the actual, theoretical, variance rather than only an estimator for it.) This statistic is algebraically totally interchangeable with its unconditional counterpart in Equation 11.4 (cf. Pearson, 1947; Barnard, 1947). Generalization of this conditional statistic for the purposes of stratified analyses leads to the form

$$X_0^2 = \frac{(\sum_j c_{1j} - \sum_j E_{c_{1j}|c_j})^2}{\sum_j V_{c_{1j}|c_j}}. \tag{11.11}$$

Given by Mantel and Haenszel (1959), this (conditional) form of the stratified null chi square is now known as *the Mantel–Haenszel statistic*. It, in turn, is *algebraically the very same as the unconditional, modified Cochran statistic* in Equations 11.7 and 11.8.

Even though the modified Cochran and Mantel–Haenszel statistics are algebraically interchangeable, and even though the Mantel–Haenszel formulation is now being used almost exclusively in epidemiologic data anlysis, it is intellectually necessary to consider whether there are good reasons to return to the earlier, Cochran, formulation. The question springs from an educational perspective: the null chi square for stratified 2 × 2 tables is now, albeit with questionable justification, the centerpiece of epidemiologic data analysis, and it is therefore good to use for this particular purpose a formulation that serves as a paradigm for other analyses. In this regard, the very first issue is *the relative merits of unconditional and conditional analytic approaches in general.* That these approaches are both usable, and even interchangeable, in the context of the *null* chi square for 2 × 2 tables is a striking exception. For chi square functions of rate difference and rate ratio, all nonnull values (for confidence limits) *must* be derived by the use of an *unconditional* approach (Chapters 12 and 13). For odds ratio the conditional approach is appropriate but unnecessary, as the very same formulations can be derived unconditionally (and this is done in Chapter 14); and where the determinant and outcome measures are both quantitative (a case of an R × C table), the generalization of the conditional approach to 2 × 2 tables is theoretically improper (Chapter 16). Not only does the Cochran approach represent the generally applicable, solely sufficient, unconditional approach, but it is also instructive as to the use of weighting, which is applicable in stratified analyses involving 2 × C (or R × 2) tables (Chapter 15) or quantitative observations (Chapter 16). The unconditional approach is also intuitively more attractive to most analysts. For these reasons and others (Equation 11.9 etc.), it seems that *the Cochran formulation of the null chi square for a set of 2 × 2 tables (Equations 11.7 and 11.8) should replace the currently popular Mantel–Haenszel formulation (Equation 11.11) in the teaching and practice of epidemiologic data analysis.*

11.1.2.2. LR Statistics

Although the statistic for a single 2 × 2 table (Equation 11.4) is ideal for testing the "null hypothesis" ($R_1 = R_0$) regardless of what comparative parameter at issue is, its generalization to several 2×2 tables in the form presented above (Equations 11.7, 11.8, and 11.11) is theoretically optimal for odds ratio analysis only (Birch, 1964; Radhakrishna, 1965), with the alternative for the null state $(R_{1j} = R_{0j})$ taken as a constant nonnull value of the comparative parameter over the strata (the case of no modification of the comparative parameter by the strata). This point may also be argued by noting that the "efficient score" approach, which generally provides for efficient statistics (see, for example, Cox and Hinkley, 1974), leads to the Cochran–Mantel–Haenszel statistic in the context of odds ratio only (Miettinen and Nurminen, 1985).

The pursuit of optimality for rate difference and rate ratio involves serious problems in terms of the "score statistic" approach (Miettinen and Nurminen, 1985), but the likelihood ratio approach is workable in this context. The basic idea (see, for example, Cox and Hinkley, 1974) in the context of a single 2×2 table implies the null chi square (1 df)

$$X_0^2 = 2 \log \frac{\Pr(c_1, c_0 \mid R_1 = r_1, R_0 = r_0)}{\Pr(c_1, c_0 \mid R_1 = R_0 = r)}. \tag{11.12}$$

The numerator of the likelihood ratio (Section 9.7) in this statistic involves unrestricted maximization of the likelihood: the exact probability (binomial) of both c_1 and c_0 is computed by the use of the best-fitting (probability-maximizing) value for the respective theoretical rates, and the joint probability is then derived as the product of those two probabilities. By contrast, the denominator involves the maximum of the likelihood on the null constraint of $R_1 = R_0$. The specific form of this statistic is

$$X_0^2 = 2 \log \frac{r_1^{c_1}(1 - r_1)^{S_1 - c_1} r_0^{c_0}(1 - r_0)^{S_0 - c_0}}{r^{c_1}(1 - r)^{S_1 - c_1} r^{c_0}(1 - r)^{S_0 - c_0}}$$

$$= 2 \log \frac{r_1^{c_1}(1 - r_1)^{S_1 - c_1} r_0^{c_0}(1 - r_0)^{S_0 - c_0}}{r^c(1 - r)^{S - c}}$$

$$= 2[c_1 \log r_1 + (S_1 - c_1) \log (1 - r_1) + c_0 \log r_0 \tag{11.13}$$

$$+ (S_0 - c_0) \log (1 - r_0) - c \log r$$

$$- (S - c) \log (1 - r)].$$

These last formulations require that $0^0 = 1$ and $0 (\log 0) = 0$.

EXAMPLE 11.5. Recall Example 11.1, with $r_1 = 19/204$, $r_0 = 5/205$, $r = 24/409$, and the ordinary null chi square equal to 8.7. The likelihood ratio statistic in Equation 11.13 gives $X_0^2 = 9.3$, a result that is in good conformity with the previous one. Both of these approaches are theoretically fine, as was noted, in the sense that it does not matter what comparative parameter is at issue, as no stratification is involved.

For stratified analysis the counterpart of the statistic in Equation 11.12 is

$$X_0^2 = 2 \sum_j \log \frac{\Pr(c_{1j}, c_{0j} \mid R_{1j} = \hat{\hat{R}}_{1j}, R_{0j} = \hat{\hat{R}}_{0j})}{\Pr(c_{1j}, c_{0j} \mid R_{1j} = R_{0j} = r_j)} \tag{11.14}$$

where $\hat{\hat{R}}_{1j}$ and $\hat{\hat{R}}_{0j}$ represent, for the jth stratum, the pair of values for the theoretical rates such that they maximize the joint probability for c_{1j} and c_{0j} within the constraint that the interrelation of R_{1j} and R_{0j} satisfies the maximum likelihood (*ML*) point estimate of the comparative parameter at issue based on combining the information over all the strata (on the assumption of no modification). Such restricted *ML* estimation of the compared parameters for the analysis of rate difference, rate ratio, and odds ratio are delineated in Chapters 12, 13, and 14, respectively.

Evidently, the numerator of the likelihood ratio, and thus *the null chi square itself, depends on the comparative parameter at issue*, in contradistinction to the Cochran–Mantel–Haenszel statistic.

For computational purposes the statistic may be taken (cf. Equation 11.13) as

$$
\begin{aligned}
X_0^2 &= 2 \sum_j \log \frac{\hat{\hat{R}}_{1j}^{c_{1j}}(1 - \hat{\hat{R}}_{1j})^{S_{1j} - c_{1j}} \hat{\hat{R}}_{0j}^{c_{0j}}(1 - \hat{\hat{R}}_{0j})^{S_{0j} - c_{0j}}}{r_j^{c_j}(1 - r_j)^{S_j - c_j}} \\
&= 2 \{ \sum_j [c_{1j} \log \hat{\hat{R}}_{1j} + (S_{1j} - c_{1j}) \log (1 - \hat{\hat{R}}_{1j}) \\
&\quad + c_{0j} \log \hat{\hat{R}}_{0j} + (S_{0j} - c_{0j}) \log (1 - \hat{\hat{R}}_{0j})] \\
&\quad - \sum_j [c_j \log r_j + (S_j - c_j) \log (1 - r_j)] \}.
\end{aligned}
\tag{11.15}
$$

EXAMPLE 11.6.   Recall Examples 11.3 and 11.4, dealing with null X^2 for the allopurinol data in Table 11.3, and yielding, for X_0^2, the values 19.5 and 12.2, respectively, with the Gaussian modeling presumably better justified for the latter. The *LR*-based statistic given above—which is rather immune to the skewness problem that led to $X_0^2 = 19.5$—gives $X_0^2 = 12.3$ for *RD*, 14.5 for *RR*, and 14.1 for *OR*(odds ratio) (see Examples 12.6, 13.5, and 14.6). The chi square value for *RR* is a bit larger than that for *OR*, because the empirical rate ratio values for the two strata (2.5 and 3.4) are a bit more alike than the empirical odds ratio values (2.5 and 4.7). For *RD* the null chi square is distinctly the smallest, owing to the small degree of stability that the empirical values of this parameter show between the strata (7.9 and 24%). (For tests of constancy of *RD, RR,* and *OR* over the two strata, see Examples 12.9, 12.10, 13.8, 13.9 and 14.8, respectively.)

As Example 11.6 illustrates, the null chi square (and thus the null *P*-value) might best be computed specifically for the comparative parameter at issue.

TABLE 11.4.

Layout and notation for data from individually matched series with dichotomous observation (1 or 0)[a]

One-to-one matching:			Observation on Reference Subject		
			1	0	Total
Observation on	1		f_{11}	f_{10}	$f_{1.}$
index subject	0		f_{01}	f_{00}	$f_{0.}$
	Total		$f_{.1}$	$f_{.0}$	$f_{..}$

R-to-one matching:			Number of Reference Subjects with Observation = 1			
			R	$\cdots$	0	Total
Observation on	1		f_{1R}	$\cdots$	f_{10}	$f_{1.}$
index subject	0		f_{0R}	$\cdots$	f_{00}	$f_{0.}$
	Total		$f_{.R}$	$\cdots$	$f_{.0}$	$f_{..}$

[a] f_{ij} is the number of matched groups with i index and j reference subjects giving observation = 1.

In case-referent studies the concern is with OR, and thus the Cochran–Mantel–Haenszel statistic, or its LR counterpart given above, is the appropriate statistic to use. When census data are at hand (Section 4.1), OR is not the comparative parameter of interest (Appendix A.2.4); thus, instead of the Cochran–Mantel–Haenszel statistic or its LR counterpart (for OR), it might be preferable to give the result from the LR approach for RD, RR, or both.

11.1.3. Matched Series

Stratified testing subsumes testing in the context of individually *matched* series. Most of the principles presented above still apply, but the flavor of the analysis and the applicability of the LR-based null X^2 are influenced by the multitude of strata and the small number of potential constellations of observations within them.

Consider first the extreme case of *pairwise* (one-to-one) matching, for example, the situation in which for each treated patient a single and specific untreated reference subject is obtained. Each matched pair represents a distinct stratum, so that $S_{1j} = S_{0j} = 1$ and $S_j = 2$. Moreover, there are only four possible outcomes for a stratum. Thus, the data may be reduced to a layout such as that presented in Table 11.4: there are a total of f_{11} pairs (strata) with both members a case ($r_{1j} = 1$, $r_{0j} = 1$, $c_j = 2$); f_{10} pairs with the index subject a case and the reference subject a noncase ($r_{1j} = 1$, $r_{0j} = 0$, $c_j = 1$); and so on.

Hence, for the modified Cochran null X^2 statistic in Equation 11.7 we have $W_j = (1/1 + 1/1)^{-1} = 1/2$ for all j; the f_{11} strata with $c_{1j} = c_{0j} = 1$ make no contribution to either the numerator of the statistic ($rd_j = 0$) or the denominator [$r_j(1 - r_j) = 0$]; from the f_{00} strata with $c_{1j} = c_{0j} = 0$ the contributions are also zero [$rd_j = 0$, $r_j(1 - r_j) = 0$]; the f_{10} strata with $c_{1j} = 1$ and $c_{0j} = 0$ contribute $f_{10}(1/2)(1 - 0) = (1/2)f_{10}$ to the square root of the numerator, and $f_{10}(1/2)(1/2) (1 - 1/2)2/1 = (1/4)f_{10}$ to the denominator; and finally, the f_{01} strata with $c_{1j} = 0$ and $c_{0j} = 1$ contribute $-(1/2)f_{01}$ and $(1/4)f_{01}$, respectively. Thus,

$$X_0^2 = \frac{(f_{10} - f_{01})^2}{f_{10} + f_{01}}. \tag{11.16}$$

This formulation was derived, in a different way, by McNemar (1947), and it is known as "the McNemar statistic."

When the number of reference subjects obtained for each index subject is some *general* number R, then $S_{1j} = 1$, $S_{0j} = R$, and $W_j = (1/1 + 1/R)^{-1} = R/(1 + R)$; and the frequency f_{uv} (Table 11.4) represents the number of strata with $r_{1j} = u$, $r_{0j} = v/R$, and $r_j = (u + v)/(1 + R)$. Thus, the Cochran–Mantel–Haenszel null chi square statistic (Equations 11.7, 11.8, and 11.11) takes on the form

$$
\begin{aligned}
X_0^2 &= \frac{R}{1 + R} \frac{[\sum_j (rd_j)]^2}{\sum_j r_j(1 - r_j)(1 + R)/R} \\
&= \frac{[Rf_{1\cdot} - \sum_v f_{\cdot v}v]^2}{\sum_{u,v} f_{uv}(u + v)(1 + R - u - v)}.
\end{aligned}
\tag{11.17}
$$

(Cf. Miettinen, 1969 and Pike and Morrow, 1970.)

The transformation directed to a more nearly Gaussian null distribution of X_0 (Equation 11.9) is of no real interest for matched pairs because of the symmetry of the design ($S_{1j} = S_{0j}$). For asymmetrical designs ($R > 1$) it can be important. We rewrite the basic statistic (Equation 11.17) as

$$X_0^2 = \frac{[f_{1\cdot}/f_{\cdot\cdot} - \sum_v f_{\cdot v}v/(Rf_{\cdot\cdot})]^2}{\dfrac{\sum_{u,v} f_{uv}(u + v)(1 + R - u - v)}{(Rf_{\cdot\cdot})^2}} \tag{11.18}$$

(cf. Equation 11.8). Then, evidently, the angular version is

$$X_0^2 = \frac{\{\sin^{-1} (f_{1\cdot}/f_{\cdot\cdot})^{1/2} - \sin^{-1} [\sum_v f_{\cdot v}v/(Rf_{\cdot\cdot})]^{1/2}\}^2}{\dfrac{1}{4}\dfrac{\sum_{u,v} f_{uv} (u + v)(1 + R - u - v)}{(Rf_{\cdot\cdot})^2 r^*(1 - r^*)}} \tag{11.19}$$

where $r^* = (f_{1\cdot} + \sum_v f_{\cdot v}v)/[(1 + R)f_{\cdot\cdot}]$ (cf. Equation 11.9).

TABLE 11.5.

Distribution of matched quintuples of cases of ectopic pregnancy and four reference subjects according to history of induced abortion (Panayotou *et al.*, 1972)

		Number of Reference Subjects with Positive History					
		4	3	2	1	0	Total
History of case	+	1	0	3	5	3	12
	−	0	0	0	1	5	6
	Total	1	0	3	6	8	18

EXAMPLE 11.7.   Consider the data in Table 11.5. They have to do with rates of positive history for induced abortion, comparing cases of ectopic pregnancy and reference subjects, as opposed to rates of illness, comparing two categories of a determinant. Yet, the test procedures presented above are applicable to the rates of positive history (cf. Section 17.1). For the statistic in Equation 11.18 the overall rates in the numerator, mutually standardized (cf. Equation 11.8) are $12/18 = 0.677$ and $[8(0) + 6(1) + 3(2) + 0(3) + 1(4)]/[4(18)] = 16/[4(18)] = 0.222$. The corresponding overall rate is $(12 + 16)/[(1 + 4)18] = 0.311$, a value close enough to 0.5 to imply that the statistic without transformation (Equation 11.18) should give a result similar to that derived from the angular statistic (Equation 11.19), even though $R > 1$. The summation element in the denominator from $u = 0$ is $5(0 + 0)(1 + 4 - 0 - 0) + 1(0 + 1)(1 + 4 - 0 - 1) + \ldots = 4$, and from $u = 1$ it is $3(1 + 0)(1 + 4 - 1 - 0) + \ldots = 60$; the total thus is 64. Thus, incidentally, the conditional estimate of the unit (Bernoulli) variance of the histories is $\{64/[(1 + R)R]\}/f_{..} = 0.178$, and the unconditional estimate is $r^* (1 - r^*) = 0.311(1 - 0.311) = 0.214$, with the discrepancy a reflection of the correlatedness of the series. The basic statistic thus takes on the value $X_0^2 = (0.677 - 0.222)^2/\{64/[4(18)]^2\} = 16.8$. For the angular statistic, the numerator involves $\sin^{-1}(0.677)^{1/2} = 55.4° = 55.4(\pi/180)\text{rad} = 0.966\text{rad}$, and $\sin^{-1}(0.222) = 0.491\text{rad}$. Thus, $X_0^2 = (0.966 - 0.491)^2/\{(1/4)64/[4^2(18)^2 0.214]\} = 15.6$.

The null chi square formulations given above were applications of the Cochran–Mantel–Haenszel null chi square to the situation of individually matched series. Thus, they are really directed to testing the "null hypothesis" that OR is 1 (and that other comparative parameters are at their null value) against the alternative that OR has some other, common value over the matching categories.

Approaching the null chi square for OR in terms of the LR statistic (Equation 11.15), we note first that for OR only tables with $0 < r_j < 1$ are informative, so that only discordant pairs need to be considered in the context of *matched pairs*. The null chi square in Equation 11.15 in the analysis of matched pairs for *OR* assumes the form

$$X^2_{OR=1} = 4[f_{10} \log \hat{\hat{R}}_1 + f_{01} \log \hat{\hat{R}}_0$$

$$-(f_{10} + f_{01}) \log \left(\frac{1}{2}\right) \tag{11.20}$$

$$= 4[f_{10} \log (2\hat{\hat{R}}_1) + f_{01} \log (2\hat{\hat{R}}_0)].$$

Curiously, the values $\hat{\hat{R}}_1$ and $\hat{\hat{R}}_0$ for the discordant pairs—the maximum likelihood values for R_1 and R_0 for these strata—correspond to *OR* estimate $\hat{OR} = (f_{10}/f_{01})^2$, which is the square of what is usually the *ML* estimator (Miettinen, 1970a). Further, whereas those rate inputs are

$$\hat{\hat{R}}_1 = 1 - \hat{\hat{R}}_0,$$

$$\hat{\hat{R}}_0 = \frac{(\hat{OR})^{1/2} - 1}{\hat{OR} - 1}, \tag{11.21}$$

even the use of $\hat{OR} = f_{10}/f_{01}$ gives rather poor results.

EXAMPLE 11.8.   Suppose that $f_{10} = 8$ and $f_{01} = 2$. The exact upper-tail mid-*P* (Equation 10.26) from the binomial model is 0.033. The McNemar statistic (Equation 11.16) gives $X^2_0 = (8 - 2)^2/(8 + 2) = 3.6$, and its corresponding upper-tail *P*-value is 0.03 (Appendix 12), and the corresponding exact binomial mid-*P* (Equation 10.26) is 0.03 as well. The *LR* statistic given above, with $\hat{OR} = 8/2$ (given $\hat{R}_1 = 2/3$, $\hat{R}_0 = 1/3$), takes on the value $X^2_0 = 6.0$, and with $\hat{OR} = (8/2)^2$ its value is 7.7.

As these theoretical and numerical considerations illustrate, the unconditional *LR* approach to null chi square (Equation 11.15) involves problems in the context of matched pairs and, by extension, more generally in situations in which the intrastratum information is sparse (cf. Breslow and Day, 1981).

11.2.   TWO DENSITIES

For the situation in which the compared rates are incidence densities, the basic layout and notation are given in Table 11.6.

The empirical rate difference is

$$rd = \frac{c_1}{T_1} - \frac{c_0}{T_0}, \tag{11.22}$$

and its null variance is

$$V_{rd|RD=0} = R \left(\frac{1}{T_1} + \frac{1}{T_0}\right) \tag{11.23}$$

TABLE 11.6.

**Data layout and notation for comparative analysis
(unstratified) of two density-type rates, analogous to that
given for proportions in Table 11.1**

	Category of Determinant			
	$D = 1$	$D = 0$	Other	Total
Cases	c_1	c_0	c'	$c + c'$
Population time	T_1	T_0	T'	$T + T'$

(cf. Equations 10.30 and 11.2). The estimate (unbiased) of the latter takes
the form of

$$\hat{V}_{rd \mid RD=0} = r\left(\frac{1}{T_1} + \frac{1}{T_0}\right). \tag{11.24}$$

With these inputs, the form of the basic chi square statistic for the null point
remains

$$X_0^2 = \frac{(rd)^2}{\bar{V}_{rd \mid RD=0}} \tag{11.25}$$

(cf. expression 11.4). The angular transformations of the square roots of the
component rates reduce to no transformation at all. A density-type rate can
be construed as an extreme of a proportion, with the proportion approaching
zero; and as the corresponding square root also approaches zero, its arc sin,
in radians, becomes interchangable with the angle itself ($R^{1/2}$). Thus, the
employment of the variance-stabilizing (and thereby also "Gaussianizing")
transformation leads (cf. Equation 11.5) to

$$X_0^2 = \frac{(r_1^{1/2} - r_0^{1/2})^2}{(1/4)(1/T_1 + 1/T_0)}. \tag{11.26}$$

For the stratified null X^2, the weights are

$$W_j = \left(\frac{1}{T_1} + \frac{1}{T_0}\right)^{-1} \tag{11.27}$$

(cf expression 11.6). The statistic itself can be put in the form

$$X_0^2 = \frac{(r_1^* - r_0^*)^2}{r^*/\sum_j W_j}, \tag{11.28}$$

where, as before, r_1^*, r_0^*, and r^* are the rates for the index category, the reference category, and the combination of the two categories, all mutually standardized according to the weights indicated above (cf. Equation 11.8). The variance-stabilizing transformation leads (cf. Equation 11.9) to

$$X_0^2 = \frac{[(r_1^*)^{1/2} - (r_0^*)^{1/2}]^2}{(1/4)/\sum_j W_j}. \tag{11.29}$$

The formulations for matched series in the context of proportion-type rates have no counterparts for incidence-density data; one matches persons (units of observation), not units of person-time.

12

Comparative Analysis of Two Rates II:

CHI SQUARE FUNCTION FOR RATE DIFFERENCE

The null chi square, considered in the preceding chapter, constitutes an insufficient statistic (summary of the evidence) for hypothesis testing, let alone for estimation (cf. Section 9.5.1). By contrast, the presentation of *chi square as a function of the comparative parameter of interest implies all "frequentist" statistics (asymptotic) of interest*—the null *P*-value, the point estimate, and all interval estimates (Section 9.8). In addition, the statistic of interest to the Bayesian, *the LR function, is but a trivial transform of the chi square function*, given that the latter is based on the variance-stabilizing transformation (Section 10.1.2).

In this and subsequent chapters, the chi square functions for comparative analyses of two rates are introduced. These functions are specific for particular types of comparative parameter, and in this chapter the concern is with rate difference.

12.1. CONTRAST-BASED X^2 FUNCTION OF RD

12.1.1. Unstratified Series

For an unstratified rate difference (RD), the basic chi square (X^2) function may be based on the contrast between r_1 and r_0 and taken as

$$X^2_{RD} = \frac{(rd - RD)^2}{\hat{V}_{rd|RD}} \tag{12.1}$$

(cf. Equations 11.4 and 10.4). Here the variance estimator is, in the context of *proportion-type rates*,

$$\hat{V}_{rd|RD} = \tilde{V}_{rd}$$
$$= \left[\frac{\tilde{R}_1(1 - \tilde{R}_1)}{S_1} + \frac{\tilde{R}_0(1 - \tilde{R}_0)}{S_0} \right] \frac{S}{S - 1}, \tag{12.2}$$

where the tildes designate *estimators conditional on the particular value of the comparative parameter at issue (RD)*. Naturally,

$$\tilde{R}_1 = \tilde{R}_0 + RD. \tag{12.3}$$

$\tilde{R}_0$, in turn, is the solution of the following likelihood equation based on two independent binomials:

$$\frac{c_1 - S_1(\tilde{R}_0 + RD)}{(\tilde{R}_0 + RD)(1 - \tilde{R}_0 - RD)} + \frac{c_0 - S_0\tilde{R}_0}{\tilde{R}_0(1 - \tilde{R}_0)} = 0, \tag{12.4}$$

subject to $0 \le \tilde{R}_0 \le 1$ and $0 \le \tilde{R}_0 + RD \le 1$. The solution can be found iteratively. Alternatively, a closed-form solution can be employed. The equation can be written as

$$\sum_{k=0}^{3} L_k \tilde{R}_0^k = 0, \tag{12.5}$$

with

$$L_3 = S,$$
$$L_2 = (S_1 + 2S_0)(RD) - S - c,$$
$$L_1 = [S_0(RD) - S - 2c_0](RD) + c,$$
$$L_0 = (RD)(1 - RD)c_0,$$

with $c = c_1 + c_0$, as before. The solution, based on the guidelines given, for example, by Bronshtein and Semendyayev (1973) and satisfying the range constraints for $\tilde{R}_1$ and $\tilde{R}_0$, is

$$\tilde{R}_0 = 2p\cos(a) - \frac{L_2}{3L_3}, \tag{12.6}$$

where $a = (1/3)[\pi + \cos^{-1}(q/p^3)]$, $p = \pm [L_2^2/(3L_3)^2 - L_1/(3L_3)]^{1/2}$, $q = L_2^3/(3L_3)^3 - L_2L_1/(6L_3^2) + L_0/(2L_3)$, and the sign of p coincides with that of q. (Cf. Miettinen and Nurminen, 1985.)

If the rates are *incidence densities*, the variance estimator is

$$\tilde{V}_{rd} = \frac{\tilde{R}_0 + RD}{T_1} + \frac{\tilde{R}_0}{T_0}, \tag{12.7}$$

with $\tilde{R}_0$ the solution of

$$\frac{c_1 - T_1(\tilde{R}_0 + RD)}{\tilde{R}_0 + RD} + \frac{c_0 - T_0\tilde{R}_0}{\tilde{R}_0} = 0, \tag{12.8}$$

with $\tilde{R}_0 \geq 0$. This equation is only quadratic, and the solution has the closed form of

$$\tilde{R}_0 = \frac{-B + (B^2 - 4AC)^{1/2}}{2A}, \tag{12.9}$$

where $A = T$, $B = -c + T(RD)$, and $C = -c_0(RD)$ (cf. Miettinen and Nurminen, 1985).

Although the X^2 function given above (Equation 12.1) is a theoretically coherent basic function for the determination of asymptotic confidence bounds (cf. Equation 10.4), the usual approach is still to take the function as

$$\begin{aligned} X_{RD}^2 &= \frac{(rd - RD)^2}{\hat{V}_{rd}} \\ &= \frac{(rd - RD)^2}{r_1(1 - r_1)/S_1 + r_0(1 - r_0)/S_0} \end{aligned} \tag{12.10}$$

for proportion-type rates, and, correspondingly, as

$$X_{RD}^2 = \frac{(rd - RD)^2}{r_1/T_1 + r_0/T_0} \tag{12.11}$$

TABLE 12.1.

For the data $c_1/S_1 = 0/10$ and $c_0/S_0 = 0/20$, technical solutions of the likelihood equation (Equation 12.4) for $\tilde{R}_0$; actual estimates of R_1, R_0, and variance of rd; and chi square corresponding to RD

RD	Solutions of Likelihood Equation for $\tilde{R}_0$			Estimates			Chi Square
				$\tilde{R}_0$	$\tilde{R}_1$	$\tilde{V}_{rd}$	
-0.30	0.000	0.300	1.200	0.300	0.000	0.011	8.29
-0.20	0.000	0.200	1.133	0.200	0.000	0.008	4.83
-0.10	0.000	0.100	1.066	0.100	0.000	0.005	2.15
-0.005	0.000	0.005	1.003	0.005	0.000	0.000	0.10
0.005	0.000	-0.005	0.996	0.000	0.005	0.001	0.05
0.01	0.000	-0.010	0.993	0.000	0.010	0.001	0.10
0.10	0.000	-0.099	0.933	0.000	0.100	0.009	1.07
0.20	0.000	-0.200	0.866	0.000	0.200	0.017	2.42
0.30	0.000	-0.300	0.800	0.000	0.300	0.022	4.14
0.40	0.000	-0.400	0.733	0.000	0.400	0.025	6.44

for incidence densities. These latter formulations, when set equal to χ^2_α, yield the usual confidence bounds of

$$RD_{\alpha/2}, RD_{1-\alpha/2} = rd \mp \chi_\alpha \left[\frac{r_1(1-r_1)}{S_1} + \frac{r_0(1-r_0)}{S_0} \right]^{1/2} \quad (12.12)$$

for proportions, and

$$RD_{\alpha/2}, RD_{1-\alpha/2} = rd \mp \chi_\alpha \left(\frac{r_1}{T_1} + \frac{r_0}{T_0} \right)^{1/2} \quad (12.13)$$

for incidence densities.

EXAMPLE 12.1. Suppose the index and reference rates (c_i/S_i) are 0/10 and 0/20, respectively. The classical approach (Equation 12.10) makes all confidence intervals (Equation 12.12) reduce to the point zero, regardless of the confidence level $(1 - \alpha)$. This is distinctly unattractive (cf. Example 10.3). The use of the approach advocated here starts with the solution of Equation 12.4 for $\tilde{R}_0$, corresponding to various values of RD. With the extreme data at issue the proper solution of the equation is $\tilde{R}_0 = 0$ for $RD > 0$ and $\tilde{R}_0 = |RD|$ for $RD < 0$. This is obvious intuitively, and it is also seen by examining the solutions of the third-degree equation from which $\tilde{R}_0$ is derived (Equation 12.4). Those solutions, for various values of RD in the range of $-0.30 \leq RD \leq 0.40$ are given in Table 12.1. The table also gives the choice of $\tilde{R}_0$ such that both $\tilde{R}_0$ and $\tilde{R}_1 (= \tilde{R}_0 + RD)$ remain within the 0–1 range, together with $\tilde{V}_{rd}$ and X^2_{RD} itself. In the range of $RD > rd = 0$, the X^2 function is (0

Chi Square as a function of RD; c_1/S_1 = 0/10, c_0/S_0 = 0/20

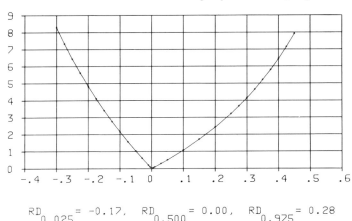

$$RD_{0.025} = -0.17, \quad RD_{0.500} = 0.00, \quad RD_{0.975} = 0.28$$

Figure 12.1. For the data c_1/S_1 = 0/10 and c_0/S_0 = 0/20, chi square as a function of RD. See Example 12.1.

$-RD)^2/\{[(RD(1-RD)/10+0(1-0)/20]30/29\} = 10(RD)/[(1-RD)30/29]$, and the upper 95% bound, the solution of $10(RD)/[(1-RD)30/29] = 3.84$, is $RD_{0.975} = 0.28$. The corresponding lower bound is the solution of $(0-RD)^2/\{0(1-0)/10+[(-RD)(1+RD)/20]30/29\} = 3.84$, and it is $RD_{0.025} = -0.17$. The X^2 function itself is shown in Figure 12.1.

EXAMPLE 12.2. Now consider the other extreme: c_1/S_1 = 10/10 and c_0/S_0 = 20/20. Technical solutions of the likelihood equation (Equation 12.4) for various values of RD are given in Table 12.2, and the X^2 function is shown graphically in Figure 12.2. The latter is the mirror image of that in Figure 12.1, with reference to $RD = rd = 0$.

EXAMPLE 12.3. Suppose that c_1/S_1 = 8/10 and c_0/S_0 = 5/20. For the likelihood equation (Equation 12.4), technical solutions for various values are given in Table 12.3. When $RD = 0.00$, for example, the proper solution is $\tilde{R}_0 = 0.433$, which corresponds to $\tilde{R}_1 = 0.433$ and $X_0^2 = 7.9$. The X^2 function is depicted in Figure 12.3. The function ordinarily used as the basis of interval estimation of RD (Equation 12.10) gives, for $RD = 0$, the value of $X_0^2 = (0.8 - 0.25)^2/[0.8(0.2)/10 + 0.25(1 - 0.25)/20] = 11.9$, a value much larger than the 7.9 obtained above. However, the Pearson–Barnard null X^2 in Equation 11.4 takes on the value $X_0^2 = (0.80 - 0.25)^2/\{[(13/30)(30 - 13)/30](30/29)(1/10 + 1/20)\} = 7.9$, with which the realization of X_{RD}^2 at $RD = 0$ is strictly consonant, here and in general.

In the examples presented above, the various technical solutions of the likelihood equation were considered to develop insight only. The single right solution, given in the tables for each value of RD, may be computed directly

TABLE 12.2.

For the data $c_1/S_1 = 10/10$ and $c_0/S_0 = 20/20$, technical solutions of the likelihood equation (Equation 12.4) for $\tilde{R}_0$; actual estimates of R_1, R_0, and variance of rd; and chi square corresponding to RD

RD	Solutions of Likelihood Equation for $\tilde{R}_0$			Estimates			Chi Square
				$\tilde{R}_0$	$\tilde{R}_1$	$\tilde{V}_{rd}$	
−0.40	0.266	0.999	1.400	1.000	0.600	0.025	6.44
−0.30	0.200	0.999	1.300	1.000	0.700	0.022	4.14
−0.20	0.133	0.999	1.200	1.000	0.800	0.017	2.42
−0.01	0.006	0.999	1.010	1.000	0.990	0.001	0.10
−0.005	0.003	1.000	1.004	1.000	0.995	0.001	0.05
0.005	−0.003	0.997	0.997	0.995	1.000	0.000	0.10
0.10	−0.066	0.899	1.000	0.900	1.000	0.005	2.15
0.20	−0.133	0.800	0.999	0.800	1.000	0.008	4.83
0.30	−0.200	0.700	1.000	0.700	1.000	0.011	8.29

from Equation 12.6, as was noted; and in practice, the latter is the approach of choice.

Since the approach suggested here gives distinctly better results (confidence limits) than the approach currently employed (Equations 12.10 and 12.12; see Examples 12.1, 12.2, and 12.3 and especially Miettinen and Nurminen, 1985), it is worth the necessary implementation on a computer. Indeed, given the modern ease of computing and still unabated pain and other costs of data collection, considerations of computational practicality no

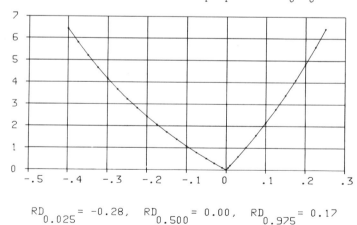

Figure 12.2. For the data $c_1/S_1 = 10/10$ and $c_0/S_0 = 20/20$, chi square as a function of RD. See Example 12.2.

TABLE 12.3.

For the data c_1/S_1 = 8/10 and c_0/S_0 = 5/20, technical solutions of the likelihood equation (Equation 12.4) for $\bar{R}_0$; actual estimates of R_1, R_0, and variance of rd; and chi square corresponding to *RD*

RD	Solutions of Likelihood Equation for $\bar{R}_0$			Estimates			Chi Square
				$\bar{R}_0$	$\bar{R}_1$	$\bar{V}_{rd}$	
0.00	0.000	0.433	1.000	0.433	0.433	0.038	7.94
0.20	−0.089	0.361	0.827	0.361	0.561	0.037	3.27
0.40	−0.200	0.300	0.666	0.300	0.700	0.033	0.69
0.50	0.594	−0.261	0.267	0.267	0.767	0.029	0.09
0.55	−0.294	0.250	0.560	0.250	0.800	0.026	0.00
0.60	0.230	−0.327	0.529	0.230	0.830	0.024	0.11
0.80	0.131	0.434	−0.466	0.131	0.931	0.013	4.99

longer are a defensible factor in favor of a distinctly inferior approach, neither in this context nor in others.

In this context it is to be noted that exact *P*-value functions (and thus exact confidence limits) are not left without consideration here for reasons of computational challenges, but because they do not exist, even in principle, for rate difference or for rate ratio (Barndorff-Nielsen, 1976).

As an alternative to the chi square function presented above, the chi square function of *RD* can reasonably be based on the *LR* function, as $X^2_{RD} = 2 \log(LR_{RD})$. This function, apparently somewhat inferior to that

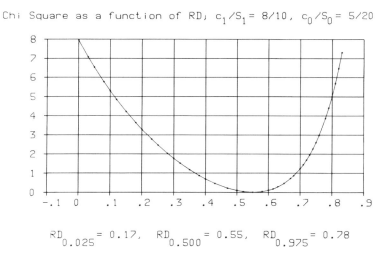

Chi Square as a function of RD; c_1/S_1 = 8/10, c_0/S_0 = 5/20

$RD_{0.025}$ = 0.17, $RD_{0.500}$ = 0.55, $RD_{0.975}$ = 0.78

Figure 12.3. For the data c_1/S_1 = 8/10 and c_0/S_0 = 5/20, chi square as a function of *RD*. See Example 12.3.

Chi Square as a function of RD

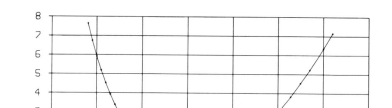

$$RD_{0.025} = 0.07, \quad RD_{0.500} = 0.15, \quad RD_{0.975} = 0.26$$

Figure 12.4. For the data in Table 11.3 ($c_{11}/S_{11} = 5/38$, $c_{01}/S_{01} = 36/681$, $c_{12}/S_{12} = 10/29$, and $c_{02}/S_{02} = 58/576$), chi square as a function of RD. See Example 12.4.

specified by Equations 12.1–12.4 (Miettinen and Nurminen, 1985), is considered in Section 12.3.

12.1.2. Stratified Series in General

In the context of stratified series the basic X^2 function of RD, as an extension of Equations 12.1 and 11.8, may be given the form

$$X^2_{RD} = \frac{(r_1^* - r_0^* - RD)^2}{\sum_j W_j^2 \tilde{V}_{rdj}/(\sum_j W_j)^2}, \tag{12.14}$$

where $r_i^* = \sum_j W_j r_{ij}/\sum_j W_j$. The variance estimators for proportion-type rates, conditional on RD, may be taken as

$$\tilde{V}_{rdj} = \left[\frac{\tilde{R}_{1j}(1 - \tilde{R}_{1j})}{S_{1j}} + \frac{\tilde{R}_{0j}(1 - \tilde{R}_{0j})}{S_{0j}} \right] \frac{S_j}{S_j - 1}, \tag{12.15}$$

where $\tilde{R}_{1j} = \tilde{R}_{0j} + RD$, and $\tilde{R}_{0j}$ is the solution of Equation 12.4 applied to the jth stratum. The weights are now derived (as measures proportional to inverses of the variances of the $\{rd_j\}$) on the assumption that $R_{0j}(1 - R_{0j})$, and hence $R_{1j}(1 - R_{1j})$, is constant over the strata:

$$W_j = \left[\frac{1}{S_{1j}} + \frac{R_0^*(1 - R_0^*)}{R_1^*(1 - R_1^*)S_{0j}} \right]^{-1}, \tag{12.16}$$

TABLE 12.4.

For the data in Table 11.3, analysis for rate difference (*RD*); the stratum-specific
estimates $\tilde{R}_1$ and $\tilde{R}_0$, their respective weighted averages $\tilde{R}_1^*$ and $\tilde{R}_0^*$, and the
contrast-based chi square (X^2) are shown for various values of *RD*

	Males		Females				
RD	$\tilde{R}_1$	$\tilde{R}_0$	$\tilde{R}_1$	$\tilde{R}_0$	$\tilde{R}_1^*$	$\tilde{R}_0^*$	X^2
0.000	0.0570	0.0570	0.1124	0.1124	0.0811	0.0811	19.5
0.040	0.0941	0.0541	0.1483	0.1083	0.1176	0.0776	7.64
0.060	0.1134	0.0534	0.1668	0.1068	0.1366	0.0766	4.53
0.065	0.1182	0.0532	0.1715	0.1065	0.1413	0.0763	3.93
0.066	0.1192	0.0532	0.1725	0.1065	0.1423	0.0763	3.81
0.125	0.1770	0.0520	0.2288	0.1038	0.1994	0.0744	0.27
0.150	0.2017	0.0517	0.2530	0.1030	0.2239	0.0739	0.00
0.175	0.2264	0.0514	0.2773	0.1023	0.2484	0.0734	0.21
0.264	0.3146	0.0506	0.3643	0.1003	0.3361	0.0721	3.82
0.265	0.3156	0.0506	0.3653	0.1003	0.3371	0.0721	3.88
0.300	0.3503	0.0503	0.3997	0.0997	0.3717	0.0717	6.34

where $\tilde{R}_0^* = \sum_j W_j \tilde{R}_{0j}/\sum_j W_j$, and $\tilde{R}_1^* = \tilde{R}_0^* + RD$. This definition is, admittedly, somewhat circular. In practice one may compute first approximations to $\tilde{R}_1^*$ and $\tilde{R}_0^*$ by using the null weights, $W_j = (1/S_{1j} + 1/S_{0j})^{-1}$. These provide for first approximations for the nonnull weights given above. In the second cycle, the latter are used in the approximations to R_1^* and R_{0j}^*. Once convergence has been achieved (a couple of iterations usually suffice), those weights are applied in the computation of r_1^*, r_0^*, and the denominator for the X^2 corresponding to a particular value of *RD*. The whole process is then repeated for other values of *RD*.

EXAMPLE 12.4. Recall Example 11.3, in which the null X^2 value of 19.5 was derived for the data in Table 11.3. Since $S_{0j} \gg S_{1j}$ for each stratum, W_j is approximately equal to S_{1j} regardless of *RD*. Computed in detail, with *RD* = 0, we obtain $W_1 = 36.0$ and $W_2 = 27.6$; with *RD* = 0.30, $W_1 = 37.4$ and $W_2 = 28.6$. Against *RD* = 0, the realization of the X^2 function (Equation 12.14) is 19.5, as in Example 11.3. The X^2 function is depicted in Figure 12.4, which also shows numerically the *RD* values corresponding to P = 0.025, 0.500, and 0.975, respectively. Numerical representation of the function is given in Table 12.4.

If the rates represent incidence densities, the variance estimators are

$$\tilde{V}_{rd_j} = \frac{\tilde{R}_{1j}}{T_{1j}} + \frac{\tilde{R}_{0j}}{T_{0j}}, \tag{12.17}$$

with $\tilde{R}_{1j} = \tilde{R}_{0j} + RD$, but $\tilde{R}_{0j}$ is computed from Equation 12.9. The other modification is that the weights are

$$W_j = \left[\frac{1}{T_{1j}} + \frac{\tilde{R}_0^*/R_1^*}{T_{0j}} \right]^{-1} \qquad (12.18)$$

with $\tilde{R}_1^* = \sum_j W_j \tilde{R}_{ij} / \sum_j W_j$. Their computation requires the same kind of iterative procedure as was outlined for the case of proportion-type rates.

12.1.3. Matched Series

If the compared series have been individually matched, the extension of the null X^2 (Equation 11.18) to a function of RD involves some points of interest. The weights (Equation 12.16) are evidently identical among the strata (matched sets). Therefore, $r_1^* = f_1/f_{..}$ and $r_0^* = \sum_v f_{.v} v/(Rf_{..})$, as in the null X^2; and the weights for the denominator of the X^2 function (Equation 12.14) may be set equal to unity. Thus,

$$X_{RD}^2 = \frac{[f_1/f_{..} - \sum_v f_{.v} v/(Rf_{..}) - RD]^2}{\sum_{u,v} f_{uv} \tilde{V}_{rd\,|\,u,v}/f_{..}^2}. \qquad (12.19)$$

The variance element takes the form

$$\tilde{V}_{rd\,|\,u,v} = \left[\tilde{R}_1(1 - \tilde{R}_1) + \frac{\tilde{R}_0(1 - \tilde{R}_0)}{R} \right] \frac{1 + R}{R} \qquad (12.20)$$

(cf. Equation 12.2), with $\tilde{R}_1 = \tilde{R}_0 + RD$, and with $\tilde{R}_0$ the solution of

$$\frac{u - \tilde{R}_0 - RD}{(\tilde{R}_0 + RD)(1 - \tilde{R}_0 - RD)} + \frac{v - R\tilde{R}_0}{\tilde{R}_0(1 - \tilde{R}_0)} = 0 \qquad (12.21)$$

(cf. Equation 12.4). Solutions of this equation are tabulated in Appendix 13, which gives $\tilde{R}_0$ and $\tilde{V}_{rd}$ (Equation 12.20) for the various possible combinations of u and v for particular matching ratios (R) in the range from 1 to 5, corresponding to a sequence of values of RD in the range from -0.5 to 0.5. It is worthy of particular note that these variance estimators do not reduce to zero for the "uninformative" sets in which either $u = 1$ and $v = R$, or $u = 0$ and $v = 0$, except in the null situation of $RD = 0$.

Examination of matched *pairs* in these terms may be illustrative. The numerator of the X^2 function is $(f_1/f_{..} - f_{.1}/f_{..} - RD)^2$. In the denominator, the f_{11} pairs with $u = 1$ and $v = 1$ correspond to $\tilde{R}_1 = 1$ and $\tilde{R}_0 = 1 - RD$ in the range of $RD > 0$, and the corresponding variance estimate is $2(RD)(1 - RD)$. In the $RD < 0$ range, $\tilde{R}_1 = 1 + RD$ and $\tilde{R}_0 = 1$, so that $\tilde{V}_{rd\,|\,1,1} = -2(RD)(1 + RD)$. For the f_{00} pairs with $u = v = 0$, $\tilde{R}_1 = RD$

and $\tilde{R}_0 = 0$ in the $RD > 0$ range with $\tilde{V}_{rd|1,1} = 2(RD)(1 - RD)$, while in the $RD < 0$ range, $\tilde{V}_{rd|1,1} = -2(RD)(1 + RD)$. For both the f_{10} pairs with $u = 1$ and $v = 0$, and the f_{01} pairs with $u = 0$ and $v = 1$, $\tilde{R}_1 = (1/2)(1 + RD)$ and $\tilde{R}_0 = (1/2)(1 - RD)$. Thus, the X^2 function is

$$X_{RD}^2 = \frac{(f_1./f.. - f._1/f.. - RD)^2}{[(f_{11} + f_{00})\tilde{V}_{rd|u=v} + (f_{10} + f_{01})\tilde{V}_{rd|u\neq v}]/f..^2}. \quad (12.22)$$

where $\tilde{V}_{rd|u=v} = 2|RD|(1 - |RD|)$ and $\tilde{V}_{rd|u\neq v}$ $(1 + RD)(1 - RD)$. Evidently, at the null point $(RD = 0)$ this function becomes the McNemar statistic (Equation 11.16).

12.2. *LR*-BASED X^2 FUNCTION OF *RD*

If the X^2 function is formed with angular transformation, the *LR* function, a simple transform of the X^2 function, can be (analogously with Equation 10.17) taken as

$$LR_{RD} = \exp[-\tfrac{1}{2}(X_{RD}^2 - X_{RD=0}^2)]. \quad (12.23)$$

If the transformation is not used, it is necessary to employ the counterpart of the function in Equation 10.16, with the variance ratio based on the denominators of the X^2 statistic at $RD = 0$ and RD, respectively.

The *LR* function of *RD* can also be computed directly, by the use of binomial probabilities of the c_{ij} ($i = 1,0; j = 1 \ldots$) instead of the Gaussian densities for X. Thus,

$$
\begin{aligned}
LR_{RD} &= \frac{\widehat{Pr}(\{c_{ij}\} \mid RD = \hat{RD})}{\widehat{Pr}(\{c_{ij}\} \mid RD)} \\
&= \frac{\max_{RD}\widehat{Pr}(\{c_{ij}\} \mid RD)}{\widehat{Pr}(\{c_{ij}\} \mid RD)} \\
&= \exp(\max_{RD} \textstyle\sum_j \tilde{U}_j - \sum_j \tilde{U}_j),
\end{aligned}
\quad (12.24)
$$

where $\tilde{U}_j = c_{1j} \log \tilde{R}_{1j} + (S_{1j} - c_{1j})\log(1 - \tilde{R}_{1j}) + c_{0j} \log \tilde{R}_{0j} + (S_{0j} - c_{0j}) \log (1 - \tilde{R}_{0j})$. (For computational purposes it is necessary to define $0[\log(0)] = 0$, insofar as $r_j = 0$ or $r_j = 1$ for one or more strata.) The maximum of $\sum_j \tilde{U}_j$ over values of *RD* must be found iteratively.

Just as a X^2 function defines its corresponding *LR* function (Equation 12.23), this exact *LR* function implies an asymptotic X^2 function:

$$X_{RD}^2 = 2 \log(LR_{RD}). \quad (12.25)$$

This is, indeed, the X^2 function whose null value is given by Equation 11.15.

The performance of this LR-based X^2 function in the context of unstratified data seems, in light of computer simulations, somewhat inferior to that of the X^2 function in Equation 12.1 (Miettinen and Nurminen, 1985). Moreover, in the context of matched series (strata with very sparse intrastratum information) the LR-based X^2 is capable of quite poor results (Section 12.1.3). However, given that the amounts of intrastratum information are appreciable, the results from this X^2 function should generally be essentially interchangeable with those from Equation 12.1 and its stratified counterpart in Equation 12.14.

EXAMPLE 12.5. Recall Example 12.1, which is concerned with the data $r_1 = 0/10$, $r_0 = 0/20$. For a two-sided 95% interval, the X^2 function in Example 12.1 gave $RD_{0.025} = -0.17$ and $RD_{0.975} = 0.28$. Consider the upper bound ($RD = 0.28$). It corresponds to $\tilde{R}_1 = 0.28$ and $\tilde{R}_0 = 0.00$, and the likelihood-maximizing values are $\hat{R}_1 = \hat{R}_0 = 0.00$. Thus, at $RD = 0.28$, the LR-based X^2 function takes on the value $2 \log[1/(1 - 0.28)^{10}] = 6.6$, instead of the target value of 3.84. From this LR approach, $RD_{0.975} = 0.17$.

EXAMPLE 12.6. Recall Example 12.4, dealing with the stratified allopurinol data in Table 11.3. The X^2 function (contrast-based) derived in that example and presented numerically in Table 12.4 was replicated in terms of the LR-based X^2 function given above. The point estimates ($RD_{0.50}$)—the values of RD corresponding to the value zero for the two X^2 functions, respectively—are both equal to 0.15. For $RD_{0.025}$ the two functions give 0.07 and 0.05 (LR-based), respectively; the null X^2 values are 19.5 and 12.3 (LR-based), respectively (cf. Examples 11.3, 11.4, and 11.6).

12.3. SIMPLE ANALYSIS FOR *RD*

In the presentation of data analysis for rate difference given above, the accent was on theoretically attractive asymptotic procedures (exact procedures being unavailable even in principle). That those procedures are demanding computationally was viewed as basically a nonissue in the context of modern electronic calculators and computers. Thus the adopted view was that, given modern computational technology and the cost of epidemiologic data collection, the analysis of data in today's environment is to be done in a way that is the best justifiable theoretically (cf. Section 12.1).

When modern technology for data analysis is not available, the classical need for simple procedures persists. In these situations of no access to computer-plotted chi square functions involving heavy calculations, one usually resorts to computing, by the use of a hand calculator, a null chi square ($X^2_{RD=0}$), a point estimate ($RD_{0.50}$), and one confidence interval (usually a two-sided 95% interval, $RD_{0.025}$ and $RD_{0.975}$).

In these terms, the null X^2 is still the *CMH null statistic* in Equation 11.8 or its *angular counterpart* in Equation 11.9. The point estimator may be taken as

$$RD_{0.50} = r_1^* - r_0^*, \qquad (12.26)$$

with, as before (Equation 12.14),

$$r_i^* = \frac{\sum_j W_j r_{ij}}{\sum_j W_j},$$

but with the simplification of involving the null weights

$$W_j = \left(\frac{1}{S_{1j}} + \frac{1}{S_{0j}} \right)^{-1}$$

(cf. Equation 11.8). Thus, although a simplicity-accenting analysis of stratified data shares the calculation for the null point with the X^2 function delineated in Section 12.1.2 [the point ($RD = 0$, X_0^2)], the values of the point estimates coincide in the context of unstratified series only.

For a two-sided $100(1 - \alpha)\%$ confidence interval, the simplest formulation is based on the null X^2 and the point estimate involved in it—the *test-based interval* (Miettinen, 1976a). Its structure is simply

$$RD_{\alpha/2}, RD_{1-\alpha/2} = RD_{0.50} \left(1 \mp \frac{\chi_\alpha}{X_0} \right), \qquad (12.27)$$

where $RD_{0.50}$ is as defined above; χ_α is the square root of the $100(1 - \alpha)$ centile of the chi square distribution with $1 df$, or the $100(1 - \alpha/2)$ centile of the standard Gaussian distribution ($\chi_\alpha = 1.96$ for a 95% interval); and X_0 is the square root of the null chi square in Equation 11.8 or Equation 11.9.

In addition to extreme simplicity, this formulation of confidence limits for *RD* has the theoretical attraction that where the null X^2 gives $P = \alpha/2$ or $P = 1 - \alpha/2$, one of the limits equals the null value ($RD = 0$).

An alternative approach to interval estimation is also worth consideration, despite its somewhat greater complexity, namely the *standard-error-based interval*

$$RD_{\alpha/2}, RD_{1-\alpha/2} = RD_{0.50} \mp \chi_\alpha (\text{SE}_{RD_{0.50}}), \qquad (12.28)$$

with $RD_{0.50}$ based on Equation 12.26, and with the standard error of this point estimate computed as

$$\text{SE}_{RD_{0.50}} = \frac{\{\sum_j W_j^2 [r_{1j}(1 - r_{1j})/(S_{1j} - 1) + r_{0j}(1 - r_{0j})/(S_{0j} - 1)]\}^{1/2}}{\sum_j W_j}.$$

$$(12.29)$$

This approach tends to give theoretically good results in the vicinity of the point estimate. In the context of unstratified (single-stratum) data this "local" good performance is assured; with stratified data it requires reasonably close constancy of the empirical rate difference over the strata. This requirement tends not to be met in the context of scanty amounts of intrastratum information, matched pairs being the extreme case in general.

Given these two simple approaches to interval estimation, and their properties as outlined, there is a need for suitable principles for choosing between them. The first principle in this area is that one need *not* derive both limits of a two-sided interval by the use of a single approach. In these terms one may adopt the broad principle that any limit that is closer to the null value ($RD = 0$) than to the point estimate is better if it is test-based (Equation 12.27) than if it is standard error based (Equation 12.28). Otherwise, the latter approach may be preferable, especially if the stratum-specific empirical values of *RD* are reasonably constant over the strata.

EXAMPLE 12.7.   Consider again the allopurinol data in Table 11.3, recalling Examples 11.3 and 11.4. The values of the mutually standardized empirical rates, with weights designed to maximize comparative efficiency, in the null situation, were calculated to be $r_1^* = 0.224$ and $r_0^* = 0.074$. Thus the point estimate $RD_{0.50}$ is $r_1^* - r_0^* = 0.224 - 0.074 = 0.150$, which coincides with the previous result (Table 12.4), and the value of the null chi square (Equation 11.9) was calculated to be 12.2 (Example 11.4). The test-based 95% two-sided confidence limits (Equation 12.27) are $0.15[1 \mp 1.96/(12.2)^{1/2}] = 0.07$, 0.23. The standard error of the point estimate (Equation 12.29) is $\{(36.0)^2[(5/38)(1 - 5/38)/(38 - 1) + (36/681)(1 - 36/681)/(681 - 1)] + (27.6)^2[(10/29)(1 - 10/29)/(29 - 1) + (58/576)(1 - 58/576)/(576 - 1)]\}^{1/2}/(36.0 + 27.6) = 0.051$. Thus the 95% SE-based limits (Equation 12.28) are $0.15 \mp 1.96(0.051) = 0.05, 0.25$, as opposed to the test-based limits 0.07 and 0.23 given above. The choice between the two lower bounds is not obvious, as both are intermediate between $RD = RD_{0.50}$ and $RD = 0$, and thus averaging of the two might be appropriate, while the upper bound is preferably taken from the SE based approach (since that bound is closer to $RD = RD_{0.50}$ than to $RD = 0$). The "deluxe" 95% interval ranges from 0.07 to 0.26 (Figure 12.4 and Example 12.4), but its lower bound is presumably too high, and perhaps its upper bound as well, due to rightward skewness of the respective sampling distributions (cf. Example 11.4).

12.4. ANALYSIS FOR MODIFICATION OF *RD*

In the preceding sections we considered the derivation of a chi square function as the summary of evidence, or elements of it, in the sense of the null X^2 and the values of *RD* at which $X_{RD}^2 = 0$ ($RD_{0.50}$) and $X_{RD}^2 = \chi_\alpha^2$ ($RD_{\alpha/2}$, $RD_{1-\alpha/2}$). These statistics address *RD* as a singular, even if unknown, parameter of nature. Therefore, their presentation is sensible only insofar as it is indeed reasonable to entertain such constancy, in light of a priori considerations together with the data at hand.

When the potential modifier is *dichotomous*, such as gender, the evidence in the data regarding modification includes a point estimate for the difference between the stratum-specific theoretical rate differences (RD_1 and RD_2) and a chi square value corresponding to the null situation of identity of those differences ($RD_1 = RD_2$), but there is little interest in confidence limits for the *RD* difference (*RDD*).

The point estimate of *RDD* is naturally taken as the empirical value

$$rdd = rd_1 - rd_2. \tag{12.30}$$

The null X^2 (and confidence limits) might be derived, in rough terms, on the basis of the standard error of *rdd*, which is

$$\mathrm{SE}_{rdd} = \left[\sum_j \sum_i \frac{r_{ij}(1 - r_{ij})}{S_{ij} - 1} \right]^{1/2}, \tag{12.31}$$

where $i = 1, 0$ and $j = 1, 2$. In these terms, of course, $X_0^2 = (rdd/\mathrm{SE}_{rdd})^2$.

A better null X^2 involves a variance estimate derived on the basis not of r_{ij} but of $\hat{R}_{ij}$ corresponding to $RD_1 = RD_2 = RD_{0.50}$, the point estimate of *RD* from an analysis stratified by the potential modifier. In these terms the proper null variance for *rdd* is

$$\hat{V}_{rdd} = \sum_j \left[\frac{\hat{R}_{1j}(1 - \hat{R}_{1j})}{S_{1j}} + \frac{\hat{R}_{0j}(1 - \hat{R}_{0j})}{S_{0j}} \right] \frac{S_j}{S_j - 1} \tag{12.32}$$

EXAMPLE 12.8.   Recall Example 12.4, dealing with the rate of drug-attributed rash in terms of the gender-stratified data in Table 11.3. The analysis in that example involved the assumption that the theoretical rate difference is constant over gender. The empirical value for males was 5/38 − 36/681 = 0.0787, while for females it was 0.2441. Thus the empirical values for RD_1 and RD_2 are quite different, by a factor of 3, with $rdd = -0.165$, so that the X^2 for $RD_1 = RD_2$ is of interest. The standard error for this value is $[5/38(1 - 5/38)/(38 - 1) + \ldots]^{1/2} = 0.107$. Thus, the null X^2 for constancy of *RD* over gender is 2.4. For a more proper null variance we read values of $\hat{R}_{ij}$ from Table 12.4, from the line for $RD = 0.15 = RD_{0.50}$ (as $X^2_{RD=0.15} = 0.00$). We find $\hat{R}_{11} = 0.202$, $\hat{R}_{01} = 0.0517$, $\hat{R}_{12} = 0.253$, and $\hat{R}_{02} = 0.103$. With these entries, together with S_{ij} as above, $S_1 = 719$, and $S_2 = 602$, Equation 12.32 gives $\hat{V}_{rdd} = 0.0132$, and the corresponding null X^2 value is $(0.165)^2/0.0132 = 2.1$, rather than 2.4.

When the two categories of a potential modifier of the binary kind involve *confounding* by extraneous factors, the modifier-specific evidence is usually presented in terms of the point estimate $(RD_{0.50})_j$, $j = 1, 2$, together with its associated standard error SE_j or 95% confidence interval; and if the latter is available, the SE can be derived by dividing the width of the interval by $2(1.96) = 3.92$. In this case it is appropriate to take

$$SE_{rdd} = [(SE_1)^2 + (SE_2)^2]^{1/2} \qquad (12.33)$$

(cf. Equation 12.31) for the denominator of the X^2 statistic.

If the scale of the potential modifier is more than dichotomous and is either quasi-quantitative or *quantitative*, the evaluation still starts from the stratum-specific empirical values for RD: rd_1, rd_2, and so on. For the SE-based null X^2 the counterpart (extension) in this situation involves fitting a weighted regression line

$$RD = A + BM, \qquad (12.34)$$

where M is the potential modifier. The fitted slope is

$$b = \frac{\sum_j W_j(m_j - \bar{m})(rd_j)}{\sum_j W_j(m_j - \bar{m})^2}, \qquad (12.35)$$

where $W_j = (1/S_{1j} + 1/S_{0j})^{-1}$, m_j is the value of M for the jth stratum, and $\bar{m} = \sum_j W_j m_j / \sum_j W_j$. The standard error of this slope is

$$SE_b = \frac{\{\sum_j [W_j(m_j - \bar{m})]^2 (SE_{rd_j})^2\}^{1/2}}{\sum_j W_j(m_j - \bar{m})^2}, \qquad (12.36)$$

with $(SE_{rd_j})^2 = r_{1j}(1 - r_{1j})/(S_{1j} - 1) + r_{0j}(1 - r_{0j})/(S_{0j} - 1)$.

A better null X^2 is again obtained by replacing $(SE_{rd_j})^2$ by $\hat{V}_{rd_j} = [\hat{R}_{1j}(1 - \hat{R}_{1j})/S_{1j} + \hat{R}_{0j}(1 - \hat{R}_{0j})/S_{0j}]S_j/(S_j - 1)$ (cf. Equation 12.32).

For a potential modifier measured on a *nominal* scale with three or more categories, the null X^2 of choice might be one based on the likelihood ratio:

$$X^2_{RD_j=RD} = 2 \sum_j \left[c_{1j} \log \frac{r_{1j}}{\hat{R}_{1j}} + (S_{1j} - c_{1j}) \log \frac{1 - r_{1j}}{1 - \hat{R}_{1j}} \right. $$
$$\left. + c_{0j} \log \frac{r_{0j}}{\hat{R}_{0j}} + (S_{0j} - c_{0j}) \log \frac{1 - r_{0j}}{1 - \hat{R}_{0j}} \right]. \qquad (12.37)$$

Here, as above, $\hat{R}_{1j}$ and $\hat{R}_{0j}$ are the estimates of R_{1j} and R_{0j} obtained on the restriction that $\hat{R}_{1j} - \hat{R}_{0j} = RD_{0.50}$, the point estimate of RD from an analysis stratified by the covariate, ideally the value that maximizes the likelihood restricted by $RD_j \equiv RD$ (Section 12.2). This statistic is referred to tables of chi square distribution with $J - 1$ df (J being the number of strata at issue).

It should not be used when the intrastratum amounts of information are small.

EXAMPLE 12.9. Recall Example 12.8, including the values of $\hat{\hat{R}}_{ij}$. The statistic given above, when applied to those data, yields the chi square (1 df) value 2.5 against the null hypothesis of no difference in *RD* between males and females.

Alternatively, again, modifier-specific point estimates $(RD_{0.50})_j$, $j = 1, \ldots$, and their associated standard errors SE_j may be available—with the latter possibly deduced from the corresponding confidence intervals (see above). With these inputs the counterpart of the X^2 statistic in Eq. 12.37 is

$$X^2_{RDj \equiv RD} = \sum_j \left[\frac{(RD_{0.50})_j - RD_{0.50}}{SE_j} \right]^2, \qquad (12.38)$$

where $RD_{0.50} = \sum_j W_j (RD_{0.50})_j / \sum_j W_j$ with $W_j = 1/(SE_j)^2$. As above, the result is referred to a tabulation of the χ^2 distribution with $J - 1$ *df*.

13

Comparative Analysis of Two Rates III:

CHI SQUARE FUNCTION FOR RATE RATIO

13.1. CONTRAST-BASED X^2 FUNCTION OF RR

13.1.1. Unstratified Series

When the parameter of interest is the rate ratio (RR), the basic X^2 function for the unstratified situation may be formulated in the spirit of Fieller's theorem (Fieller, 1944):

$$X^2_{RR} = \frac{[r_1 - (RR)r_0]^2}{\hat{V}_{r_1|RR} + (RR)^2 \hat{V}_{r_0|RR}}. \tag{13.1}$$

The variance estimators for proportion-type rates are of the form

$$\begin{aligned} \hat{V}_{r_i|RR} &= \tilde{V}_{r_i} \\ &= \frac{\tilde{R}_i(1 - \tilde{R}_i)}{S_i} \frac{S}{S - 1}. \end{aligned} \tag{13.2}$$

Of course,

$$\tilde{R}_1 = \tilde{R}_0(RR). \tag{13.3}$$

$\tilde{R}_0$ is solved from the likelihood equation

$$\frac{c_1 - S_1\tilde{R}_0(RR)}{1 - \tilde{R}_0(RR)} + \frac{c_0 - S_0\tilde{R}_0}{1 - \tilde{R}_0} = 0, \tag{13.4}$$

subject to $0 \le \tilde{R}_0 \le 1$ and $0 \le \tilde{R}_0(RR) \le 1$. In contrast to the likelihood equation in the context of *RD* (Equation 12.4), this equation is only quadratic, and the solution that satisfies the range criteria for $\tilde{R}_1$ and $\tilde{R}_0$ is

$$\tilde{R}_0 = \frac{-B - (B^2 - 4AC)^{1/2}}{2A}, \tag{13.5}$$

where $A = S(RR)$, $B = -[c_1 + S_1(RR) + c_0(RR) + S_0]$, and $C = c$. For incidence densities,

$$\tilde{V}_{r_i} = \frac{\tilde{R}_i}{T_i}, \tag{13.6}$$

with $\tilde{R}_1 = \tilde{R}_0(RR)$, and with

$$\tilde{R}_0 = \frac{c}{T_1(RR) + T_0}. \tag{13.7}$$

(Cf. Miettinen and Nurminen, 1985).

An alternative approach of some interest is to write

$$X^2_{RR} = \frac{[\log(rr) - \log(RR)]^2}{\hat{V}_{\log(rr)\,|\,RR}}. \tag{13.8}$$

Here, in contrast to the X^2 function in Equation 13.1, it is necessary to employ a Taylor series approximation in the variance estimator:

$$\hat{V}_{\log(rr)\,|\,RR} = \tilde{V}_{\log(rr)} = \frac{\tilde{V}_{r_1}}{R_1^2} + \frac{\tilde{V}_{r_0}}{R_0^2}. \tag{13.9}$$

Specifically, for proportion-type rates,

$$\tilde{V}_{\log(rr)} = \left(\frac{1 - \tilde{R}_1}{S_1\tilde{R}_1} + \frac{1 - \tilde{R}_0}{S_0\tilde{R}_0}\right)\frac{S}{S - 1}, \tag{13.10}$$

and for incidence densities it is

$$\tilde{V}_{\log(rr)} = \frac{1}{T_1\tilde{R}_1} + \frac{1}{T_0\tilde{R}_0}. \tag{13.11}$$

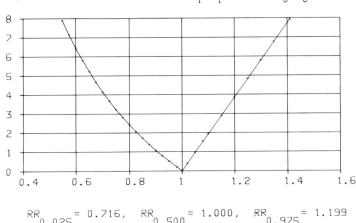

Chi Square as a function of RR; $c_1/S_1 = 10/10$, $c_0/S_0 = 20/20$

$RR_{0.025} = 0.716$, $RR_{0.500} = 1.000$, $RR_{0.975} = 1.199$

Figure 13.1. For the data $c_1/S_1 = 10/10$ and $c_0/S_0 = 20/20$, chi square as a function of *RR*. See Example 13.1.

It remains commonplace to use the log-transformation approach together with unrestricted estimation of variance, that is, to take the X^2 function as

$$X_{RR}^2 = \frac{[\log(rr) - \log(RR)]^2}{\hat{V}_{\log(rr)}}, \tag{13.12}$$

with

$$\hat{V}_{\log(rr)} = \frac{1 - r_1}{S_1 r_1} + \frac{1 - r_0}{S_0 r_0}$$

$$= \frac{1 - r_1}{c_1} + \frac{1 - r_0}{c_0},$$

in lieu of the restricted unbiased estimator in Equation 13.10 (see, for example, Katz et al., 1978). This is not in keeping with first principles (Section 10.1.1), and it can give poor results.

EXAMPLE 13.1. Suppose that $c_1/S_1 = 10/10$ and $c_0/S_0 = 20/20$. With these data, $\hat{V}_{\log(rr)}$ (Equation 13.12) is zero, so that X_{RR}^2 (Equation 13.8) is infinity at all $RR \neq 1$ and, thereby, all confidence bounds converge at $RR = 1$. The values of $\tilde{R}_0$ from Equation 13.5 are $1/RR$ and 1. For the range of $RR > 1$, we take $\tilde{R}_0 = 1/RR$; for $RR < 1$ we set $\tilde{R}_0 = 1$. Thus, for $RR > 1$, the X^2 function in Equation 13.8 takes the form $[\log(RR)]^2/\{[(1 - 1/RR)/(20/RR)]30/29\}$, and the function in Equation 13.1 becomes $(1 - RR)^2/\{[RR(1 - 1/RR)/20]30/29\}$. For $RR_{0.975}$ ($X^2 = 3.84$) the respective values are 1.25 and 1.20, not 1.00. For $RR < 1$, with $\tilde{R}_1 = RR$ and $\tilde{R}_0 = 1$, the corresponding X^2 functions are $[\log(RR)]^2/\{[(1 - RR)/(10RR)]30/29\}$ and $(1 - RR)^2/\{[RR(1 - $

TABLE 13.1.

For the data $c_1/S_1 = 8/10$ and $c_0/S_0 = 5/20$, estimates of R_0 (Equation 13.5), R_1, and variance of contrast in Equation 13.1, together with chi square corresponding to RR

	Estimates			Chi
RR	$\tilde{R}_0$	$\tilde{R}_1$	$\tilde{V}_{r_1-(RR)r_0}$	Square
1.0	0.433	0.433	0.038	7.94
1.4	0.408	0.571	0.050	4.06
2.0	0.353	0.706	0.069	1.31
3.0	0.264	0.792	0.107	0.02
3.2	0.250	0.800	0.116	0.00
3.6	0.226	0.812	0.133	0.08
4.0	0.205	0.820	0.150	0.27
6.0	0.140	0.841	0.238	2.06
8.0	0.106	0.849	0.327	4.40
10.0	0.085	0.853	0.417	6.94

$RR)/10]30/29\}$, respectively. For $RR_{0.025}$ they yield the values of 0.59 and 0.72, respectively, not 1.00. The X^2 function is shown in Figure 13.1.

EXAMPLE 13.2 Suppose now that $c_1/S_1 = 8/10$ and $c_0/S_0 = 5/20$ (as in Example 12.3). Solutions of the likelihood equation for $\tilde{R}_0$ (Equation 13.5) are shown in Table 13.1 for various values of the parameter (RR). The resulting X^2 function is shown in Figure 13.2. At $RR = 1$ its realization is

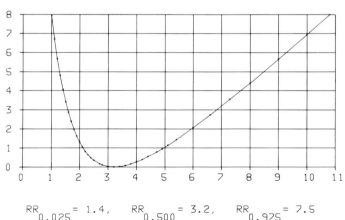

Figure 13.2. For the data $c_1/S_1 = 8/10$ and $c_0/S_0 = 5/20$, chi square as a function of RR. See Example 13.2.

7.9, which is strictly consonant with the basic null X^2 (see Example 12.3). The function based on log transformation together with restricted estimation of variance (Equation 13.8) gives, at $RR = 1$, $X_0^2 = [\log(0.8/0.25)]^2/[(17/13)(1/10 + 1/20)30/29] = 6.7$. If the ordinary, unconditional maximum likelihood estimator of the variance (Equation 13.12) is used, the null realization is $X_0^2 = [\log(0.8/0.25)]^2/[0.2/8 + 0.75/5] = 7.7$.

Theory suggests, and computer simulations confirm, that the function in Equation 13.1 is superior to the one now in common use (Equation 13.12), and it seems somewhat superior to the LR-based X^2 function as well (Section 13.2) (see Miettinen and Nurminen, 1985).

13.1.2. Stratified Series in General

The X^2 function of a crude (unconditional) RR (Equation 13.1) extends to the case of stratified series in a manner analogous to that presented for RD in Section 12.1.2. The generalized function is of the form of

$$X_{RR}^2 = \frac{[r_1^* - (RR)r_0^*]^2}{\tilde{V}_{r_1^*} + (RR)^2 \tilde{V}_{r_0^*}}, \tag{13.13}$$

where, as before, $r_i^* = \sum_j W_j r_{ij}/\sum_j W_j$ and the tildes designate estimators restricted on the parameter at issue (RR). Specifically, the variance estimators for proportion-type rates, again with no Taylor series approximation involved, are

$$\tilde{V}_{r_i^*} = \frac{\sum_j W_j^2 [\tilde{R}_{ij}(1 - \tilde{R}_{ij})/S_{ij}] \, S_j/(S_j - 1)}{(\sum_j W_j)^2}, \tag{13.14}$$

with $\tilde{R}_{1j} = \tilde{R}_{0j}(RR)$, and $\tilde{R}_{0j}$ is computed from the data for the jth stratum according to Equation 13.5. In this context the weights, analogous to those in Equation 12.16 for RD, are

$$W_j = \left[\frac{1}{S_{1j}} + \frac{(RR)(1 - R_0^*)}{(1 - R_1^*)S_{0j}} \right]^{-1} \tag{13.15}$$

with $\tilde{R}_0^* = \sum_j W_j \tilde{R}_{0j}/\sum_j W_j$, and $\tilde{R}_1^* = \tilde{R}_0^*(RR)$. The derivation of these weights requires an iterative procedure such as the one discussed in the context of Equation 12.16. If the rates represent incidence densities,

$$\tilde{V}_{r_i^*} = \frac{[\sum_j W_j^2 \tilde{R}_{ij}/T]}{(\sum_j W_j)^2}, \tag{13.16}$$

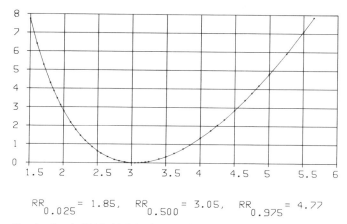

Chi Square as a function of RR

$$RR_{0.025} = 1.85, \quad RR_{0.500} = 3.05, \quad RR_{0.975} = 4.77$$

Figure 13.3. For the data in Table 11.3 ($c_{11}/S_{11} = 5/38$, $c_{01}/S_{01} = 36/681$, $c_{12}/S_{12} = 10/29$, and $c_{02}/S_{02} = 58/576$), chi square as a function of *RR*. See Example 13.3.

with $\tilde{R}_{1j} = \tilde{R}_{0j}(RR)$ and $\tilde{R}_{0j}$ computed according to Equation 13.7 from the data for the *j*th stratum. In this context the weights take on the form

$$W_j = \left(\frac{1}{T_{1j}} + \frac{RR}{T_{0j}} \right)^{-1}. \tag{13.17}$$

EXAMPLE 13.3. Recall the allopurinol data in Table 11.3, which were considered in Examples 11.3, 11.4, 12.4, 12.6, and 12.7. The evidence as to rate ratio is summarized in Figure 13.3 and Table 13.2. It deserves note that the function, which involves no transformation, is rather closely log-symmetrical around the point estimate (cf. Figure 13.4).

13.1.3. Matched Series

For individually matched series the X^2 function in Equation 13.13 can be written as

$$X_{RR}^2 = \frac{[f_1./f.. - (RR) \sum_v f._v/(Rf..)]^2}{\sum_{u,v} f_{uv} \tilde{V}_{r1-(RR)r0|u,v}/f..^2} \tag{13.18}$$

(cf. Equation 12.19 and Table 11.4). The variance estimator is

$$\tilde{V}_{r1-(RR)r0|u,v} = \{[\tilde{R}_1(1 - \tilde{R}_1) + (RR)^2\tilde{R}_0(1 - \tilde{R}_0)/R](1 + R)/R\}\,|_{u,v}. \tag{13.19}$$

TABLE 13.2.

For the data in Table 11.3, analysis for rate ratio (RR); shown are, for various values of RR, the stratum-specific estimates $\tilde{R}_1$ and $\tilde{R}_0$ together with their respective weighted averages $\tilde{R}_1^*$ and $\tilde{R}_0^*$, and the contrast-based chi square (X^2)

	Males		Females				
RR	$\tilde{R}_1$	$\tilde{R}_0$	$\tilde{R}_1$	$\tilde{R}_0$	$\tilde{R}_1^*$	$\tilde{R}_0^*$	X^2
1.00	0.0570	0.0570	0.1124	0.1124	0.0811	0.0811	19.5
1.50	0.0834	0.0556	0.1655	0.1103	0.1191	0.0794	7.74
1.80	0.0986	0.0548	0.1962	0.1090	0.1411	0.0784	4.29
1.85	0.1011	0.0547	0.2012	0.1088	0.1447	0.0782	3.86
2.00	0.1085	0.0542	0.2161	0.1081	0.1553	0.0777	2.77
2.90	0.1500	0.0517	0.3003	0.1036	0.2156	0.0743	0.04
3.00	0.1543	0.0514	0.3091	0.1030	0.2219	0.0740	0.00
3.10	0.1586	0.0512	0.3177	0.1025	0.2281	0.0736	0.01
3.25	0.1649	0.0507	0.3304	0.1017	0.2373	0.0730	0.07
4.75	0.2218	0.0467	0.4410	0.0928	0.3181	0.0670	3.78
4.80	0.2235	0.0466	0.4441	0.0925	0.3204	0.0668	3.98
5.50	0.2462	0.0448	0.4851	0.0882	0.3514	0.0639	7.10

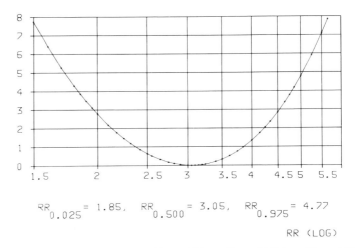

Figure 13.4.   For the data in Table 13.3 ($c_{11}/S_{11} = 5/38$, $c_{01}/S_{01} = 36/681$, $c_{12}/S_{12} = 10/29$, and $c_{02}/S_{02} = 58/576$), chi square as a function of RR. See Example 13.3.

Here $\tilde{R}_1 = \tilde{R}_0(RR)$, and $\tilde{R}_0$ is computed according to Equation 13.5, with $c_1 = u$, $S_1 = 1$, $c_0 = v$, $S_0 = R$, $c = u + v$, and $S = 1 + R$. Values of $\tilde{R}_0$ and the variance estimator itself (Equation 13.19) are tabulated in Appendix 13, for various combinations of u and v for particular matching ratios (R) in the range from 1 to 5, corresponding to a sequence of values of RR in the range from 0.2 to 5.

In the context of matched pairs the X^2 function does not reduce to anything as simple as in the context of RD (Equation 12.22). The f_{11} pairs with $u = 1$ and $v = 1$ are associated with a variance element of either $2(RR - 1)$ or $2(RR)(1 - RR)$, according as $RR > 1$ or $RR < 1$. The f_{10} pairs with $u = 1$ and $v = 0$ each correspond to a variance estimate equal to RR as long as $RR < 2$; for $RR > 2$ it is $2(RR - 1)$. For each of the f_{01} pairs with $u = 0$ and $v = 1$ the variance estimate equals RR as long as $RR > \frac{1}{2}$; for $RR < \frac{1}{2}$ it equals $2(RR)(1 - RR)$. From the f_{00} pairs with $u = 0$ and $v = 0$ the variance contributions are zero for all values of RR. In spite of these complexities, it is easy to observe that in the null situation $(RR = 1)$ the X^2 function again reduces to the null X^2, the McNemar statistic (Equation 11.16).

13.2. *LR*-BASED X^2 FUNCTION OF *RR*

What was said about the *LR* function of *RD* in Section 12.2 applies with full analogy to *RR*. Thus, given a contrast-based chi square function of *RR*, the "local" *LR* function may be taken as

$$LR_{RR} = \exp[-\tfrac{1}{2}(X^2_{RR} - X^2_{RR=1})], \qquad (13.20)$$

an expression which involves the assumption that the variance of the Gaussian density of X is constant over the range of *RR* considered, including $RR = 1$.

The exact *LR* function is here

$$LR_{RR} = \exp(\max_{RR} \Sigma_j \tilde{U}_j - \Sigma_j \tilde{U}_j) \qquad (13.21)$$

with, as in the context of *RD*, $\tilde{U}_j = c_{1j} \log \tilde{R}_{1j} + (S_{1j} - c_{1j})\log(1 - \tilde{R}_{1j}) + c_{0j} \log \tilde{R}_{0j} + (S_{0j} - c_{0j})\log(1 - \tilde{R}_{0j})$, but these estimators of R_1 and R_0 involve the *RR* constraint and are, thus, based on Equations 13.3 and 13.5. Strata with $r_j = 0$ are noncontributory to this *LR* function, and since they can cause computational problems, they may best be deleted from the analysis. As with *RD*, the maximum of $\Sigma_j \tilde{U}_j$ over *RR* (which will correspond to a value close to r_1^*/r_0^*) is to be found iteratively.

Naturally, as in the context of *RD*, the exact *LR* function of *RR* gives rise to an asymptotic X^2 function of *RR*:

$$X^2_{RR} = 2 \log(LR_{RR}). \qquad (13.22)$$

As to the performance of this function, the discussion regarding RD (Section 12.2) applies here as well.

EXAMPLE 13.4. Recall Example 12.5 for RD, and Example 13.1 for RR. The former involved the data $r_1 = 0/10$ and $r_0 = 0/20$, which are uninformative for RR, and the latter involved the corresponding informative data $r_1 = 10/10$, $r_0 = 20/20$. The 95% two-sided interval, based on the X^2 function in Equation 13.1, was found to range from 0.72 to 1.20. The lower bound ($RR_{0.025} = 0.72$) corresponds to $\tilde{R}_1 = 0.72$, $\tilde{R}_0 = 1.00$ (and thus to $RD_{0.025} = -0.28$; cf. Example 12.5). Thus, as in Example 12.5, the corresponding value of the LR-based chi square statistic is 6.6, instead of 3.84. The latter function gives $RR_{0.025} = 0.83$ (corresponding to $RD_{0.025} = -0.17$; cf. Example 12.5).

EXMPLE 13.5. Consider again the stratified allopurinol data in Table 11.3, recalling the corresponding X^2 function presented in Figures 13.3 and 13.4 and in Table 13.2. The LR-based X^2 function gives $RR_{0.50} = 3.1$ (as does the contrast-based X^2 function), the 95% interval is $RR_{0.25} = 1.8$, $RR_{0.975} = 4.8$ (as before), and the null X^2 value is 14.8 (as opposed to 12.3 from the LR-based X^2 function for RD) (cf. Example 12.6).

13.3. SIMPLE ANALYSIS FOR *RR*

When the comparative parameter is RR, the simple approach to analysis is closely analogous to that for RD (Section 12.3).

The null X^2 for RR, just as for RD, is the CMH null statistic in Equation 11.8 or its angular counterpart in Equation 11.9.

The point estimator, analogously with that for RD (Equation 12.26), may be taken as

$$RR_{0.50} = \frac{r_1^*}{r_0^*}, \tag{13.23}$$

with $r_i^* = \sum_j W_j r_{ij} / \sum_j W_j$ and $W_j = (1/S_{1j} + 1/S_{0j})^{-1}$. As with RD, this point estimator may provide a value somewhat different from that corresponding to the minimum (zero) value of the X^2 function in Equation 13.13. With RR as with RD, discrepancies are prone to appear when the point estimate and S_{1j}/S_{0j} vary appreciably over the strata.

The test-based $100(1 - \alpha)\%$ two-sided confidence interval, owing to the skewness of the sampling distribution of the point estimates, is here derived with the use of log transformation:

$$RR_{\alpha/2}, RR_{1-\alpha/2} = \exp[\log(RR_{0.50})(1 \mp \chi_\alpha/X_0)] \tag{13.24}$$
$$= (RR_{0.50})^{1 \mp \chi_\alpha/X_0}.$$

The corresponding SE-based interval is

$$RR_{\alpha/2}, RR_{1-\alpha/2} = \exp[\log(RR_{0.50}) \mp \chi_\alpha(SE_{\log(RR_{0.50})})], \quad (13.25)$$

with

$$SE_{\log(RR_{0.50})} = \left[\frac{\sum_j W_j^2 r_{1j}(1 - r_{1j})}{(r_1^* \sum_j W_j)^2(S_{1j} - 1)} + \frac{\sum_j W_j^2 r_{0j}(1 - r_{0j})}{(r_0^* \sum_j W_j)^2(S_{0j} - 1)}\right]^{1/2} \quad (13.26)$$

The choice between these two types of limit for *RR* depends on considerations identical to those pertaining to *RD*, except that relative distances from $RR_{0.50}$ and $RR = 1$ are measured on the log scale.

EXAMPLE 13.6. Recall Example 12.7, which was concerned with stratified analysis for *RD*. The null X^2 was $X_0^2 = 12.2$, and this value applies to *RR* analysis as well. The point estimate there was $r_1^* - r_0^* = 0.224 - 0.074$, and here it is $RR_{0.50} = r_1^*/r_0^* = 0.224/0.074 = 3.0$, agreeing with that given in Figure 13.3 (Example 13.3). Test-based 95% limits for *RR* are $RR_{0.025}$, $RR_{0.975} = \exp\{\log(3.0)[1 \mp 1.96/(12.1)^{1/2}]\} = 1.6, 5.6$. For the other approach, the SE of $\log(RD_{0.50})$ is $\{[(36.0)^2(5/38)(1 - 5/38)/(38 - 1) + (27.6)^2(10/29)(1 - 10/29)/(29 - 1)]/[0.224(36.0 + 27.6)]^2 + [(36.0)^2(36/681)(1 - 36/681)/(681 - 1) - (27.6)^2(58/576)(1 - 58/576)/(576 - 1)]/[0.074(36.0 + 27.6)]^2\}^{1/2} = 0.24$. Thus, the SE-based interval is $\exp[\log(3.0) \mp 1.96(0.24)] = 1.9, 4.8$. (Cf. Figure 13.3.)

13.4. ANALYSIS FOR MODIFICATION OF *RR*

Analogously with analyses for *RD* the analyses presented above for *RR* involve the presumption that this comparative parameter is constant (or nearly so) over various categories of the types of subject involved. And again, it may be desirable to examine the extent to which the data themselves are at variance with this presumption.

When the scale of the potential modifier is dichotomous, the empirical measure corresponding to rate difference difference (*rdd*) is rate ratio ratio (*rrr*):

$$rrr = \frac{rr_1}{rr_2}. \quad (13.27)$$

For a rough null X^2 (and confidence limits, if desired), one might consider log(*rrr*) and its standard error. For the latter, the first-order Taylor series approximation is (cf. Equation 13.12)

$$SE_{\log(rrr)} = \left[\sum_j \sum_i \frac{1 - r_{ij}}{c_{ij}} \right]^{1/2}. \tag{13.28}$$

A better null X^2 based on log(*rrr*) involves (cf. Equation 12.32)

$$\hat{V}_{\log(rrr)} = \sum_j \sum_i \frac{1 - \hat{\tilde{R}}_{ij}}{S_{ij} \hat{\tilde{R}}_{ij}}, \tag{13.29}$$

where $\hat{\tilde{R}}_{ij}$ is the value of $\tilde{R}_{ij}$ corresponding to $RR_1 = RR_2 = RR_{0.50}$ from an analysis stratified by the potential modifier.

EXAMPLE 13.7.   Recall Example 12.8, dealing with potential *RD* modification by gender in the context of the allopurinol-rash data in Table 11.3. The *rr* for the male stratum was $(5/38)/(36/681) = 2.49$, whereas for the female stratum it was 3.42. Thus the *rrr* was 0.728, or $(0.728)^{-1} = 1.374$, and the corresponding logarithms are ∓ 0.317. The asymptotic *SE* for each of these is $[(1 - 5/38)/5 + \ldots]^{1/2} = 0.506$. Thus the SE-based null X^2 (for $RR_1 = RR_2$) is $(0.317/0.506)^2 = 0.4$. The *ML* estimate of *RR* was 3.05 (Example 13.5), and its associated values $\hat{\tilde{R}}_{ij}$ for $\tilde{R}_{ij}$ can be read from Table 13.2. In these terms the variance estimate for log(*rrr*) is $(1 - 0.157)/[38(0.157)] + \ldots = 0.260$, rather than $(0.506)^2 = 0.256$, as given above, and the corresponding null chi square is 0.4, as above.

If, for the two categories of the potential modifier, point estimates and $100 (1 - \alpha)\%$ confidence limits (based perhaps on stratified or multivariate analysis) are available, then one may take the *SE* as

$$SE_{\log(rrr)} = \left\{ \sum_{j=1}^{2} \left[\log\left(\frac{RR_{1-\alpha/2}}{RR_{\alpha/2}} \right)_j / (2\chi_\alpha) \right]^2 \right\}^{1/2} \tag{13.30}$$

(cf. Eq. 12.33).

In the context of a potential modifier that is measured on a quasi-quantitative or quantitative scale, an appropriate approach, as with *RD*, is again one of weighted regression. For the logarithm of *RR*, the fitted regression slope is

$$b = \frac{\sum_j W_j (m_j - \bar{m}) \log(rr_j)}{\sum_j W_j (m_j - \bar{m})^2}, \tag{13.31}$$

where, as in the case of *RD*, $W_j = (1/S_{1j} + 1/S_{0j})^{-1}$, m_j is the value or score of the potential modifier for the jth stratum, and $\bar{m} = \sum_j W_j m_j / \sum_j W_j$. The *SE* for this slope is

$$SE_b = \frac{\{\sum_j [W_j(m - \bar{m})]^2 (SE_{\log(rr_j)})^2\}^{1/2}}{\sum_j W_j(m_j - \bar{m})^2}, \qquad (13.32)$$

with, based on Taylor series approximation,

$$SE_{\log(rr_j)} = \frac{1 - r_{1j}}{c_{1j}} + \frac{1 - r_{0j}}{c_{0j}}.$$

Preferably, analogously with *RD*, the empirical rates are replaced by their *ML* estimates restricted in terms of $RR_j \equiv RR$, that is by $\hat{R}_{1j}$ and $\hat{R}_{0j}$.

In the context of nominal-scale stratification, an *LR*-based statistic of the sort given in Equation 12.37 is again appropriate.

EXAMPLE **13.8.** Application of the *LR*-based statistic in Equation 12.37 to the problem in Example 13.7, with the $\hat{R}_{ij}$ based on *RR* as in that example, yields a chi square (1 df) value of 0.4.

When the input consists of stratum-specific point and interval estimates, the test statistic may be taken as

$$X^2_{RR_j \equiv RR} = \sum_j \left[\frac{\log (RR_{0.50})_j - \log (RR_{0.50})}{SE_j} \right]^2, \qquad (13.33)$$

where $\log (RR_{0.50}) = \sum_j W_j \log (RD_{0.50})_j / \sum_j W_j$ with $W_j = 1/(SE_j)^2$, and SE_j is derived, stratum-specifically, as in Equation 13.30. (The number of *df* is $J - 1$, as before.)

14

Comparative Analysis of Two Rates IV:

CHI SQUARE FUNCTION FOR ODDS RATIO

For two rates, the comparative parameter in absolute terms is the rate difference, and the basic relative measure is the rate ratio. Other relative parameters, such as the etiologic fraction, are derivatives of the rate ratio. The odds ratio is of no interest per se (Section A.2.4), but only as an auxiliary parameter in the analysis of case-referent studies (Section A.2.4 and Section 17.2).

14.1. SCORE-BASED X^2 FUNCTION OF OR

14.1.1. Unstratified Series

In the context of rate difference and ratio we had the simple relations of $R_1 = R_0 + RD$ and $R_1 = R_0(RR)$, respectively. Their counterpart for odds ratio (OR) is nonlinear:

$$R_1 = \frac{(OR)R_0}{1 + (OR - 1)R_0}.$$ (14.1)

The contrast-based X^2 function, when formulated in analogy with that in Equation 13.1 for RR, is

$$X^2_{OR} = \frac{[r_1 - f(r_0)]^2}{\hat{V}_{r_1 \mid OR} + \hat{V}_{f(r_0) \mid OR}},$$ (14.2)

where

$$f(r_0) = \frac{(OR)r_0}{1 + (OR - 1)r_0}.$$

The first element in the variance estimator is, naturally,

$$\hat{V}_{r_1 \mid OR} = \tilde{V}_{r_1}$$ (14.3)

$$= \frac{\tilde{R}_1(1 - \tilde{R}_1)}{S_1} \frac{S}{S - 1}$$

(cf. Equation 13.2), where

$$\tilde{R}_1 = \frac{(OR)\tilde{R}_0}{1 + (OR - 1)\tilde{R}_0}.$$ (14.4)

For $\tilde{R}_0$ the likelihood equation, based on two independent binomials as before, has as the pertinent solution

$$\tilde{R}_0 = \frac{-B + (B^2 - 4AC)^{1/2}}{2A},$$ (14.5)

where $A = S_0(OR - 1)$, $B = c_1 + (S_1 - c_1)(OR) - c_0(OR - 1) + S_0$, and $C = -c$. (For notation, see Table 11.1.) This estimator of R_0 permits the computation of $\hat{V}_{r_1 \mid OR}$ by the use of Equations 14.3 and 14.4. The second variance element in the X^2 function (Equation 14.2) needs to be dealt with in terms of a Taylor series approximation, because of the nonlinearity of $f(r_0)$. The approximation (first-order) is

$$\hat{V}_{f(r_0) \mid OR} = \frac{(OR)^2}{[1 + (OR - 1)\tilde{R}_0]^4} \tilde{V}_{r_0}$$ (14.6)

where $\tilde{V}_{r_0} = [\tilde{R}_0(1 - \tilde{R}_0)/S_0]S/(S - 1)$ (cf. Equation 14.3).

It is apparent that the solutions for $\tilde{R}_0$, on the surface, are indeterminate and infinity in the context of $OR = 1$. It is easy to show, however, that as

OR approaches unity, the value of $\tilde{R}_0$ converges to $r = c/S$, and the X^2 function becomes the Pearson–Barnard null X^2 in Equation 11.4, as it should.

As an alternative approach, one might wish to take the X^2 function as

$$X_{OR}^2 = \frac{[\log(or) - \log(OR)]^2}{\hat{V}_{\log(or)\,|\,OR}}, \tag{14.7}$$

with the variance estimator again involving Taylor series approximation:

$$\hat{V}_{\log(or)\,|\,OR} = \{[S_1\tilde{R}_1(1 - \tilde{R}_1)]^{-1} \\ + [S_0\tilde{R}_0(1 - \tilde{R}_0)]^{-1}\} \frac{S}{S-1}. \tag{14.8}$$

Instead of this restricted and unbiased formulation of the variance estimator, the unrestricted ML estimator (Woolf, 1955) remains in common use. The structure of this latter estimator is, evidently,

$$\hat{V}_{\log(or)} = [S_1 r_1(1 - r_1)]^{-1} + [S_0 r_0(1 - r_0)]^{-1} \\ = \frac{1}{c_1} + \frac{1}{S_1 - c_1} + \frac{1}{c_0} + \frac{1}{S_0 - c_0}. \tag{14.9}$$

EXMPLE 14.1. Recall the data of $r_1 = 10/10$ and $r_0 = 20/20$ (Examples 12.2 and 13.1), and those of $r_1 = 0/10$ and $r_0 = 0/20$ (Example 12.1). It is easy to see that the basic statistic (Equation 14.2) takes on the indeterminate value of $0/0$ with each of these two sets of data for all values of OR. Since the empirical OR is indeterminate, the statistic in Equation 14.7 has an indeterminate numerator, and the denominator is infinite in constrained as well as unconstrained terms. Thus the function in Equation 14.2 leads to the recognition (correct) that the data are uninformative about OR (though not about RD or RR), whereas the statistic in Equation 14.7 does not.

EXAMPLE 14.2. Consider $c_1/S_1 = 10/10$ and $c_0/S_0 = 5/20$. The log-transformation approach (Equation 14.7) is still infeasible, because $\log(or)$ is infinite (and so is the Woolf variance in Equation 14.9). By contrast, the function in Equation 14.2 can be derived. Consider the point $OR = 2$. The corresponding solution for $\tilde{R}_0$ (Equation 14.5) is 0.443. Thus, by Equation 14.4, $\tilde{R}_1 = 2(0.443)/[1 + (2 - 1)0.443] = 0.614$. For the X^2 at $OR = 2$ (Equation 14.2) the numerator is $(1 - 0.400)^2 = 0.360$. For the denominator, $\tilde{V}_{r_1} = 0.0245$ (Equation 14.3) and the other element (Equation 14.6) is 0.235. Thus, the value of X_{OR}^2 at $OR = 2$ is $0.360/(0.0245 + 0.235) = 1.4$. One might wish to check such calculations by the use of the property that $S_1\tilde{R}_1 + S_0\tilde{R}_0 = c$. Here, $10(0.614) + 20(0.443) = 15.00$, as it should. (The relation obtains for OR but not for RD or RR.)

TABLE 14.1.

For the data $c_1/S_1 = 8/10$ and $c_0/S_0 = 5/20$, the estimates of R_0 (Equation 14.5), R_1, and variance of contrast in Equation 14.2, together with chi square corresponding to OR

OR	$\tilde{R}_0$	$\tilde{R}_1$	$\tilde{V}_{r_1 - f(r_0)}$	Chi Square
1	0.433	0.433	0.038	7.94
2	0.376	0.547	0.039	4.09
3	0.344	0.612	0.038	2.40
10	0.261	0.779	0.026	0.04
12	0.250	0.800	0.024	0.00
15	0.238	0.824	0.021	0.05
40	0.196	0.907	0.011	1.54
60	0.184	0.931	0.008	2.89
90	0.175	0.950	0.006	4.94
120	0.170	0.961	0.004	6.98

EXAMPLE 14.3. Recall the data $c_1/S_1 = 8/10$ and $c_0/S_0 = 5/20$ (Examples 12.3 and 13.2). Some elements of the X^2 function based on Equation 14.2 are given numerically in Table 14.1. It may be instructive to compare the contrast-based X^2 functions for RD (Example 12.3), RR (Example 13.2), and OR based on those data. All three take on the value zero at $(\tilde{R}_1, \tilde{R}_0) = (r_1, r_0) = (0.80, 0.25)$, as a reflection of a general feature. All three also reduce to the null X^2 (Equation 11.4) corresponding to $\tilde{R}_1 = \tilde{R}_0 = r = c/S$. However, $RD_{0.025}$ corresponds to $(\tilde{R}_1, \tilde{R}_0) = (0.541, 0.372)$, $RR_{0.025}$ to $(\tilde{R}_1, \tilde{R}_0) = (0.581, 0.405)$, and $OR_{0.025}$ to $(\tilde{R}_1, \tilde{R}_0) = (0.556, 0.372)$. Thus it is necessary to evaluate the three X^2 functions separately, despite the shared realizations corresponding to the empirical and null values of the parameters, respectively.

The X^2 function for OR has been approached still differently by Cornfield (1956). His argument, just as that of the null X^2 presented by Mantel and Haenszel (1959), is conditional on the marginal rate $r = c/S$. In this text, only the unconditional approach is used, to maintain a unified, didactically focused outlook. Nothing is lost by this imposed simplicity; conditional arguments do not provide anything that is not obtainable unconditionally for asymptotic comparisons of rates. At the same time the conditional approach involves limitations in this realm and, particularly, in generalizations beyond the comparison of two rates (cf. Section 11.1.2.1). For the null X^2, the equivalence of these two approaches has been discussed by Pearson (1947) and Barnard (1947).

The Cornfield chi square function of OR can be derived unconditionally by the use of the "efficient score" approach, with "Fisher information." The underlying principle is that instead of "scores" such as $r_1 - f(r_0)$ in

Equation 14.2, the "efficient score" to consider is the derivative, with respect to the parameter at issue, of the "likelihood," which is the probability of the observed data as a function of the parameter at issue (see, for example, Cox and Hinkley, 1974). This "score" has, asymptotically, a Gaussian distribution; its expectation (exact) is zero and its variance (exact) is the Fisher information, that is, the second derivative of the log likelihood evaluated at the theoretical value of the parameter at issue. Applied to OR analysis, this approach leads to a X^2 function of the following form:

$$X_{OR}^2 = \frac{\left[\dfrac{r_1 - \tilde{R}_1}{\tilde{R}_1(1 - \tilde{R}_1)} - \dfrac{r_0 - \tilde{R}_0}{\tilde{R}_0(1 - \tilde{R}_0)} \right]^2}{\left[\dfrac{1}{S_1 \tilde{R}_1(1 - \tilde{R}_1)} + \dfrac{1}{S_0 \tilde{R}_0(1 - \tilde{R}_0)} \right] \dfrac{S}{S - 1}}$$

$$= \frac{[S_1(r_1 - \tilde{R}_1)]^2}{\left[\dfrac{1}{S_1 \tilde{R}_1(1 - \tilde{R}_1)} + \dfrac{1}{S_0 \tilde{R}_0(1 - \tilde{R}_0)} \right]^{-1} \dfrac{S}{S - 1}}$$

(14.10)

(Miettinen and Nurminen, 1985). In this equation the meanings of $\tilde{R}_1$ and $\tilde{R}_0$ are the same as in Equations 14.4 and 14.5. It coincides with the Cornfield function with the exception of two theoretical improvements: it employs the unbiased (as opposed to ML) estimator of variance, and it is free of "Yates' correction." By virtue of these two features, this function gives the Pearson–Barnard statistic in Equation 11.4 for the null situation ($OR = 1$), as it should (and as does the function in Equation 14.2).

This function is no more difficult to compute than that in Equation 14.2.

EXAMPLE 14.4. Consider Table 14.1, and the point $OR = 90$. For the statistic in Equation 14.2 we have $r_1 = 8/10$, $f(r_0) = 90(5/20)/[1 + (90 - 1)5/20]$, $\hat{V}_{r_1 | OR = 90} = [0.950(1 - 0.950)/10]30/29$, and $\hat{V}_{f(r_0) | OR = 90} = \{(90)^2/[1 + (90 - 1)(0.175)]^4\}[0.175(1 - 0.175)/20]30/29$; and with these inputs the value of the X^2 function in Equation 14.2 at $OR = 90$ is 4.94 (cf. Table 14.1). For the Cornfield X^2 function in Equation 14.10, the first formulation therein, the numerator is $\{(8/10 - 0.950)/[0.950(1 - 0.950)] - (5/20 - 0.175)/[0.175(1 - 0.175)]\}^2$, and the denominator is $\{1/[10(0.950)(1 - 0.950)] + 1/[20(0.175)(1 - 0.175)]\}30/29$. The result is, thus, $X_{OR = 90}^2 = 5.33$. (That this value is somewhat larger than the value of 4.94 given above indicates that the score-based X^2 function is somewhat steeper here than the one in Equation 14.2, yielding somewhat narrower confidence limits, as would be expected of the *efficient* score.)

Given the theoretical virtues of score statistics in general, and the lack of computational problems with this approach in the context of OR, the approach of choice to asymptotic OR analysis is represented by the function in Equation 14.10.

As for this issue in the contexts of RD and RR, two points are worthy of note. First, in contrast to OR, exact variances can be estimated for those comparative parameters using the approach recommended. Second, the score-statistic approach to RD and RR involves serious problems with "nuisance parameters," and this renders the score-statistic approach unsuitable for RD and RR (see Miettinen and Nurminen, 1985).

Finally, it is to be remembered that, in contrast to RD and RR, OR lends itself to exact computation of the P-value function (Barndorff-Nielsen, 1976). In such calculations, use can be made of published programs (Thomas, 1975).

14.1.2. Stratified Series in General

Apart from the theoretical virtues of the score-based chi square function in Equation 14.10, it has the attractiveness of very ready generalizability to stratified data. Thus, the stratified counterpart of the first formulation of the function in Equation 14.10 is

$$X_{OR}^2 = \frac{\left\{ \sum_j W_j \left[\frac{r_{1j} - \tilde{R}_{1j}}{\tilde{R}_{1j}(1 - \tilde{R}_{1j})} - \frac{r_{0j} - \tilde{R}_{0j}}{\tilde{R}_{0j}(1 - \tilde{R}_{0j})} \right] \right\}^2}{\sum_j W_j^2 \left[\frac{1}{S_{1j}\tilde{R}_{1j}(1 - \tilde{R}_{1j})} + \frac{1}{S_{0j}\tilde{R}_{0j}(1 - \tilde{R}_{0j})} \right] \frac{S_j}{S_j - 1}}. \quad (14.11)$$

with

$$W_j = \frac{S_{1j}S_{0j}[(1 - \tilde{R}_{1j})\tilde{R}_{0j}]^2}{S_{1j}\tilde{R}_{1j}(1 - \tilde{R}_{1j}) + S_{0j}\tilde{R}_{0j}(1 - \tilde{R}_{0j})}.$$

But for the second formulation in Equation 14.10 the generalization takes an even simpler, yet algebraically strictly equivalent, form:

$$X_{OR}^2 = \frac{[\sum_j S_{1j}(r_{1j} - \tilde{R}_{1j})]^2}{\sum_j \left[\frac{1}{S_{1j}\tilde{R}_{1j}(1 - \tilde{R}_{1j})} + \frac{1}{S_{0j}\tilde{R}_{0j}(1 - \tilde{R}_{0j})} \right]^{-1} \frac{S_j}{S_j - 1}} \quad (14.12)$$

(for derivation of these, see Miettinen and Nurminen, 1985). Both of these expressions are equivalent to the generalization that Gart (1971) gave to the Cornfield function for unstratified data—again with the distinction that the formulations shown above employ unbiased rather than ML estimation of the variances and omit "Yates' correction" for noncontinuity.

For illustrations of these calculations, see Sections 14.2 and 17.2.

14.1.3. Matched Series

If the series are individually matched (with matching ratio R), the elements in the stratified X^2 function of OR (Equation 14.12) assume simpler forms, as before.

In the context of matched *pairs* (for notation, see Table 11.4) the function in Equation 14.12 assumes the form

$$X_{OR}^2 = \frac{[f_{10}(1 - \tilde{R}_1) - f_{01}\tilde{R}_1]^2}{2(f_{10} + f_{01}) \left[\dfrac{1}{\tilde{R}_1(1 - \tilde{R}_1)} + \dfrac{1}{\tilde{R}_0(1 - \tilde{R}_0)} \right]^{-1}}, \quad (14.13)$$

where, as before, $\tilde{R}_1$ is computed according to Equation 14.4 and $\tilde{R}_0$ according to Equation 14.5, here with $S_1 = S_0 = 1$, $c = 1$, and either $c_1 = 1$ and $c_0 = 0$ or $c_1 = 0$ and $c_0 = 1$, so that

$$\tilde{R}_1 = 1 - \tilde{R}_0,$$

$$\tilde{R}_0 = \frac{(OR)^{1/2} - 1}{OR - 1}.$$

Since $\tilde{R}_1 = 1 - \tilde{R}_0$, the function shown above can be recast as

$$X_{OR}^2 = \frac{[f_{10}\tilde{R}_0 - f_{01}(1 - \tilde{R}_0)]^2}{(f_{10} + f_{01})\tilde{R}_0(1 - \tilde{R}_0)}. \quad (14.14)$$

At $OR = 1$, $\tilde{R}_0$ appears, on the surface, to be indeterminate, but in point of fact the limit value is $\frac{1}{2}$, and at this point the function replicates the McNemar statistic (without "Yates' correction") in Equation 11.16. It is also evident that the X^2 function assumes its minimum ($X^2 = 0$) at the point where $\tilde{R}_0 = f_{01}/(f_{10} + f_{01})$, and the corresponding value of OR (the point estimator, $OR_{0.50}$) is f_{10}/f_{01}, which is the familiar *ML* estimator (see Miettinen, 1970a).

In the general context of R-to-one matching, the relevant frequencies for OR are $f_{u,v}$ with $u + v = c_j \neq 1 + R$ and $u + v = c_j \neq 0$ (for notation, see Table 11.4). In this general case the function in Equation 14.12 assumes the form

$$X_{OR}^2 = \frac{[\sum_{u,v} f_{u,v}(R\tilde{R}_{0(u,v)} - v)]^2}{\sum_{u,v} f_{u,v} \left\{ \dfrac{1}{\tilde{R}_{1(u,v)}[1 - \tilde{R}_{1(u,v)}]} + \dfrac{1}{R\tilde{R}_{0(u,v)}[1 - \tilde{R}_{0(u,v)}]} \right\}^{-1} \dfrac{1 + R}{R}},$$

$$(14.15)$$

where R is the matching ratio, $\tilde{R}_{1(u,v)} = u + v - R\tilde{R}_{0(u,v)}$, and $\tilde{R}_{0(u,v)}$ is solved by the use of Equation 14.5, with $A = R(OR - 1)$, $B = u + (1 - u)(OR) - v(OR - 1) + R$, and $C = -(u + v)$. This function has the form

$$X_{OR}^2 = \frac{[\sum_{u,v} f_{u,v}g_R(u, v \mid OR)]^2}{\sum_{u,v} f_{u,v}h_R(u, v \mid OR)}, \quad (14.16)$$

and values of the two functions involved, $g_R(\ )$ and $h_R(\ )$, are tabulated in Appendix 14, separately for $R = 1$–5, and for each value of R, for all the relevant combinations of u and v at a whole sequence of values of *OR*.

EXAMPLE 14.5. Recall Example 11.7 and the associated data in Table 11.5, with the matching ratio (R) equal to 4. The relevant frequencies are $f_{u,v} = f_{1,2} = 3$, $f_{u,v} = f_{1,1} = 5$, $f_{u,v} = f_{1,0} = 3$, and $f_{u,v} = f_{0,1} = 1$. Consider computation of the value of the chi square function (Equation 14.16) at *OR* $= 5$. From Appendix 14, for $R = 4$ and *OR* $= 5$, we find that for $u = 1$ and $v = 2$ (corresponding to $f_{1,2} = 3$) the g function in the numerator takes on the value 0.147, and the h function in the denominator equals 0.139. Both of these are multiplied by $f_{1,2} = 3$, the former for the numerator sum, and the latter for the denominator sum. Carrying out these calculations for the other relevant values of u and v as well, leads to $X_{OR}^2 = 4.3$.

14.2. *LR*-BASED X^2 FUNCTION OF *OR*

Analogously with *RD* and *RR* analyses, chi square functions of *OR* translate to an approximate *LR* function:

$$LR_{OR} = \exp\left[-\tfrac{1}{2}\left(X_{OR}^2 - X_{OR=1}^2\right)\right]. \tag{14.17}$$

The exact *LR* function is also completely analogous to those for *RD* and *RR*. Thus,

$$LR_{OR} = \exp\left(\max_{OR} \sum_j \tilde{U}_j - \sum_j \tilde{U}_j\right), \tag{14.18}$$

with $\tilde{U}_j = c_{1j} \log \tilde{R}_{1j} + (S_{1j} - c_{1j})\log(1 - \tilde{R}_{1j}) + c_{0j} \log \tilde{R}_{0j} + (S_{0j} - c_{0j})\log(1 - \tilde{R}_{0j})$ (cf. Equation 13.21). Here, of course, the values of $\tilde{R}_{1j}$ and $\tilde{R}_{0j}$ are based on Equations 14.4 and 14.5, respectively. In the context of *RR*, strata with $r_j = c_j/S_j = 0$ were noncontributory, but here strata with $r_j = 1$ are to be ignored as well. As with *RD* and *RR*, the maximum of $\sum_j \tilde{U}_j$ is found iteratively. It will be close to the Mantel–Haenszel (1959) estimate presented in Section 14.3.

And again, the exact *LR* function gives rise to an asymptotic X^2 function:

$$X_{OR}^2 = 2 \log(LR_{OR}). \tag{14.19}$$

This function is unlikely to be more accurate than the score statistic in Equations 14.11 and 14.12.

EXAMPLE 14.6. Consider again the stratified allopurinol data in Table 11.3, considered in Example 13.5 for *RR*. Even though census data like these are not of substantive interest in terms of *OR*, it is of comparative statistical

TABLE 14.2.

For the data in Table 11.3, analysis for odds ratio (OR); shown are, for various values of OR, the stratum-specific estimates $\tilde{R}_1$ and $\tilde{R}_0$, together with the corresponding score- and LR-based values of chi square

OR	Males		Females		Chi Square	
	$\tilde{R}_1$	$\tilde{R}_0$	$\tilde{R}_1$	$\tilde{R}_0$	Score	LR
1.00	0.057	0.057	0.112	0.112	19.5	14.1
1.80	0.095	0.055	0.180	0.109	5.46	4.74
2.00	0.103	0.054	0.195	0.108	3.95	3.52
3.40	0.156	0.052	0.283	0.104	0.08	0.08
3.70	0.166	0.051	0.298	0.103	0.00	0.00
4.00	0.175	0.050	0.313	0.102	0.05	0.05
6.70	0.246	0.046	0.418	0.097	3.53	3.71
7.40	0.261	0.046	0.440	0.096	4.86	5.12
10.00	0.310	0.043	0.505	0.093	10.3	10.9

interest to consider those same data for OR analysis as well. Table 14.2 shows, for various values of OR, the restricted estimates $\tilde{R}_1$ and $\tilde{R}_0$ for each of the two strata, and also the corresponding values of the score-X^2 (Equations 14.11 and 14.12) and the LR-X^2 (Equation 14.19).

14.3. SIMPLE ANALYSIS FOR OR

As with RD and RR, the null X^2 may be taken as the CMH statistic in Equation 11.8 or its angular counterpart in Equation 11.9. Indeed, it is in the context of OR that this statistic is theoretically optimal, in contrast to RD and RR, as was noted in Section 11.1.2.2.

For simple point estimation of OR, a very useful statistic is that suggested by Mantel and Haenszel (1959):

$$OR_{0.50} = \frac{\sum_j c_{1j}(S_{0j} - c_{0j})/S_j}{\sum_j (S_{1j} - c_{1j})c_{0j}/S_j}. \tag{14.20}$$

The corresponding test-based $100(1 - \alpha)\%$ confidence interval is (Miettinen, 1976a)

$$OR_{\alpha/2}, OR_{1-\alpha/2} = \exp[\log(OR_{0.50})(1 \mp \chi_\alpha/X_0) \tag{14.21}$$
$$= (OR_{0.50})^{1 \mp \chi_\alpha/X_0}.$$

14.4. ANALYSIS FOR MODIFICATION OF *OR*

The evidence in the data regarding modification of *OR* may be summarized in terms completely analogous to those presented for *RR* in Section 13.4. The only point of note is that here we have, for a dichotomous covariate and the associated empirical odds ratio ratio (*orr*),

$$\text{SE}_{\log(orr)} = \{\sum_j \sum_i [r_{ij}(1 - r_{ij})S_{ij}]^{-1}\}^{1/2} \qquad (14.22)$$

where $i = 1, 0$ and $j = 1, 2$ (cf. Equation 14.9).

EXAMPLE 14.7.   Examples 12.8, 13.7 and 13.8 dealt with possible modification by gender of *RD* and *RR*, respectively, in the context of the allopurinol-rash data in Table 11.3. Even though these data do not call for *OR* analysis, such an analysis is statistically instructive when compared with the *RD* and *RR* analyses. For the male stratum the empirical odds ratio (*or*$_1$) was $(5/33)/(36/645) = 2.71$, and for the female stratum, $or_2 = 4.70$. Thus, $\log(orr) = \log(2.71/4.70)^{\pm 1} = \pm 0.549$. To the square of the SE of this, the contribution from the male stratum is $[5(33)/38]^{-1} + [36(645)/681]^{-1} = 0.260$, and from the female stratum it is 0.172, and the SE itself is, thus, 0.657. Then, $X^2_{OR_1 = OR_2} = (0.549/0.657)^2 = 0.7$. For the better variance estimate for $\log(orr)$ we replace the r_{ij} in the calculation given above by the values of $\hat{R}_{ij}$ corresponding to the *ML* estimate $OR_{0.50} = 3.7$. These values (Table 14.2) give $\bar{V}_{\log(orr)} = [38(0.166)(1 - 0.166)]^{-1} + \ldots = 0.423$, and correspondingly, $X^2_{OR_1 = OR_2} = (0.549)^2/0.423 = 0.7$. The *LR*-based X^2 takes on the value $2\{5 \log[(5/38)/0.166] + \ldots\} = 0.6$.

15

Comparative Analysis of Several Rates

NULL CHI SQUARE

When more than two rates are to be compared with one another, pairwise comparisons, discussed in previous chapters, may suffice.

However, when the compared rates represent categories of an ordinal- or quantitative-scale determinant, a null chi square that draws from all the rates is often desirable. Moreover, when the determinant is quantitative, one is commonly concerned to quantify the occurrence relation.

For these purposes, extensions of the procedures of pairwise comparison are needed, and they are the subject of this chapter.

15.1. BASIC NULL X^2

As noted, we are concerned with rates specific for categories of an ordinal or a quantitative determinant. If the determinant D is ordinal, simple numerical scores are assigned to its categories. For example, if D involves the categories of "no," "mild," "moderate," and "heavy" exposure, these might be scored as $D = 0$, $D = 1$, $D = 2$, and $D = 3$, respectively. In

TABLE 15.1.
Comparison of several rates (unstratified): Data layout and notation[a]

A. Cohort incidence, prevalence, or case-referent data

	Category of Determinant		
	... $D = d_i$	... Other	Total
Cases	c_i	c'	$c + c'$
Noncases	$S_i - c_i$	$S' - c'$	$S - c + S' - c'$
Subjects	S_i	S'	$S + S'$

B. Incidence density data

	Category of Determinant		
	... $D = d_i$	... Other	Total
Cases	c_i	c'	$c + c'$
Population time	T_i	T'	$T + T'$

[a] Cf. Tables 11.1 and 11.6.

general, an ordinal D is taken to have quasi-quantitative realizations $D = d_i$, $i = 1, \ldots$.

The layout and notation for unstratified data are given in Table 15.1.

Cochran (1954) approached the cohort incidence and prevalence data in Table 15.1 in terms of a straight-line model for the rate R of case occurrence. His approach applies to case-referent data also, even though the proportion of cases out of the number of subjects does not have the interpretation of an occurrence rate. This approach means fitting to the data the model

$$R = A + BD. \tag{15.1}$$

For the parameter of relation (B), Cochran used the least-squares point estimator, or the empirical regression slope

$$b = \frac{\sum_i S_i(d_i - \bar{d})r_i}{\sum_i S_i(d_i - \bar{d})^2}, \tag{15.2}$$

which involves $r_i = c_i/S_i$, and $\bar{d} = \sum_i S_i d_i / S$.

The null variance of b may be estimated as

$$\hat{V}_{b|B=0} = \frac{\sum_i [S_i(d_i - \bar{d})]^2 r(1 - r)[S/(S - 1)]/S_i}{[\sum_i S_i(d_i - \bar{d})^2]^2}$$

$$= \frac{r(1 - r)S/(S - 1)}{\sum_i S_i(d_i - \bar{d})^2}, \tag{15.3}$$

where $r = c/S$. (Cochran actually used the *ML* estimator of the null variance of r_i, that is, S in place of the $S - 1$ in the unbiased estimator given above.)
    In these terms the null X^2 is

$$X_0^2 = \frac{b^2}{\hat{V}_{b \mid B = 0}}$$

$$= \frac{[\sum_i S_i(d_i - \bar{d})r_i]^2}{r(1 - r)[S/(S - 1)] \sum_i S_i(d_i - \bar{d})^2}.$$

(15.4)

It may be instructive to approach this test formulation from another angle, namely, by comparing the mean values of the determinant between the cases and the noncases. The empirical means are

$$\bar{d}_1 = \frac{\sum_i c_i d_i}{c},$$

$$\bar{d}_0 = \frac{\sum_i (S_i - c_i)d_i}{S - c}.$$

(15.5)

Thus, the empirical mean difference (of D between cases and noncases) is

$$md = \bar{d}_1 - \bar{d}_0$$

$$= \sum_i d_i \left(\frac{c_i}{c} - \frac{S_i - c_i}{S - c} \right)$$

$$= \frac{\sum_i S_i(d_i - \bar{d})r_i}{Sr(1 - r)},$$

(15.6)

with $\bar{d}$ the overall mean of d (as in Equation 15.2). The null variance of the mean difference may be computed as

$$\hat{V}_{md \mid MD = 0} = \hat{V}_{D \mid MD = 0} \left(\frac{1}{c} + \frac{1}{S - c} \right).$$

(15.7)

For this, the estimator of the unit variance of D may be derived from the pooled (marginal) distribution as

$$\hat{V}_{D \mid MD = 0} = \frac{1}{S - 1} \sum_i S_i(d_i - \bar{d})^2.$$

(15.8)

The test statistic is, then,

$$X_0^2 = \frac{(md)^2}{\hat{V}_{md \mid MD = 0}},$$

(15.9)

which is *algebraically identical with that in Equation 15.4.*

For data representing *incidence densities* the statistic in Equation 15.4 is replaced by

$$X_0^2 = \frac{[\sum_i T_i(d_i - \bar{d})r_i]^2}{r \sum_i T_i(d_i - \bar{d})^2},$$

(15.10)

where $r = c/T$ (for notation see Table 15.1).

As for stratified data, we may apply the principle Cochran used in the context of differences between proportions (Section 11.1.2.1): as each stratum provides an elementary estimate of the comparative parameter of interest (here, b_j for B), one computes a weighted average of those elementary estimates, with weights inversely proportional to the respective null variances. Specifically, the null X^2 may be taken as

$$X_0^2 = \frac{(\sum_j W_j b_j / \sum_j W_j)^2}{\sum_j W_j^2 \hat{V}_{b_j | B = 0} / (\sum_j W_j)^2}$$

$$= \frac{(\sum_j W_j b_j)^2}{\sum_j W_j^2 \hat{V}_{b_j | B = 0}},$$

(15.11)

where b_j is derived according to Equation 15.2 (from the data specific for the jth stratum). If the data reduce to $2 \times C$ tables (Table 15.1), the variances are computed according to Equation 15.3, and the weights are therefore taken, under the assumption that $R_j(1 - R_j)$ is constant over the strata, as

$$W_j = \sum_i S_{ij}(d_i - \bar{d}_j)^2.$$

(15.12)

In these terms the statistic becomes

$$X_0^2 = \frac{[\sum_j \sum_i S_{ij}(d_i - \bar{d}_j)r_{ij}]^2}{\sum_j [r_j(1 - r_j)S_j/(S_j - 1)] \sum_i S_{ij}(d_i - \bar{d}_j)^2}$$

(15.13)

This statistic can also be derived on the basis of the differences between cases and noncases in the mean value of the determinant (Equation 15.6), using the weights $W_j = [1/c_j + 1/(S_j - c_j)]^{-1}$ (cf. Equation 15.7). Mantel (1963) derived it using an argument that is conditional on the marginal frequencies in the $2 \times C$ tables involved.

If the data represent *incidence densities* (Table 15.1), the counterpart of the statistic in Equation 15.13 is

$$X_0^2 = \frac{[\sum_j \sum_i T_{ij}(d_i - \bar{d}_j)r_{ij}]^2}{\sum_j r_j \sum_i T_{ij}(d_i - \bar{d}_j)^2}.$$

(15.14)

TABLE 15.2.

Distribution of cases of acute myeloid leukemia and a sample of the study base (reference series) according to the level of an index of gamma radiation exposure, by age (Flodin et al., 1981)

Age (yr)	Series	Exposure Level			Total
		1	2	3	
20–49	Cases	1	2	7	10
	Base sample	15	8	21	44
	Total	16	10	28	54
50–69	Cases	3	4	11	18
	Base sample	32	21	42	95
	Total	35	25	53	113
70+	Cases	8	3	3	14
	Base sample	63	20	22	105
	Total	71	23	25	119

EXAMPLE 15.1.   Flodin et al. (1981) studied the occurrence of acute myeloid leukemia in relation to background radiation (*inter alia*), using the case-referent approach. The data are summarized in Table 15.2. The categories of the exposure index may be treated quasi-quantitatively with scores 1, 2, and 3 assigned to categories of increasingly high exposure. In the first stratum $\bar{d}_1 = [16(1) + 10(2) + 28(3)]/54 = 2.22$, whereas $\bar{d}_2 = 2.16$ and $\bar{d}_3 = 1.61$. To the square root of the numerator of the test statistic (Equation 15.13) the first stratum contributes $(1 - 2.22)1 + (2 - 2.22)2 + (3 - 2.22)7 = 3.80$, and from the second and third strata the contributions are 5.12 and 0.46, respectively. Thus, the numerator of the statistic is $(3.80 + 5.12 + 0.46)^2 = 88.0$. To the denominator the first stratum contributes $\{10(44)/[54(53)]\}[16(1 - 2.22)^2 + 10(2 - 2.22)^2 + 28(3 - 2.22)^2] = 6.35$, whereas the second and third strata contribute 11.5 and 8.2, respectively. The value of the denominator thus is $6.35 + 11.5 + 8.2 = 26.0$, and the statistic itself takes on the value of $88.0/26.0 = 3.4$.

15.2. ANGULAR NULL X^2

The usual formulation of the null X^2, considered in Section 15.1, involves two problems. First, the least-squares procedure shares the efficiency properties of the *ML* approach only insofar as the distributions of the component rates are Gaussian. Second, the weights are efficient only to the extent that the unit variances are uniform over the strata.

Both of these deficiencies can be remedied, to some extent, by the use of the variance-stabilizing arc-sine (angular) transformation of the rates involved (cf. Chapter 11). This means taking the basic model as

$$\sin^{-1} R^{1/2} = A + BD \tag{15.15}$$

(cf. Equation 15.1). For the slope the least-squares estimator from unstratified data is

$$b = \frac{\sum_i S_i(d_i - \bar{d}) \sin^{-1} r_i^{1/2}}{\sum_i S_i(d_i - \bar{d})^2} \tag{15.16}$$

(cf. Equation 15.2). Since the variance of $\sin^{-1} r_i^{1/2}$ is $1/(4S_i)$, the variance of b is

$$\hat{V}_b = \frac{1/4}{\sum_i S_i(d_i - \bar{d})^2} \tag{15.17}$$

(cf. Equation 15.3). Thus the null X^2 for a single $2 \times C$ table is

$$\begin{aligned} X_0^2 &= \frac{b^2}{\hat{V}_b} \\ &= \frac{[\sum_i S_i(d_i - \bar{d}) \sin^{-1} r_i^{1/2}]^2}{(1/4) \sum_i S_i(d_i - \bar{d})^2} \end{aligned} \tag{15.18}$$

(cf. Equation 15.4). In the context of incidence density data its counterpart is (cf. Equation 15.10)

$$X_0^2 = \frac{[\sum_i T_i^{1/2}(d_i - \bar{d}) c_i^{1/2}]^2}{(1/4) \sum_i T_i(d_i - \bar{d})^2} . \tag{15.19}$$

In the context of *stratified* data the weights can now be taken as the inverses of the actual variances of the stratum-specific estimates. In these terms the formulation in Equation 15.11 reduces to

$$X_0^2 = \frac{(\sum_j W_j b_j)^2}{\sum_j W_j}, \tag{15.20}$$

with, for $2 \times C$ tables,

$$W_j = 4 \sum_i S_{ij}(d_i - \bar{d}_j)^2 \tag{15.21}$$

(cf. Equation 15.17). The detailed form of the statistic for a set of $2 \times C$ tables is, then,

$$X_0^2 = \frac{[\sum_j \sum_i S_{ij}(d_i - \bar{d}_j)\sin^{-1}r_{ij}^{1/2}]^2}{(1/4) \sum_j \sum_i S_{ij}(d_i - \bar{d}_j)^2} \tag{15.22}$$

(cf. Equation 15.13). For incidence-density data the corresponding statistic is (cf. Equation 15.14).

$$X_0^2 = \frac{[\sum_j \sum_i T_{ij}^{1/2}(d_i - \bar{d}_j)c_{ij}^{1/2}]^2}{(1/4) \sum_i \sum_j T_{ij}(d_i - \bar{d}_j)^2} \tag{15.23}$$

EXAMPLE 15.2.   Consider again the data in Example 15.1. From the first stratum, the contribution to the square root of the numerator of the statistic in Equation 15.22 is as follows: $16(1 - 2.22)\sin^{-1}(1/16)^{1/2} + 10(2 - 2.22)\sin^{-1}(2/10)^{1/2} + 28(3 - 2.22)\sin^{-1}(7/28)^{1/2}$. The value of $\sin^{-1}(1/16)^{1/2}$ is 0.2527rad, and the entire contribution is 5.48. The second and third stratum contribute 7.35 and 0.78, respectively. Thus, the numerator of the statistic is 185, the denominator is 51.2, and $X_0^2 = 3.6$.

16

Analysis of Means
of Quantitative Observations

In the previous chapters the concern has been with all-or-none (Bernoulli) observations, that is, with observations that take on two realizations only, usually coded 1 and 0, respectively. In these terms, a proportion-type rate can be regarded as the mean of Bernoulli observations, given that cases are coded as 1 and noncases as 0. The basic model is that the number of cases has a binomial distribution in the context of proportions and a Poisson distribution when the rate is an incidence density (Chapter 10).

In this chapter we turn to the situation in which the observations are quantitative rather than binary.

16.1. SINGLE MEAN

If S subjects are observed with respect to a characteristic Y, the usual model is that those observations represent a simple random sample from a "superpopulation" in which Y has a Gaussian distribution with some mean M and variance V_y:

$$Y = G(M, V_Y). \tag{16.1}$$

Inherent in this model is the assumption that the variance V_Y is independent of the mean M, that is, one generally assumes "homoscedasticity."

It is a corollary of such a model that the distribution of the empirical mean $(m = \bar{y})$ is Gaussian, specifically

$$m = G\left(M, \frac{V_Y}{S}\right).$$
(16.2)

The model also implies that the chi square function is

$$X_M^2 = \frac{(m - M)^2}{V_Y/S}.$$
(16.3)

This function is generally unusable, however, because the variance is unknown. (In the context of binary outcomes the mean implies the variance, so that this problem does not arise.) Nevertheless, unless the number of subjects (S) is very small (a couple of dozen or less), one may use

$$X_M^2 = \frac{(m - M)^2}{\hat{V}_Y/S},$$
(16.4)

with

$$\hat{V}_Y = \frac{1}{S - 1} \sum_s (Y_s - m)^2,$$
(16.5)

the subscript referring to individual subjects $(s = 1, \ldots, S)$.

This function is actually justifiable (by the use of the Central Limit Theorem) even if the distribution of Y is not Gaussian, given that the number of subjects is large enough. This point is important, inasmuch as the distribution of the observations (Y) often is far from Gaussian. When the number of subjects is very small, the Gaussian model for the distribution of means (Equation 16.2) tends not to apply.

Thus the X^2 function in Equation 16.4 tends to be adequate whenever Gaussian distribution of the empirical means can be assumed. In the exceptional situations in which the number of subjects is very small, and in which the Gaussian model for the distribution of the individual observations is known to be correct enough to justify a Gaussian model for the small-sample mean, a refinement of Equation 16.4 is needed. The use of the estimated variance in lieu of the actual one means, in very small samples, that the distribution of the statistic is not closely chi square (1 df) but F, with 1 and $S - 1$ df:

$$F_M = \frac{(m - M)^2}{\hat{V}_Y/S}.$$
(16.6)

This F statistic is the square of the t statistic with $S - 1$ df:

$$F_M = t_M^2 \tag{16.7}$$
$$= \left[\frac{m - M}{(\hat{V}_Y)^{1/2}} \right]^2.$$

EXAMPLE 16.1.   As an indication of how much difference there is between the results from the X^2 function (Equation 16.4) on one hand and the F function (Equation 16.6), or the t function (Equation 16.7) on the other, consider the case of $S = 20$ and the values of M that satisfy $(m - M)^2/(\hat{V}_Y/20) = 3.84$. Since this value (3.84) is the 95th centile of the χ^2 distribution (1 df), the equivalence implies that the corresponding M values can be taken as the 95% two-sided confidence limits in terms of the chi square formulation. From F tables, under 1 and 19 df, one finds that the 95th centile is 4.38, and the 90th centile is 2.99. From t tables, which are more detailed than F tables, one can read that -1.96 and 1.96 (whose squares equal 3.84) correspond to the 3.3th and the 96.7th centiles, respectively. Thus, what from the X^2 function would appear to be a 95% interval is, in point of fact, a 93.4% interval, insofar as the Gaussian model for the distribution of the mean is correct. The difference is a minor one, particularly in the face of the usual uncertainties about the model in small-sample situations.

These functions imply that the null statistic is usually properly taken as

$$X_0^2 = \frac{(m - M_0)^2}{\hat{V}_Y/S}, \tag{16.8}$$

while in some instances of scanty data a better justification can be given to

$$t_0 = \frac{m - M_0}{(\hat{V}_Y/S)^{1/2}}. \tag{16.9}$$

The homoscedasticity assumption inherent in the functions—insofar as it is tenable—provides for solving them for two-sided $100(1 - \alpha)\%$ confidence limits of the form

$$M_{\alpha/2}, M_{1-\alpha/2} = m \mp \chi_\alpha \left(\frac{\hat{V}_Y}{S} \right)^{1/2} \tag{16.10}$$
$$= m \left(1 \mp \frac{\chi_\alpha}{X_0} \right)$$

or

$$M_{\alpha/2}, M_{1-\alpha/2} = m \mp t_{\alpha/2} \left(\frac{\hat{V}_Y}{S} \right)^{1/2}$$

$$= m \left(1 \mp \frac{t_{\alpha/2}}{t_0} \right). \tag{16.11}$$

As a special case of these, evidently, the point estimator is

$$M_{0.50} = m. \tag{16.12}$$

Given a null value $M = M_0$, the model implies the LR function

$$LR_M = \exp\left[-\tfrac{1}{2}(X_M^2 - X_0^2) \right]. \tag{16.13}$$

In contrast to the analysis of a single rate or comparative analyses of rates where functions of this same type were considered, this type of function does not inherently involve the issue of inconstancy of variance over values of the parameter at issue. The usual model, considered above, involves the assumption that the variance of Y does not depend on the mean (M) of Y. In reality, generally, variance of a quantitative measure tends to increase with increasing mean (over some determinant of M).

It is instructive to note that this LR function is implicit in the basic ("exact") model together with the exact LR function, in contrast to the case of a single rate.

16.2. TWO MEANS

16.2.1. Null X^2 or t^2

When two empirical means (m_1 and m_0) are compared, there tends to be a strong preoccupation with the null proposition of no difference in the theoretical means and, thus, with the value of the test statistic at the null point (cf. Chapter 11).

The null test statistic is commonly taken as

$$t_0 = \frac{m_1 - m_0}{[\hat{V}_Y(1/S_1 + 1/S_0)]^{1/2}}, \tag{16.14}$$

referring its value to tables of the t distribution with $S_1 + S_2 - 2$ df. The usual, unbiased estimator of the unit variance is

$$\hat{V}_Y = \frac{SS_1 + SS_0}{S_1 + S_0 - 2}, \tag{16.15}$$

where SS_1 is the sum of squared deviations of the observations in the first (index) series from the mean value (m_1) in that series, and SS_0 is the analogous "sum of squares" for the other (reference) series.

As noted, one could just as well use the square of the statistic given above,

$$F_0 = \frac{(m_1 - m_0)^2}{\hat{V}_Y(1/S_1 + 1/S_0)},\qquad(16.16)$$

referring its value to tables of the F distribution with 1, $S_1 + S_2 - 2$ df (cf. Section 16.1).

Moreover, as noted, it is reasonable to think of the F statistic as a chi square (1 df) taking

$$X_0^2 = \frac{(m_1 - m_0)^2}{\hat{V}_Y(1/S_1 + 1/S_0)},\qquad(16.17)$$

except when S_1 or S_2 is quite small (cf. Section 16.1).

For the X^2, a somewhat different formulation is implicit in the test recommended for $2 \times C$ tables by Cochran (1954) and by Mantel (1963). That test can be construed as a comparison of means of quantitative observations (Section 15.1), but it uses the *marginal* estimator of the unit variance (V_Y) in place of the *intragroup* estimator given in Equation 16.14. This approach has the justification that in the null situation the distinction should be moot. The use of the marginal estimator makes, however, the test less "powerful" in nonnull situations. Barnard (1947) rejected the use of the marginal estimator—on the grounds of validity—as a "well-known fallacy." It is to be noted, however, that Barnard addressed expressly and singularly the case of Gaussian observations, whereas Cochran and Mantel were more catholic in their concerns, placing no constraints on the distribution of the polytomous observation variate.

If the data are stratified by a covariate, an extension is needed for the formulations given above. This is achieved readily by the use of the principle Cochran applied in the context of Bernoulli observations (Section 11.1.2). The resulting statistic is

$$X_0^2 = \frac{[\sum_j W_j(md_j)]^2}{\sum_j W_j(\hat{V}_Y)_j},\qquad(16.18)$$

where md_j is the empirical mean difference for the jth stratum ($md_j = m_{1j} - m_{0j}$),

$$W_j = \left(\frac{1}{S_{1j}} + \frac{1}{S_{0j}}\right)^{-1},\qquad(16.19)$$

and $(\hat{V}_Y)_j$ is the unit variance estimator derived according to Equation 16.15 from the data of the jth stratum.

The homoscedasticity assumption in the model here, in contrast to the situation Cochran considered, actually suggests a somewhat different formulation of the null X^2:

$$X_0^2 = \frac{[\sum_j W_j(md_j)]^2}{\hat{V}_Y \sum_j W_j}, \tag{16.20}$$

in which the unit variance is estimated not separately for each stratum but by pooling the information over the strata. This variance estimator is

$$\hat{V}_Y = \frac{\sum_j \sum_i SS_{ij}}{S - 2J}, \tag{16.21}$$

where $S = \sum_i \sum_j S_{ij}$, the total number of subjects, J is the number of strata, and SS is "sum of squares."

In the analysis of rates there was a duality between null X^2 based on rd and its null expectation and variance on one side and that based on the exact LR on the other side. Here we do not have this duality, because of the assumption that Y is Gaussian (rather than Bernoulli), and that variance of m_{ij} involves a unit variance that is common over the categories defined by i and j. Here the statistic given above can be derived as two times the logarithm of the maximum of the exact LR.

16.2.2. X^2 or t^2 Function of Mean Difference

The null statistic may be extended to a X^2 function of the theoretical mean difference (MD), as follows:

$$\begin{aligned} X_{MD}^2 &= \frac{(md - MD)^2}{\hat{V}_{md}} \\ &= X_0^2 \left(1 - \frac{MD}{md}\right)^2. \end{aligned} \tag{16.22}$$

In this expression, md is the empirical mean difference ($m_1 - m_0$) in the context of unstratified data; with stratified data it is the weighted average

$$md = \frac{\sum_j W_j(md_j)}{\sum_j W_j}, \tag{16.23}$$

with W_j as given in Equation 16.19. The variance estimator for unstratified data is

$$\hat{V}_{md} = \hat{V}_Y \left(\frac{1}{S_1} + \frac{1}{S_0} \right), \qquad (16.24)$$

as in the null statistics in Equations 16.16 and 16.17. For stratified data it is

$$\hat{V}_{md} = \frac{\hat{V}_Y}{\sum_j W_j}, \qquad (16.25)$$

with $\hat{V}_Y$ derived according to Equation 16.21, as above.

If the data are scanty, and if the distribution of Y can be assumed to be Gaussian, it is necessary to think in terms of the t distribution ($S - 2J$ df):

$$t_{MD}^2 = t_0^2 \left(1 - \frac{MD}{md} \right)^2, \qquad (16.26)$$

where t_0^2, just as X_0^2, is $(md)^2/\hat{V}_{md}$; only the translation of the function to the corresponding P-value function is now based on the t distribution.

The $100(1 - \alpha)\%$ two-sided confidence limits are, accordingly, either

$$MD_{\alpha/2}, MD_{1-\alpha/2} = (md) \left(1 \mp \frac{\chi_\alpha}{\chi_0} \right) \qquad (16.27)$$

or

$$MD_{\alpha/2}, MD_{1-\alpha/2} = (md) \left(1 \mp \frac{t_{\alpha/2}}{t_0} \right). \qquad (16.28)$$

The LR function of MD is, naturally,

$$LR_{MD} = \exp[-\tfrac{1}{2}(t_{MD}^2 - t_0^2)]. \qquad (16.29)$$

16.3. SEVERAL MEANS

16.3.1. Null X^2 or t^2

Just as with several rates, the comparison of several means of a quantitative characteristic takes on a special flavor if the compared values represent categories of an ordinal or quantitative determinant. In these instances pairwise contrasts will not do. Instead, the concern is to capture the aggregate information from the relation of the means of the observations to the determinant.

The null X^2 for unstratified data is based on the regression slope of the relation. The fitted, or empirical, slope is

$$b = \frac{\sum_i S_i (d_i - \bar{d}) m_i}{\sum_i S_i (d_i - \bar{d})^2} \tag{16.30}$$

(cf. Equation 15.2). As before (Section 15.1), this entails numerical scoring of the categories of an ordinal determinant.

The estimator of the null variance of b is, in classical terms,

$$\hat{V}_{b|B=0} = \hat{V}_b \tag{16.31}$$

$$= \frac{\hat{V}_{Y|D}}{\sum_i S_i (d_i - \bar{d})^2},$$

with $\hat{V}_{Y|D}$ the estimator of the variance of the observation variate Y *conditionally on the determinant* D, that is, of the variance around the regression line; in other words, it is the estimator of the "residual" variance of the observation variate. Its magnitude is

$$\hat{V}_{Y|D} = (1 - r^2) \hat{V}_Y \frac{S - 1}{S - 2}. \tag{16.32}$$

In this, r^2 is the square of the sample correlation coefficient between Y and D,

$$r^2 = \frac{[\sum_i S_i (d_i - \bar{d}) m_i]^2}{\sum_i S_i (d_i - \bar{d})^2 \, [\sum_i S_i (m_i - m)^2 + \sum_i SS_i]}, \tag{16.33}$$

where $SS_i = \sum_s (Y_{is} - m_i)^2$. $\hat{V}_Y$, in turn, is the unconditional, or marginal, estimator of the variance of Y,

$$\hat{V}_Y = \frac{1}{S - 1} \sum_s (Y_s - m)^2. \tag{16.34}$$

In these formulations m denotes the overall mean of Y,

$$m = \frac{\sum_i S_i m_i}{\sum_i S_i} \tag{16.35}$$

$$= \frac{\sum_s Y_s}{S}.$$

The null t statistic ($S - 2$ df) is, then,

$$t_0 = \frac{b}{(\hat{V}_b)^{1/2}}$$

$$= \frac{\sum_i S_i(d_i - \bar{d})m_i}{\{(1 - r^2)\hat{V}_Y[(S - 1)/(S - 2)] \sum_i S_i(d_i - \bar{d})^2\}^{1/2}}.$$

(16.36)

As noted, when the number of subjects (S) is large enough to justify the Gaussian model in practice, it is also reasonable to take

$$X_0^2 = t_0^2. \tag{16.37}$$

Mantel (1963) suggested the use of

$$X_0^2 = \frac{[\sum_i S_i(d_i - \bar{d})m_i]^2}{\hat{V}_Y \sum_i S_i(d_i - \bar{d})^2}, \tag{16.38}$$

that is, that one replace the residual variance of Y (Equation 16.32) by the marginal one (Equation 16.34). This runs counter to well-established theory in regression analysis, and its consequence is unnecessary loss of "power" of the test (cf. Section 16.2.1).

If the subjects are not categorized by the determinant (into groups indexed by i), the sth subject provides the observation pair $(D, Y) = (d_s, y_s)$, and the test statistic (Equation 16.36) takes the form

$$t_0 = \frac{\sum_s(d_s - \bar{d})y_s}{(1 - r^2)\hat{V}_Y[(S - 1)/(S - 2)] \sum_s(d_s - \bar{d})^2}$$

$$= \frac{\sum_s(d_s - \bar{d})y_s}{(1 - r^2) \sum_s(d_s - \bar{d})^2 \sum_s(y_s - \bar{y})^2/(S - 2)}. \tag{16.39}$$

In this formulation, as in general,

$$\bar{d} = \frac{\sum_s d_s}{S},$$

$$\bar{y} = \frac{\sum_s y_s}{S}, \tag{16.40}$$

$$r^2 = \frac{[\sum_s(d_s - \bar{d})y_s]^2}{\sum_s(d_s - \bar{d})^2 \sum_s(y_s - \bar{y})^2}.$$

With stratified data, the weights are naturally taken as

$$W_j = \sum_i S_{ij}(d_i - \bar{d}_j)^2 \tag{16.41}$$

(cf. Equation 16.29), and the null t^2 is

$$t_0^2 = \frac{(\sum_j W_j b_j)^2}{\sum_j W_j^2 \hat{V}_{b_j}}. \tag{16.42}$$

16.3.2. X^2 or t^2 Function of Regression Slope

Generalized beyond the null point ($B = 0$), the t^2, or X^2, is

$$t_B^2 = \frac{(b - B)^2}{\hat{V}_b}$$

$$= t_0^2 \left(1 - \frac{B}{b}\right)^2. \tag{16.43}$$

In the context of stratified data this involves

$$b = \frac{\sum_j W_j b_j}{\sum_j W_j}$$

$$= \frac{\sum_j \sum_i S_{ij}(d_i - \bar{d}_j)m_{ij}}{\sum_j \sum_i S_{ij}(d_i - \bar{d}_j)^2}. \tag{16.44}$$

The two-sided $100(1 - \alpha)\%$ confidence bounds are, thus,

$$B_{\alpha/2}, B_{1-\alpha/2} = b\left(1 \mp \frac{t_{\alpha/2}}{t_0}\right)$$

$$= b\left(1 \mp \frac{X_\alpha}{X_0}\right). \tag{16.45}$$

17

Analysis of
Case-Referent Data

17.1. NULL X^2

When the data derive from a case-referent (census-sample) scheme of "harvesting" the experience of the study base, the derivation of the null X^2 poses no real novelty relative to the census approach.

The data consist of the frequency distribution of cases according to categories of the determinant, representing numerators of the compared rates (Section 4.1) and an analogous distribution of noncases from the reference series (cf. Table 15.1). If the base is dynamic, the reference subjects, as representatives of the candidate population, are inherently noncases. If the reference series is a sample of a cohort or cross-sectional base, it is in the interest of statistical efficiency to distinguish between the cases and noncases in the base sample (Miettinen, 1982b). The cases in it are to be discarded, except cases not included in the original case series, which may be added to it. Thus, regardless of the nature of the base and its sampling (sampling of the base itself vs. its noncase subdomain), for the null X^2 the data reduce to the case and noncase distributions by the determinant

$$c_0, \ldots, c_i, \ldots,$$
$$n_0, \ldots, n_i \ldots$$

$$(17.1)$$

TABLE 17.1.

Distributions of cases of death from respiratory cancer and a base sample (taken as a series of cases of death from other causes) according to history of occupational exposure to wood dust, by age (Esping and Axelson, 1980)[a]

Age (yr)	Series	Exposure +	Exposure −	Total
50–69	Cases	2	10	12
	Base sample	7	107	114
	Total	9	117	126
70+	Cases	4	9	13
	Base sample	21	235	256
	Total	25	244	269

[a] See Example 17.1.

in the unstratified situation, and

$$c_{0j}, \ldots, c_{ij} \ldots ,$$
$$n_{0j}, \ldots, n_{ij} \ldots ,$$

(17.2)

$j = 1, \ldots$, in the context of stratification.

If only two categories of the determinant are contrasted, the basic null X^2 for unstratified data is still that in Equation 11.4, even if one may not wish to think of $c_i/(c_i + n_i) = c_i/S_i$ as a rate of any substantive interest. If the series are stratified by a covariate, the Cochran–Mantel–Haenszel statistic in Equations 11.7 and 11.8 is applicable. In both unstratified and stratified situations, greater validity is commonly to be expected with the use of the corresponding angular statistics given in Equations 11.5 and 11.9, respectively.

EXAMPLE 17.1. Table 17.1 shows data on the relation of respiratory cancer to working with wood, from a case-referent study by Esping and Axelson (1980). For the two strata the amounts of comparative information are proportional to $W_1 = (1/9 + 1/117)^{-1} = 8.36$ and $W_2 = (1/25 + 1/224)^{-1} = 22.68$, respectively (Equation 11.6). Thus, the average proportion of cases among the exposed, weighted according to the amount of comparative information, is $[8.36(2/9) + 22.68 (4/25)]/(8.36 + 22.68) = 0.177$, whereas for the nonexposed it is 0.051. Thus, the numerator of the basic null X^2 (Equation 11.8) is $(0.177 − 0.051)^2 = 0.0159$. For the denominator, the estimates of the unit variances are $12(114)/[126(125)] = 0.0869$ and 0.0462, respectively. The denominator itself becomes 0.00184, so that $X_0^2 = 0.0159/0.00184 = 8.6$. For the angular statistic (Equation 11.9), the numerator involves $\sin^{-1}$

$(0.177)^{1/2} = 0.434$rad, and $\sin^{-1}(0.051)^{1/2} = 0.228$rad, and the numerator thus is 0.0425. For the denominator, the overall weighted proportion of cases is $r^* = [8.36(12/126) + 22.68(13/269)]/(8.36 + 22.68) = 0.0610$. Thus, the denominator is $(1/4)(0.00184)/[r^*(1 - r^*)] = 0.00803$. Consequently, the angular null X^2 takes on the value of $0.0425/0.00803 = 5.3$, in contrast to the value of 8.6 given above. (Cf. Example 11.4.)

For matched case-referent data the null X^2 statistics given in Equations 11.18 and 11.19 are applicable. Their application to case-referent data is illustrated in Example 11.6.

When more than two levels of an ordinal or quantitative determinant are considered, the basic null X^2 for unstratified series is that given in Equation 15.4. Its counterpart for stratified data is given by Equation 15.13 and illustrated with case-referent data in Example 15.1. The corresponding angular statistics are shown in Equations 15.18 and 15.22, respectively, with the latter illustrated with case-referent data in Example 15.2.

17.2. X^2 FUNCTION OF RR

In the context of contrasting a single index category of the determinant to its reference category, the corresponding rate ratio (RR) is readily estimable as long as the reference series is a sample of the study base itself. The condition is always satisfied when the base is a dynamic-population experience, which inherently is one of noncases, of candidates for the event at issue (Miettinen, 1976a). If the base is a cohort experience or a population cross section, the condition is satisfied whenever the reference series is drawn from the base itself rather than from its noncase subdomain (Miettinen, 1982a).

If the base population is *dynamic*, the immediately estimable RR is the incidence-density ratio (IDR). For unstratified data, the X^2 function is that given in Equation 14.10, with $r_1 = c_1/(c_1 + n_1) = c_1/S_1$ and $r_0 = c_0/(c_0 + n_0) = c_0/S_0$, and with $\tilde{R}_1$ and $\tilde{R}_0$ defined by Equations 14.4 and 14.5 (using IDR in place of OR).

For stratified series in the general sense the corresponding function is defined by Equation 14.11.

EXAMPLE 17.2. For the data in Table 17.1, the score- and LR-based X^2 functions of $OR = IDR$ (Equations 14.11 and 14.19) are listed numerically in Table 17.2. (See also Example 14.6.)

For matched case-referent data the appropriate X^2 function is given in Equations 14.15 and 14.16, and its elements are tabulated in Appendix 14. An illustration of calculations of case-referent data is given in Example 14.5.

When the base is not a dynamic-population experience but a cohort follow-up, or cross-sectional, and when the reference series is a sample of such

TABLE 17.2.

For the data in Table 17.1, analysis for incidence density ratio ($IDR = OR$); for various values of IDR are shown the corresponding stratum-specific estimates $\tilde{R}_1$ and $\tilde{R}_0$, and also the values of score- and LR-based chi squares (Equations 14.11 and 14.19, respectively)

	Age (50–69 yr)		Age (70+ yr)		Chi Square	
IDR	$\tilde{R}_1$	$\tilde{R}_0$	$\tilde{R}_1$	$\tilde{R}_0$	Score	LR
1.0	0.095	0.095	0.048	0.048	8.73	6.28
1.5	0.132	0.092	0.068	0.046	4.16	3.41
1.6	0.139	0.092	0.072	0.046	3.61	3.02
3.8	0.256	0.083	0.135	0.039	0.03	0.02
4.0	0.264	0.082	0.140	0.039	0.00	0.00
4.5	0.283	0.081	0.150	0.038	0.02	0.02
11.0	0.446	0.068	0.243	0.028	3.75	3.88
12.0	0.463	0.067	0.253	0.027	4.49	4.63

a base population, the analysis for RR (risk ratio or prevalence ratio) takes a different form. Suppose that the numbers of cases deriving from the index and reference categories of the determinant at issue are c_1 and c_0, as before, and that for the base sample the corresponding numbers are b_1 and b_0. Then rr is naturally taken as

$$ rr = RR_{0.50} = \frac{c_1/b_1}{c_0/b_0} . \tag{17.3}$$

If the data are stratified by a set of covariates, the point estimate may be computed as (cf. Equation 14.20)

$$ RR_{0.50} = \frac{\sum_j c_{1j} b_{0j}/(c_j + b_j)}{\sum_j c_{0j} b_{1j}/(c_j + b_j)} . \tag{17.4}$$

The null chi square can be computed in the usual way, involving only the noncases in the base sample.

Confidence limits may then be derived by the use of the test-based principle (cf. Sections 13.4 and 14.4).

$$ RR_{\alpha/2}, RR_{1-\alpha/2} = (RR_{0.50})^{1 \pm \chi_\alpha/X_0} \tag{17.5}$$

17.3. SIMPLE ANALYSIS FOR RR

"Simple analysis" of case-referent data for IDR (odds ratio) is presented in Section 14.3.

EXAMPLE 17.3.   For the data in Table 17.1, the null X^2 (8.6) derived in Example 17.1 might be complemented by a point estimate and a 95% confidence interval for *IDR*. The Mantel–Haenszel point estimate (Equation 14.20) is $IDR_{0.50} = [2(107)/126 + 4(235)/269]/[7(10)/126 + 21(9)/269] = 4.13$. The corresponding 95% interval, test-based, is $\exp\{\log(4.13) [1 \mp 1.96/(8.6)^{1/2}]\}$. Thus, $IDR_{0.025}$, $IDR_{0.975} = 1.6$, 11.

When the base is not dynamic, the point estimate of *RR* can be derived according to Equation 17.4 and other confidence intervals by the use of Equation 13.24.

Simple analyses beyond the concern for *RR* have been described by Miettinen (1976a).

18

Regression Analysis

In the previous chapters, the relation of an outcome parameter to a particular determinant has been considered either unconditionally or within strata based on a single covariate or on cross classification by two or more of them. In the conditional analyses, each stratum was thought to provide an elementary estimate of a parameter of relation (rate difference, regression slope, etc.), and those elements were aggregated over the strata by averaging with weights proportional to the stratum-specific amounts of comparative information.

Such an approach to the conditional relation can be very inefficient in the absence of matching. This is evident from the basic null X^2 (Equation 11.8). The denominator, or the variance of the difference between the information-standardized rates, is the ratio of the average (weighted) of the stratum-specific estimates of the Bernoulli unit variance and the measure of the total amount of comparative information $(\sum_j W_j)$. With matching, $S_{0j}/S_{1j} = R$ and, therefore, $\sum_j W_j = \sum_j [(1/S_{1j})(1/1 + 1/R)]^{-1} = (1/S_1 + 1/S_0)^{-1}$, that is, the total amount of comparative information is inherent in the total numbers of index and reference subjects. In general, however,

$$\sum_j W_j \le \left(\frac{1}{S_1} + \frac{1}{S_0}\right)^{-1}, \tag{18.1}$$

with the inequality signifying inefficiency arising from variability of the S_0/S_1 ratio, that is, from lack of matching in the selection of subjects, in the context of stratified analysis (Section 4.3).

A partial remedy for the inefficiency of stratified analysis is analysis under a regression model. In a way, its simplifying assumptions smooth out the irregularities in the allocation ratio over the strata.

The price, however, is the possibility that the model is too unrealistic, so that validity is sacrificed for efficiency.

18.1. LINEAR REGRESSION: THE CONCEPT

The term "regression" in data analysis originally meant regression toward the mean (Galton, 1889). Subsequently "regression models" and "regression analyses" have been taken to deal with a parameter's (e.g., the mean's) relation to its quantitative determinants, in contrast to "analysis of variance," in which the "independent" variates (determinants) are indicator (0, 1) variates, and "analysis of covariance," in which there is a mixture of both types of variate. In modern terms *"regression" refers to a parameter's relation to its determinants*, regardless of their nature.

A regression model is said to be "linear" when it is of the form

$$P = A + \sum_i B_i X_i, \qquad (18.2)$$

which means that in any given type of situation, defined by the realizations of the X's, the value of the dependent parameter P is viewed as a *linear combination of the independent parameters $A, B_1, \ldots$*, the coefficients of the linear combination being the realizations for the X's.

EXAMPLE **18.1.**   Consider intraoperative mortality in open-heart surgery. Here, P designates the incidence (risk) of intraoperative death. For this parameter of occurrence one might consider the determinants congestive heart failure (CHF) and duration of cardiac bypass. The former might be represented by an indicator variate X_1, with $X_1 = 1$ if CHF, $X_1 = 0$ otherwise. For the latter the representation might be X_2 = number of minutes of bypass (pump use). The model might be taken as $P = A + B_1 X_1 + B_2 X_2$. An individual's risk P is a linear composite of A, B_1, and B_2, with the individual composite determined by how the individual is predestined to draw from the smorgasbord of nature. One, and only one, A unit is a must for everyone, regardless of X_1 and X_2. One B_1 unit is picked by those with CHF ($X_1 = 1$), and by them only. The remaining elements (B_2) are picked in a number equal to the number of minutes (X_2) one spends in bypass.

It is to be noted that "linear regression" does not mean straight-line regression. Thus, a quadratic relation between the occurrence parameter P and a subject characteristic Z, $P = A + B_1 Z + B_2 Z^2$, is linear in the sense of linear models: the value of the dependent parameter P is a linear combination of A, B_1, and B_2, with coefficients $X_0 \equiv 1$, $X_1 = Z$, and $X_2 = Z^2$, respectively.

Because the value of the dependent parameter in a linear model is expressed as the sum of the general, or "intercept," element A and the unit "effect" B_1 of X_1 taken X_1 times, and so on, it is inherently additive in an algebraic sense. (For more appropriate conceptualization of regression parameters, see Section A.2.5.)

In statistical terms the model may be *nonadditive*, however, which means that one of the statistical variates in the linear model is a product of two others, in a particular sense. The meaning is not exemplified by $X_1 = Z$, $X_2 = Z^2$, $X_3 = Z^3 = X_1 X_2$, because all of these statistical variates have to do with the dependent parameter's relation to a single subject characteristic (Z). Rather, if Z_1 and Z_2 are two distinct subject characteristics, and if X_1 and X_2 are defined in terms of Z_1 and Z_2, respectively, the inclusion of $X_3 = X_1 X_2$ in the model means that the "effects" of X_1 and X_2 ($B_1 X_1$ and $B_2 X_2$) are not additive but that a "product term" is involved in this situation.

18.2. INDEPENDENT VARIATES: SPECIFICATION AND RESULT INTERPRETATION

The comments made above indicated that the design of a multiple regression model involves, among other issues, the translation of data on subject characteristics (Z) into statistical variates (X). This can pose some challenges, especially in the context of the determinant of focal interest, and the challenges are accentuated if data on the determinant deal with a variety of aspects—level, duration, timing, and so on.

18.2.1. Determinant Representation

The issues in translating the determinant information into statistical variates are examined here in the particular context of *smoking*. Not only does this provide a concrete and familiar focus, but the resulting paradigm is complex enough to apply to practically any aspect of behavior, as well as to environmental exposures and biomedical characteristics such as diabetes. Throughout, the concern in this section is translation of the data on the determinant D to a set of statistical variates X_1, X_2, . . . , such that their coefficients in the statistical model properly address the objects of inquiry in the study.

18.2.1.1. Representation of Nominal Determinant

In simplest possible terms, the interest in smoking as a determinant of some occurrence parameter centers on a single contrast of the habit as of a particular point in time. Even in these terms the empirical scale of the determinant tends to be a trichotomy (Section 2.3), consisting of categories such as

"Nonsmoker at present" = reference category, $D = R$.
"Smoker of only cigarettes at present" = index category, $D = I$.
"Other," $D = O$.

With subjects representing the extraneous, "other" category retained in the data base, the statistical variates in this situation might best be taken as

$$X_1 = \text{Indicator of } I$$
$$X_2 = \text{Indicator of } O. \tag{18.3}$$

(An indicator variate takes on the value of one for representatives of the category that it indicates; otherwise it equals zero.) Thus, the model is $P = A + B_1X_1 + B_2X_2$. This means that the value of P in the reference category (in which $X_1 = X_2 = 0$) is denoted by A, whereas the parameter difference between the index ($X_1 = 1, X_2 = 0$) and reference ($X_1 = X_2 = 0$) categories is denoted by B_1. It is important to represent the extraneous category ($X_1 = 0, X_2 = 1$) by an indicator of its own; otherwise B_1 would contrast I with the union of R and O rather than with R per se.

Consider next smoking status D characterized in terms of the scale

"Nonsmoker at present" = reference category, $D = R$.
"Smoker of only cigarettes at present" = index domain, $D = I$, subdivided according to the type of cigarette:
   "Nonfilter cigarettes only," $D = I_1$.
   "Filter cigarettes only," $D = I_2$.
   "Other" (combination, etc.), $D = I_3$.
"Other" $D = O$.

For the study of the relation of the outcome parameter to this scale of smoking status, one faces an important choice between two alternative sets of statistical variates in the argument of the model and their corresponding sets of parameters. In one (model 1) the variates represent separate indicators for each of the index categories of interest (I_1 and I_2):

$$X_1 = \text{Indicator of } I_1.$$
$$X_2 = \text{Indicator of } I_2. \tag{18.4}$$
$$X_3 = \text{Indicator of the union of } I_3 \text{ and } O.$$

In the alternative formulation (model 2) there is an indicator for the union of the two index categories and another for a particular one of the two:

$$X_1 = \text{Indicator of the union of } I_1 \text{ and } I_2.$$
$$X_2 = \text{Indicator of } I_2. \tag{18.5}$$
$$X_3 = \text{Indicator of the union of } I_3 \text{ and } O.$$

Model 1 provides for the assessment of the *separate* effects of I_1 and I_2 (relative to R) through the respective coefficients B_1 and B_2. To see this, suppose that a linear model of the form of model 1 is fitted to data to obtain, for the dependent parameter (P), the empirical relation $p = a + \sum_1^3 b_i X_i$, together with the standard errors for a, b_1, and so on. For the absolute "effect" of I_1 (relative to R), the point estimate is b_1, considering that the fitted value of P in R is $p = a$ (as $X_1 = X_2 = X_3 = 0$), whereas in I_1 it is $a + b_1$ (as $X_1 = 1$, $X_2 = X_3 = 0$). The null P-value for this difference may be based on $X_0^2 = b_1^2/(SE_{b_1})^2$, and for a two-sided $100(1 - \alpha)\%$ confidence interval, the usual formulation is $b_1 \mp \chi_\alpha(SE_{b_1}) = b_1(1 \mp \chi_\alpha/X_0)$. For the "effect" of I_2 the analyses are completely analogous to those for I_1.

Under model 1—the *separating* model—the "null hypothesis" of no difference between the "effects" of I_1 and I_2 cannot be tested on the basis of $(b_1 - b_2)^2/[(SE_{b_1})^2 + (SE_{b_2})^2]$, because the estimates b_1 and b_2 are not statistically independent. Moreover, interval estimation of $B_1 - B_2$ (and B_1/B_2) involves a need to allow for the lack of independence.

By contrast, model 2—the *aggregating* or *nesting* model in Equation 18.5—does permit easy comparison of I_1 and I_2. Thus, testing of $B_2 = 0$ is tantamount to testing no difference between I_2 and I_1, and interval estimation of B_2 addresses this same difference. This model also provides for the assessment of the absolute "effect" of I_1 (through B_1). Moreover, the "effect" of the union of I_1 and I_2—the average of their "effects" (weighted according to the respective numbers of subjects)—can be assessed. It is embodied in B_1 upon the deletion of the term for the subdomain, $B_2 X_2$, from the model.

On the other hand, model 2 does not permit ready assessment of the absolute effect of I_2, that is, of the union subdomain for which there is an express indicator. The reason is, again, that no *single parameter* addresses this effect: for the absolute "effect" of I_2 (relative to R) the point estimate is $(a + b_1 + b_2) - a = b_1 + b_2$. The computations of the corresponding null P-value and confidence interval are marred by the subtlety in the SE of $b_1 - b_2$, owing to the lack of independence between b_1 and b_2.

In the design of a regression model it is not absolutely necessary to see to it that any contrast of interest is represented by a single parameter in the model. It is critical, though, to appreciate that when the point estimate of interest is the sum (or difference) of regression coefficients, the standard error of its point estimate is not the square root of the sum of the squares of the standard errors of the estimates involved in it, because those estimates are not statistically independent. Thus, the pursuit of a single-parameter representation is motivated by a desire to avoid addressing the covariances of the estimates of the coefficients and the associated escalation of complexity and risk of mistakes.

We have seen that a comparison of two categories of a determinant, in terms of a single regression coefficient, is not achieved by the use of the separating, *absolute* model (model 1 in Equation 18.4) but by the use of the aggregating, *comparative* model (model 2 in Equation 18.5). Specifically, it is accomplished by the use of an indicator for the union of those two categories together with an indicator for one of the component categories, with the comparative assessment a matter of analysis and inference directed to the coefficient of the latter indicator.

18.2.1.2. Representation of Ordinal or Quantitative Determinant

Consider next a status of smoking (D) characterized in terms of the scale:

"Nonsmoker at present" = reference category, $D = R$
"Smoker of only cigarettes at present" = index domain, $D = I$, subdivided according to the number of cigarettes smoked per day:
$\frac{1}{2}$ pack per day, $D = I_1$.
1 pack per day, $D = I_2$.
2 packs per day, $D = I_3$.
3 packs per day, $D = I_4$.
"Other," $D = I_5$.
"Other", $D = O$.

To study the relation of the occurrence parameter to current cigarette smoking, it is desirable to employ initially a model that treats the categories of the latter in terms of a set of *indicators*, despite the quantitativeness of the information. The reason is that such "nonparametric" representation of the empirical relation provides for a good understanding of its pattern. This insight is of value as such, and it provides empirical background for the choice of a simpler "parametric" model in the second stage of the analysis.

In the formulation of the indicator model, there is again a choice to be made between the equivalents of the two models considered previously. *Model 1* involves the following statistical variates:

$$X_i = \text{Indicator of } I_i, i = 1, \ldots, 4.$$
$$X_5 = \text{Indicator of the union of } I_5 \text{ and } O.$$
(18.6)

For *model 2* the variates here are:

$$X_1 = \text{Indicator of ``}\tfrac{1}{2}+\text{,'' that is, of the union of } I_1 \text{ to } I_4.$$
$$X_2 = \text{Indicator of ``}1+\text{.''}$$
$$X_3 = \text{Indicator of ``}2+\text{.''}$$
(18.7)
$$X_4 = \text{Indicator of ``}3\text{.''}$$
$$X_5 = \text{Indicator of the union of } I_5 \text{ and } O.$$

In terms of model 1, the "effect" of I_i (relative to R) on the dependent parameter is B_i, whereas model 2 implies the effects as sums: that of I_1 is the coefficient of its indicator, B_1; for I_2 it is $B_1 + B_2$; for I_3 it is $B_1 + B_2 + B_3$; and for I_4 it is $B_1 + B_2 + B_3 + B_4$.

The preference between those two models depends again on the thrust of the analysis. Absolute effects can be studied in terms of model 1, comparative effects in terms of model 2. Moreover, any prospect for wishing to pool adjacent categories favors model 2. For example, smokers of 2 and 3 packs per day cannot be pooled under model 1, but under model 2 this can be accomplished by deleting the $B_4 X_4$ term from the model (by a simple command at the computer console). Upon the deletion, the coefficient of X_3 represents the "effect" of smoking 2–3 packs per day relative to 1 pack.

After an initial exploration of the empirical response pattern in terms of a set of indicator variates, it may be feasible and desirable to revert to a representation of the relation in terms of quantitative variates. Commonly, the empirical dose-response pattern is quite "flat," with a "threshold," owing to deficiencies in the empirical scale of the determinant, resulting from the use of an entity that is suboptimal conceptually, and/or from errors in the information.

In the modeling of a *dose-response* pattern, one option is to be descriptive of the empirical relation, however artificial its flatness and threshold may be. The model involves an indicator of the habit or experience together with a quantitative measure of it:

X_1 = Indicator of "$\frac{1}{2}+$," that is, of the entire index domain $I_1 - I_4$—the domain in which dose response manifests itself.

X_2 = Number of packs per day (set to zero outside $I_1 - I_4$). (18.8)

X_3 = Indicator of the union of I_5 and O.

The fitted function, $p = a + \sum_1^3 b_i X_i$, takes on the value a in the reference category R, as always. In the index domain its value is $p = a + b_1 + b_2 X_2$. Therefore, the estimated "effect" of smoking approaches b_1 as the "dose" (X_2) approaches zero; that is, b_1 is the estimated threshold value. The trend in the "response" with increasing "dose" is reflected by b_2, which is, thus, the measure of empirical dose-response.

The other main option is to use the quantitative term without the indicator term, that is, a model that "forces" the response to be proportional to the "dose." This model involves, simply,

X_1 = Number of packs per day (set to zero outside $I_1 - I_4$).

X_2 = Indicator of the union of I_5 and O. (18.9)

With this model fitted, the implication is that the empirical "response" to any level of smoking is $b_1 X_1$, so that the "response" approaches zero as the "dose" does. This approach is justified and indeed desirable when the flatness and its associated threshold pattern are judged to be due to measurement errors and/or chance alone, but not when inappropriateness of the conceptual measure may be part of the reason for the empirical pattern.

18.2.1.3. Determinant Characterized in Two or More Dimensions

In the status of smoking (D), current cigarette smoking might be characterized as to two aspects, rate and manner of smoking. The overall scale might involve the categories

"Nonsmoker at present" = reference category, $D = R$.

"Smoker of only cigarettes at present" = index domain, $D = I$, characterized as to

$Rate$, in terms of number of cigarettes smoked per day.

$Manner$, in terms of

"Inhales."

"Does not inhale."

"Other," $D = O$.

If the manner of smoking is ignored, the simplest possible representation of the relation would be achieved by the variates (cf. Equation 18.9)

X_1 = Rate (number of cigarettes currently smoked per day).
X_2 = Indicator of O.
$$(18.10)$$

This formulation presupposes that the rate is coded as zero for those who are not current smokers of cigarettes only. To assure that no problem arises, it is preferable to employ the definitions

X_1 = Indicator of I × rate.
X_2 = Indicator of O.
$$(18.11)$$

The model based on these variates "forces" the model-implied "effect" to approach zero as the rate of smoking approaches zero. To express the empirical relation (that generally is "flatter," see discussion given above), one might take the variates as

X_1 = Indicator of I.
X_2 = X_1 × rate.
X_3 = Indicator of O.
$$(18.12)$$

As to the manner of smoking, its simplest representation involves a single added variate, an indicator of one of its two categories:

X_1 = Indicator of I.

$X_2 = X_1 \times$ rate.   (18.13)

$X_3 = X_1 \times$ indicator of "inhales."

X_4 = Indicator of O.

In terms of these variates, the "effects" of rate and manner (on the dependent parameter) are *additive*, that is, the "effect" of one of the characteristics of smoking is the same regardless of the level or category of the other. Thus, the "effect" of inhalation (relative to noninhalation) is B_3, regardless of the rate of smoking, and the "effect" of a particular rate (relative to "nonsmoking at present") is B_1 plus B_2 times that rate, regardless of inhalation.

Such an additive model can be unsatisfactory, because the actual "effect" of inhalation is very likely to depend on the rate of smoking. Moreover, when the actual effects are additive, the additive model may be invalid if a metameter of the natural dependent parameter (e.g., the logit metameter of a proportion) is used. To provide for such interdependence of the "effects" of the two characteristics of smoking as to their effects on the dependent parameter, a *nonadditive* model is needed. Such a model is characterized by the inclusion of a *product term* involving the two characteristics:

X_1 = Indicator of I.

$X_2 = X_1 \times$ rate.

$X_3 = X_1 \times$ indicator of "inhales."   (18.14)

$X_4 = X_2 X_3$.

X_5 = Indicator of O.

The use of this set of statistical variates implies that the "effect" of inhalation on the dependent parameter is $B_3 + B_4$ (rate) and is, thus, a function of, or *modified* by, the rate of smoking. The "effect" of a particular rate of smoking without inhalation ($X_3 = 0$) is $B_1 + B_2$ (rate), whereas with inhalation it is $(B_1 + B_3) + (B_2 + B_4)$ (rate). Thus here, as always, modification is mutual: the "effect" inhalation is modified by rate, and conversely.

Consider this model when it is fitted without transforming the variate that represents the outcome. The "null hypothesis" of additivity of the actual "effects" of the rate and mode of smoking may be tested by the use of $X_0^2 = (b_4)^2/(\mathrm{SE}_{b_4})^2$. By deleting the $B_4 X_4$ term, the model is not only additive in the statistical sense, but it also represents additivity of effects in the scientific sense.

If the model described above is fitted for $Y' = \ln(Y)$, $B_4 = 0$ corresponds to additivity of the "effects" on the logarithm of the median of Y, since B_4

= 0 means that the "effect" of the rate of smoking on the mean of $\ln(Y)$ is the same for both modes of smoking and, conversely, the "effect" of the mode of smoking on the mean of $\ln(Y)$ is the same at all levels of smoking.

If the outcome is binary and a logistic regression model defined by Equation 18.14 is fitted, additivity of the "effects" on the rate at issue (as against its logit) also requires the product term, that is, it implies $B_4 \neq 0$ (cf. Greenland, 1979).

The model described above has, when viewed broadly, the structure

$$P = A + B_1X_1 + B_5X_5. \tag{18.15}$$

The X_1 variate indicates the index domain I, which is the domain of express interest, relative to the reference domain R. The reference category is always left without any indicator; it is implicit in the simultaneous zero realization of the indicator of the index category (X_1) and that of the extraneous category (X_5). The function of the latter is, as noted, to keep the reference category "clean," free of extraneous elements (including missing data, perhaps). The characterization of the index category in terms of its various dimensions (rate and manner of smoking) is a matter of detail within the $X_1 = 1$ domain, expressed by X_2 through X_4.

It is not always important, but it is always safer, to form the variates for those dimensions in terms of products of the indicator of the index domain (X_1) and the dimension descriptors themselves. This arrangement is immaterial, as noted, if the descriptor of the index domain is coded as zero outside the index domain. This may be the case for the rate of smoking and also for the indicator of inhalation outside the domain of smoking, but this does not mean that zeros are used in all instances of smoking falling outside *current cigarettes only* smoking. Moreover, the code entry for such a descriptor for current nonsmokers might be designed to indicate "does not apply," and for this reason it may not equal zero. Thus, the nested characterization of the index domain (the use of products with the basic indicator of that domain) is a good policy in general.

The wisdom of utilizing the nested structure for the characterization of the determinant is underscored by considering the age of onset of smoking. In contrast to the duration of the habit, age of onset is not zero for nonsmokers, and it is probably quite uncommon to code this descriptor of smoking as zero in the context of nonsmokers. Moreover, in designing the regression model one might very well fail to take note of this difference between age of onset and duration (or rate) of smoking. In light of these possibilities for error, wisdom demands a safe routine—the use of the nested formulation advocated above.

When that approach is used in the formulation of the statistical variates to describe the determinant information, the use of products of the index-domain indicator and its descriptors do not suffice. The use of the indicator term itself (B_1X_1) as an additional term is essential; without it one cannot distinguish between the "effects" of the index domain itself and those of its descriptors.

18.2.1.4. Determinant History

Up to now our concern has been with the characterization of determinant (smoking) status as of a particular point in time, and it remains to consider how *history over time* of the determinant status might be represented.

It was argued in Section 5.2 that history characterization for individual subjects in a study should be done separately for pre-set periods of time.

Consider the periods "present" and "past," for which the operational definitions might be "within the last month" and "more than one month ago," respectively. In these terms, with only qualitative consideration of cigarette smoking, the scale of smoking might be taken to consist of the following categories:

"Never smoked" = reference category, $D = R$.

"Smoker of only cigarettes = index domain, $D = I$, subdivided according to timing:

"Present only," $D = I_1$.

"Past only," $D = I_2$.

"Present and past," $D = I_3$.

"Other," $D = O$.

This viewpoint is workable in this simple situation of only two periods of time, but it is not ideal even here.

In ideal terms the scale formation is predicated on the recognition that the *different time periods represent separate determinants*: the effects of "present" and "past" smoking are distinct issues, just as cigarette and pipe smoking are. Thus, for *"present"* smoking (D_1) the scale is

"Nonsmoker at present" = reference category, $D_1 = R$.

"Smoker of only cigarettes at present" = index category, $D_1 = I$.

"Other," $D_1 = O$.

And for *"past"* smoking (D_2) it is, analogously,

"Nonsmoker in the past" = reference category, $D_2 = R$.

"Smoker of only cigarettes in the past" = index category, $D_2 = I$.

"Other," $D_2 = O$.

Each of these two scales (trichotomies) gives rise to a pair of statistical variates, an indicator of $D = I$ and another for $D = O$ (cf. Equation 18.3):

$$X_1 = \text{Indicator of } D_1 = I$$
$$X_2 = \text{Indicator of } D_1 = O \qquad (18.16)$$
$$X_3 = \text{Indicator of } D_2 = I$$
$$X_4 = \text{Indicator of } D_2 = O$$

The effects of "present" and "past" cigarette smoking—*mutually confounded* and thus requiring joint representation in the same model (Section 18.2.2)—are represented by B_1 and B_3, respectively.

This formulation has a natural extension of more than two time periods of history characterization.

18.2.2. Confounder Representation

In Section 18.2.1.4 above, the way confounding is controlled in regression analysis was introduced because that section dealt with the separation of effects (of "present" and "past" smoking). Thus, in terms of the model in 18.16, B_1 represents the effect of "present" smoking in the context of controlling "past" smoking: in the "stratum" of no "past" smoking ($X_3 = 0$) within the domain of the study ($X_2 = X_4 = 0$) the structure of the dependent parameter is $P = A + B_1X_1$, and in the "past" smoking "stratum" it is $P = A + B_1X_1 + B_3X_3$; in each, the difference in P corresponding to the contrast between $X_1 = 1$ and $X_1 = 0$ is B_1. In sharp contrast to this, the formulations for "present" smoking in Sections 18.2.1.1–18.2.1.3, which take no account of "past" smoking, leave potential confounding by "past" smoking uncontrolled.

As this example illustrates, the control of covariates in the context of multiple regression analysis is procedurally a matter of supplementing the determinant terms in the model by ones that summarize the implications of the confounders as determinants of the dependent parameter.

The representation of mere confounders (as against determinants of interest per se, as in the examples just discussed) in the model is developed with a different outlook from that used for the determinant(s) under study. With the determinant(s), the guiding concern in modeling is to provide for understanding and for ready statistical evaluation. The former goal requires the conceptualization of the reference category (if any), the index domain, and the extraneous domain of the characteristic, together with the representation of the descriptors of the index domain in a manner that truly provides for understanding their relevance. Apart from this analytic view of the characteristic, the goal of understanding—and statistical efficiency, too—demands a parsimonious representation of the structure in terms of the statistical variates in the model. Furthermore, the goal of providing for ready statistical evaluation calls for choosing among the available options one that involves a single-parameter representation of various features of the relation of the dependent parameter to the determinant. By contrast, the representation of confounders in the model is guided by the concern for *thoroughness of control*, which is moderated by the efficiency risks associated with the control of nonconfounding correlates of the determinant (Section 18.4).

To achieve thorough control one need not be particularly analytic; understanding and its associated parsimony are essentially irrelevant, and so is the choice among alternative sets of statistical variates (since statistical evaluation is not of interest). Thus, potential confounders are entered into the model quite liberally (with the reservation noted above), and in their representation the nonparametric mode of using indicator variates for various categories in lieu of simple continuous terms might be preferred. In the same spirit, insofar as continuous terms are used, allowance for curvatures (by quadratic terms, log metameters, or the like) is made without much reservation.

Thorough control of confounding entails not only liberal representation of potential confounders in the model but also an appreciation of the limitations of modeling in the control. Consideration of these limitations is particularly important in situations in which the distribution matrix is very unbalanced with respect to the confounders (Section 3.2.2.4).

Consider the control of age alone. In *stratified analysis*, even when all categories of age are technically included in the analysis, only age-specific comparative information is used, very expressly, with weighting proportional to the amount of such information. As a consequence, no use is ultimately made of those categories of age in which the determinant does not vary at all, or which for reasons of sampling aberrations do not provide comparative information. By contrast, in the corresponding regression analysis the empirical relation of age to the dependent parameter derives from the entire range of age among the study subjects. If the determinant has to do with the treatment of menopausal symptoms, for example, the comparative information is confined to a limited range of age, and the broad representation of the relation of the dependent parameter to age may not apply very well in the subdomain in which the comparative information resides.

Concern for this problem was manifest in a study by Truett et al. (1967), with a suitable solution: they applied an analogue of multiple regression analysis separately for particular ranges of age. Insofar as one wishes to avoid such separate analyses, one can at least *confine the analysis to that range of a covariate in which the determinant varies*, in those instances where the variability of the determinant is limited to a subdomain of age. Moreover, domains in which all subjects are cases (among the study subjects) are uninformative about *OR*, and those in which no cases occur (among the study subjects) are uninformative about *OR* and *RR* (but not *RD*). Thus, where these parameters of relation are the objects of study, additional restrictions of the domain of analysis may be applicable in the interest of validity of the allowance for confounders. A side benefit is a crisper concept of the domain of inference.

Censoring of this type is readily extended to a set of confounders. It means considering them separately for the purpose, and defining the appropriate range for each. Thereupon, the actual analysis, with joint control of the confounders, is carried out in the domain in which each confounder is within its restricted range.

18.2.3. Nonconfounder–Nonmodifier Representation

A confounder is a covariate that is a determinant of the outcome and is associated with the determinant in the study base (conditionally on whatever other covariates are controlled in the analysis; cf. Sections 1.5 and 2.6). The degree to which it confounds depends on the joint implication of these two relations; and the desirability of its control depends on their relative strengths.

If a given degree of confounding, even minor, results predominantly from the covariate's role as a determinant of the outcome, the principle of liberal control, discussed in the section above, obtains.

In the extreme such a covariate is only a determinant of the outcome, and has no association with the determinant. Its control, though irrelevant for validity, nevertheless reduces the residual variance of the outcome variate, and this means, in the context of census data from the base, that the control enhances the statistical efficiency of the analysis.

In the other extreme a covariate becomes a nonconfounder when it is merely a correlate of the determinant. Such a covariate bears partial information about the determinant status, and its control *reduces* the statistical efficiency of the analysis.

18.2.4. Modifier Representation

In the context of a single-variate representation of both the determinant contrast and the modifier (potential), and with no additional characteristics involved in the model, the provision for assessing modification is a simple matter. One includes a product term in the model, and modification is represented by the "nonzeroness" of the coefficient of the product term between the determinant and the covariate (Sections 18.1 and 18.2.1.3).

A potential single-variate modifier of frequent interest is the *"background" level* of the outcome parameter (cf. Section 2.5). In the exploration of this issue, a two-stage analysis is needed. In the first stage, a multiple regression model is fitted, with representation of various determinants of the outcome parameter, including the determinant under study. The latter may be represented additively only, or product terms may be included as well. For the second stage, a new data item is computed for each subject in the data base, namely the "background" score. These scores are based on the fitted function derived in the first stage, specifically this function evaluated at the reference level (d_0) of the determinant under study (D); that is, the scoring function is

$$s = a + \sum_i b_i X_i \,|\, D = d_0. \tag{18.17}$$

In the second stage, with the individual S-values in the data base, one fits the simple model which involves only

$$
\begin{aligned}
X_1 &= s, \\
X_2 &= \text{statistical variate based on } D, \\
X_3 &= X_1 X_2,
\end{aligned}
\tag{18.18}
$$

and possibly also an indicator for the extraneous range of the empirical scale of D. Modification by the "background" level is represented by B_3. An alternative, or a supplement, to this second-stage analysis is to stratify the data by the score value and then to assess the trend in the stratum-specific estimates over the range of the score (cf. Miettinen, 1976b).

When studying potential modification by a particular covariate, with other covariates included in the model, the use of the determinant–covariate product term applies insofar as the question of modification is conditional on those other covariates. This condition may not apply, however. Consider age as an example. The question of whether the slope of an outcome parameter's relation to a particular determinant depends on age is not, in general, thought of conditionally on age-related covariates such as blood pressure, menopausal status, history of coronary heart disease, or number of children. Conditioning by such factors is tantamount to depriving age of its very meaning—that of changing physiology and other characteristics. Thus, with such other covariates in the model, the product term between the determinant and "age" involves a more or less hollow number in the place of age in the sense of the actual question of modification. The problem is analogous for gender, socioeconomic status, and many other characteristics (cf. Miettinen, 1974b).

Basic insight into the solution of this problem in regression analysis derives from consideration of the experimental paradigm. The way to study age modification of drug response in experimental medicine is to randomize patients of different ages to treatments by the drug and "placebo," respectively. This allows patients of different chronologic ages to be biologically and otherwise different as well, that is, such an experiment retains the meaning of age. Thus the guiding principle for nonexperimental regression analysis is the goal of replicating the experimental results.

One solution to this problem is, thus, the use of multiple regression analysis to simulate the outcome of the experiment. It is to provide estimates of the null-expected numbers of cases for the various index categories of the determinant within strata of the modifier, so as to allow analysis of the set of *modifier-conditional observed and expected numbers of cases* (Miettinen, 1974b). To this end, an overall model would be fitted to the entire body of data (left after any appropriate censoring; see Section 18.2.2). The model would incorporate the determinant, the modifier, and the other covariates (confounders), and it may well include a product term between the determinant and the modifier. Upon fitting, the determinant is fixed at its reference value, and the resulting null function (Equation 18.17) is then applied to all subjects to compute the estimated null probability of being a case. Within each category defined by the determinant and the modifier these individual probability estimates are added up to obtain the estimated null-expected number to correspond to the empirical numbers of cases.

An alternative is, of course, to carry out the regression analysis separately within categories of the modifier so as to obtain conditional estimates of the determinant contrasts together with their associated standard errors. This would be followed by a weighted regression analysis of those conditional estimates, relating them to the modifier itself.

When more than one term represent the contrasts with respect to the modifier or the determinant, all possible determinant-modifier product terms must be entered into the model to study modification conditional on other covariates in the model. The null statistic—an F statistic with more than one degree of freedom in the numerator—tends to be inefficient here, and interpretation is difficult as well. For these reasons, such an approach to the study of modification should be avoided whenever single-variate representations of both the determinant and the modifier are at all realistic.

18.2.5. Missing Data Representation

When information is missing for some of the study subjects on one or more of the subject characteristics (Z) on which the statistical X-variates are based, the problem may call for the introduction of additional X-variates.

The "cleanest" way of coping with missing data is to *delete* from the analysis those subjects on whom information is missing on any of the relevant characteristics; this is the only approach that assures that no bias is introduced under any circumstances.

The deletion approach is, however, commonly so wasteful of information that its use is out of the question. When many characteristics are involved, a high proportion of the subjects—even all of them—can have information missing on at least one of the characteristics, even when most of the desired information is available. Thus, with 20 characteristics involved, and with 50% of the subjects having some information missing, up to 97.5% of the desired information may be available. Deletion of 50% of the subjects from the analysis, when only 2.5% of information is missing, is generally disproportionate and unnecessary.

Evidently, the approach of subject deletion to missing data is to be used very sparingly, generally only for those characteristics for which the information is missing in a very small proportion of the subjects, so that no major loss of subjects results.

An alternative that deserves consideration is the use of *pseudo-data;* a best-guess value is used in place of the actual value that is unknown. An overall mean of the characteristic is sometimes appropriate, but a group-specific (e.g., age- and gender-specific) mean is generally better; and the use of the median is better than that of the mean in instances of highly skewed empirical distribution. Best results are obtained using regression estimation of the missing values, basing the analysis on the subjects for whom the information at issue is available. The independent variates in the model are based on the other variates involved in the analysis and possibly also on characteristics not involved in the analysis. In developing these estimation equations, missing data on the other Z's might be replaced by group-specific medians. In a second stage, regression estimates might be used in place of missing data in fitting the estimation models.

The use of pseudo-data has the obvious drawback of tedium. An added problem is difficulty in the assessment of the precision of the regression results, because the standard error values that the computer supplies do not include recognition of the involvement of pseudo-information.

Yet another approach worthy of consideration is one of modeling, an approach that might be termed the *indicator method.* Suppose that information items $Z_j, j = 1, \ldots, J$, give rise to statistical variates $X_i, i = 1, \ldots, I$, and suppose, too, that Z_1 is the basis for X_1 and X_2. If information on Z_1 is missing on some of the subjects, two adjustments are made into the model:

1. An indicator of unavailability of the information is added to the set of X's, that is, X_{I+1} is added such that $X_{I+1} = 1$ if information on Z_1 is unavailable; otherwise $X_{I+1} = 0$.
2. The statistical variates in the basic model that are based on Z_1 are replaced by their respective products with $1 - X_{I+1}$. Thus, with X_1 and X_2 based on Z_1, X_1 is replaced by $(1 - X_{I+1})X_1$ and X_2 by $(1 - X_{I+1})X_2$.

The basic idea with this indicator method is to draw the regression information from those subjects on whom the information is available. Thus, with X_1 and X_2 based on Z_1, the regression estimates of the dependent parameter P involve the fixed element b_{I+1} for those whose value of Z_1 is unknown; for those with Z_1 known, the estimates of P involve the individualized elements $b_1X_1 + b_2X_2$. This is the case regardless of how X_1 and X_2 are coded for those with information on Z_1 missing. The resulting fitted regression relation is interpreted in terms of $p = a + \sum_1^I b_iX_i$. The terms corresponding to $i > I$, while used in the fitting, are not part of the end result.

This indicator method is very convenient to apply, obviously, but like the pseudo-information approach, it does not guarantee validity. In particular, *when applied to confounders, it represents partial control only*. Thus, very roughly speaking, if *C%* of the confounder information is missing, *C%* of confounding is left uncontrolled. The actual proportion of uncontrolled confounding is *C%* only if this proportion of data is missing on each confounder, and randomly as to the X-characteristics of members of the data base. Otherwise, the variation of the proportion among the individual confounders needs to be considered, in addition to the implications of nonrandomness.

18.3. DEPENDENT PARAMETER: SPECIFICATION AND RESULT INTERPRETATION

In the previous sections the concern has been with the specification and intepretation of the statistical X-variates in the context of regression models of the type $P = A + \sum_i B_i X_i$. It has been taken for granted that the left-hand side of the relation—the dependent parameter—is such that its relation to the determinant, conditionally on the confounders that are being controlled, is indeed of analytic interest.

In this section the choice of the dependent parameter is discussed as to its implications for the interpretation of the empirical occurrence relation.

18.3.1. Parameter for Binary Outcome: General Linear vs. Logistic Model

When the outcome phenomenon is of the all-or-none or binary type, it is represented in the data base by an indicator variate. This variate, Y, takes on the value of one for those subjects who experience the phenomenon, and zero for those who do not.

In the context of a binary outcome variate the essential choice regarding the outcome parameter is between two options. One is to take the parameter P simply as the theoretical rate R for the occurrence of the outcome phenomenon $Y = 1$. This means viewing the occurrence relation as

$$R = A + \sum_i B_i X_i, \tag{18.19}$$

and using a computer program for the *general linear model* to do the fitting, the built-in principle of fitting being one of "least squares."

The alternative is to take the dependent parameter as the logit of the rate, that is, to take the model as

$$\log \left(\frac{R}{1 - R} \right) = A + \sum_i B_i X_i. \tag{18.20}$$

This model is fitted by the use of a *logistic regression* program, and the principle involved is one of maximum-likelihood, the procedure being iterative.

On a completely general level, the choice between these two formulations involves, first, the considerations that the *ML* fitting involved in the logistic regression approach is not only statistically more efficient but also more costly.

As for substantive preference, consider first the case in which the determinant representation in the model is based on *indicator variates*.

If the concern in such a situation is with *RD*, the general linear model has the attractive feature that quantitative assessment of this comparative parameter can be based directly on the coefficient of the indicator of the contrast at issue (cf. Section 18.2.1). When using the logistic regression model it is necessary to derive the point estimate as

$$
\begin{aligned}
RD_{0.50} = {} & \{1 + \exp[-(a + \textstyle\sum_i b_i \bar{X}_i \,|\, D = d_1)]\}^{-1} \\
& - \{1 + \exp[-(a + \textstyle\sum_i b_i \bar{X}_i \,|\, D = d_0)]\}^{-1},
\end{aligned}
\tag{18.21}
$$

which is the difference of the rate estimates for the determinant's index category $(D = d_1)$ and reference category $(D = d_0)$ in terms of the contrast at issue. In the first element of this estimate the indicator variate that represents the contrast is set equal to one, and in the second element it is set to zero, while for both, all the other X's are set to their respective mean values. Confidence limits may be derived under either model as

$$
RD_{\alpha/2},\, RD_{1-\alpha/2} = RD_{0.50} \left(1 \mp \frac{\chi_\alpha}{\chi_0}\right),
\tag{18.22}
$$

where X_0 is the ratio of the fitted coefficient for the contrast's indicator to the standard error of this coefficient (cf. Section 12.3).

In the context of analysis for *RD* the general linear model approach has, apart from the simplicity just considered, the advantage that as it addresses differences in rate inherently, it can lend itself to the study of *RD* modification simply by the use of product terms (Section 18.2.4).

If the concern is with *RR*, in the context of indicators for determinant contrasts, with both types of model the point estimate needs to be derived in terms analogous to those in Equation 18.21. Thus, when using the general linear model, the point estimate is

$$
RR_{0.50} = \frac{a + \textstyle\sum_i b_i \bar{X}_i \,|\, D = d_1}{a + \textstyle\sum_i b_i \bar{X}_i \,|\, D = d_0},
\tag{18.23}
$$

and under the logistic regression model it is

$$RR_{0.50} = \frac{\{1 + \exp[-(a + \sum_i b_i \tilde{X}_i | D = d_1)]\}^{-1}}{\{1 + \exp[-(a + \sum_i b_i \tilde{X}_i | D = d_0)]\}^{-1}}. \qquad (18.24)$$

In either case, confidence limits may be set as

$$RR_{\alpha/2}, RR_{1-\alpha/2} = (RR_{0.50})^{1 \mp \chi_\alpha/\chi_0} \qquad (18.25)$$

(cf. Section 13.3). In addition, if the rates are low, so that RR is close to OR, the logistic regression model permits taking

$$RR_{0.50} = \exp(b_{d_1}) \qquad (18.26)$$

and other confidence limits according to Equation 18.25, with b_{d_1} the fitted value for the coefficient of the contrast indicator.

Just as for RD the theoretical basis was better for the general linear model, for RR the logistic regression model is preferable whenever the rates are low.

If the concern is with OR, as in the context of case-referent data (Section 18.4), the model of choice is that of logistic regression. For such an analysis,

$$OR_{0.50} = \exp(b_{d_1}) \qquad (18.27)$$

and, more generally,

$$OR_{\alpha/2}, OR_{1-\alpha/2} = \exp\left[b_{d_1}\left(1 \mp \frac{\chi_\alpha}{\chi_0}\right)\right]$$
$$= (OR_{0.50})^{1 \mp \chi_\alpha/\chi_0}. \qquad (18.28)$$

Even in the context of indicator representation of the determinant, the proper concern may be with none of the comparative parameters discussed above. The focus on RD or RR, with the latter studied through OR in the context of case-referent data, involves the viewpoint that, ideally, the chosen comparative parameter is invariant over the "background" rate defined by characteristics other than the contrast indicator at issue. Indeed, the choice between RD and RR as the focus of the analysis is made on the basis of this invariance consideration: *the analysis is focused on the comparative parameter that it is more reasonable to view as invariant over the "background" rate.*

This search for a parsimonious representation of the distinction in the occurrence pattern between the compared categories of the determinant at issue may lead to replacement of the *"vertical" focus* of RD and RR by the *"horizontal" one*. Thus, whereas it may be, in vertical terms, that the rate in the index category of the determinant, as a function of various covariates $R_1 = f(A + \sum_i B_i X_i | D = d_1)$, is neither RD plus nor RR times the reference rate $R_0 = f(A + \sum_i B_i X_i | D = d_0)$, it remains possible under the logistic regression model that the *horizontal* distance between the index and reference functions is constant.

Consider the simplest case, the one in which the logistic model is

$$\log\left(\frac{R}{1 - R}\right) = A + B_1 X_1 + B_2 X_2, \tag{18.29}$$

where X_1 is a covariate (perhaps a covariate score; see Equations 18.17 and 18.18), and X_2 is the indicator of the index category of the determinant.

Neither RD (vertical difference) nor RR (vertical ratio) is constant over X_1. Nevertheless, the logistic functions (of X_1) for R_1 and R_0 do have a constant *horizontal* distance; the index and reference rates are identical when evaluated at $X_1 - B_2/B_1$ and X_1, respectively, regardless of the value of X_1. Thus, under this model the effect at issue, assuming that there are no confounders other than X_1, can be thought of, parsimoniously, as the shift

$$S = -\frac{B_2}{B_1} \tag{18.30}$$

in the location of the rate as a function of X_1.

EXAMPLE 18.2.   The effect of maternal glucocorticoid administration (X_2) on the rate (risk) of "respiratory distress syndrome" (RDS) in premature neonates, with gestational age (GA $= X_1$) as the practically only confounder was studied by Breart et al. (1985). The rates of RDS over GA ranged from near 100% to near 0%. The logistic model involving GA alone provided a good fit to the rates for both the exposed ($X_2 = 1$) and the unexposed ($X_2 = 0$), and these two rate curves had closely similar slopes (b_1), so that the model in Equation 18.29 was quite appropriate, as far as could be determined from the data. Furthermore, the examination of the shift in the RDS incidence curve over GA, induced by glucocorticoid use, was regarded as a very attractive way of thinking about the effect under study.

For that shift, the point estimate can be based on the corresponding empirical coefficients,

$$S_{0.50} = -\frac{b_2}{b_1}, \tag{18.31}$$

and other confidence limits may be derived as

$$S_{\alpha/2}, S_{1-\alpha/2} = S_{0.50}\left(1 \mp \frac{\chi_\alpha}{X_0}\right), \tag{18.32}$$

where $X_0 = b_2/\mathrm{SE}_{b_2}$.

Whether the shift is indeed constant may of course be explored by adding the $X_1 X_2$ product term to the logistic model involving the variates in Equation 18.29.

This kind of analysis requires that the logistic model must apply well to the relation of R to X_1 conditionally on X_2. To assure this, one might wish to define X_1 as a metameter of the numerical value of the characteristic on which it is based, for example, its logarithm. The implications of such a transformation for the interpretation of the result must be appreciated, however. Thus, if the log transform is used and the product term seems non-contributory, the data point to constancy of the shift on the *log* scale of the covariate, and on the untransformed scale the *proportional* shift is to be thought of as apparently constant.

Thus far, the entire discussion of the relative merits of taking the dependent parameter as the rate itself or its logit has centered on that situation in which the representation of the determinant under study involves indicator variates only. Even if the determinant is inherently ordinal or quantitative, this type of modeling affords a fair representation of the outcome parameter's relation to the determinant, and so the core issue has been the relative merits of the two types of dependent parameter in terms of avoiding the need to consider modification. It may be said, as a broad summary, that the use of the rate itself as the dependent parameter in the linear model (and hence the general linear model fitting) has statistical justification only in those situations in which RD is the comparative parameter of choice, for reasons of parsimony or otherwise.

When a quantitative determinant (or a quantitative aspect of a determinant; see Section 18.2.1.3) is represented not by indicator variates but by a single, quantitative X-variate, the choice between the two types of dependent parameter for the occurrence of an all-or-none outcome phenomenon involves the additional need to have the model be true to the nature of the outcome parameter's relation to the determinant under study. To this end, the use of the logit of the rate—and thus of the logistic model—is generally preferable, especially when the theoretical rates cover a wide range in terms of the relative magnitudes of the minimum and maximum for either R itself or its complement, $1 - R$.

18.3.2. Parameter for Quantitative Outcome: Mean vs. Median

When the outcome phenomenon is quantitative, the general framework for regression analysis is that of the "general linear model."

For the purpose at hand the feature of primary note is that this model addresses the *expectation* (theoretical mean) of Y as a function (linear) of the regression parameters A, B_1, and so on (Section 18.1). When the outcome phenomenon is of the all-or-none type and is represented by an indicator variate (Y) that takes on a value of one when the phenomenon occurs, the interest in the analysis indeed is in the mean of Y, because this is the occurrence rate of interest. By contrast, when the outcome phenomenon is quantitative, and when its distribution, conditional on the determinant, is asymmetrical, the main interest may be in the *median* rather than the mean as a descriptor of the frequency distribution of the occurrence of various values.

The study of median in relation to its determinants can be brought to the framework of the general linear model by defining the dependent variate Y as a metameter of the outcome characteristic Z_Y—a transform such that the distribution of Y, conditional on the determinant, is symmetrical.

The common form of asymmetry for the outcome distribution is *skewness to the right*, and in such situations reasonable symmetry of distribution is usually achieved by the use of *logarithmic* transformation. With this transformation, the overall fitted occurrence relation is

$$\text{Median}_{Z_Y} = \exp(a + \textstyle\sum_i b_i X_i). \tag{18.33}$$

For an indicator of a determinant contrast, the coefficient b_d represents the logarithm of the *median ratio (MR)* between the index and reference categories. Thus for the *MR* itself the point estimate is

$$MR_{0.50} = \exp(b_d), \tag{18.34}$$

and other confidence limits may be derived as

$$MR_{\alpha/2}, MR_{1-\alpha/2} = \exp\left[b_d \left(1 \mp \frac{X_\alpha}{X_0} \right) \right]$$
$$= (MR_{0.50})^{1 \mp X_\alpha/X_0}, \tag{18.35}$$

where $X_0 = b_d/\text{SE}_{b_d}$. If the determinant is represented by a quantitative X-variate X_d, these formulations apply to a contrast between an index level X_{d_1} and a reference level X_{d_0} upon the replacement of b_d by $b_d(X_{d_1} - X_{d_0})$.

That this approach in the context of a quantitative determinant representation inherently leads to an *exponential* relation between the median and the determinant is often quite undesirable. To avoid this, the fitting may be based on the use of a set of indicators for categories of the determinant (Section 18.2.1.2). Then for the median in the category $D = d$ the point estimate may be taken as

$$(M_d)_{0.50} = \exp (a + \textstyle\sum_i b_i \bar{X}_i \mid D = d), \tag{18.36}$$

and for the *median difference (MD)* between categories $D = d$ and $D = d_0$, the point estimate is

$$MD_{0.50} = \exp(a + \textstyle\sum_i b_i \bar{X}_i \mid D = d)$$
$$- \exp(a + \textstyle\sum_i b_i \bar{X}_i \mid D = d_0). \tag{18.37}$$

Corresponding confidence limits may be derived as

$$MD_{\alpha/2}, MD_{1-\alpha/2} = (MD_{0.50}) \left[1 \mp \frac{\chi_\alpha (SE_{b_d})}{b_d} \right] \qquad (18.38)$$

where b_d is the fitted coefficient for the indicator for category $D = d$ (in the context of a set of category-specific indicators, with none for $D = d_0$).

This estimation of median differences might be supplemented by fitting a straight-line regression line relating the median of the outcome characteristic to the determinant:

$$M = A + BD. \qquad (18.39)$$

For the fitted weighted regression line the intercept and slope may be taken as

$$a = \bar{m} - b\bar{d}, \qquad (18.40)$$

$$b = \frac{\sum_d W_d (d - \bar{d}) m_d}{\sum_d W_d (d - \bar{d})^2},$$

where m_d is the point estimate of the median in the category $D = d$ (Equation 18.36), $\bar{m} = \sum_d W_d m_d / \sum_d W_d$, $\bar{d} = \sum_d W_d d / \sum_d W_d$, and $W_d = S_d$, the number of subjects in $D = d$. The null chi square for the slope may be based on the slope (b_d) of the determinant in a second regression analysis of the original, but involving a *single, quantitative variate*, rather than indicators, for the determinant:

$$X_0^2 = \left(\frac{b_d}{SE_{b_d}} \right)^2. \qquad (18.41)$$

Confidence limits are, then,

$$B_{\alpha/2}, B_{1-\alpha/2} = b \left(1 \mp \frac{\chi_\alpha}{X_0} \right). \qquad (18.42)$$

Instead of the log metameter of the outcome characteristic, it might be better, in the pursuit of symmetry, to employ some other transformation, square root for example. With these potential alternatives, a straight-line regression analysis for the median of the untransformed outcome measure can again be achieved in terms analogous to those for the log metameter.

18.4. REGRESSION ANALYSIS OF CASE-REFERENT DATA

When the data base consist of a series of "cases" of an all-or-none outcome together with a *simple random sample* of the study base, the empirical rates within the data base are, stochastically, proportional to the actual rates in the study base itself. Those empirical rates within the data base are of the form of empirical case-referent odds, and their ratios between the compared categories of the determinant represent RR's (Section 4.1). Thus, *logistic* regression analysis of such data provides for interpreting the fitted coefficients of contrast indicators as estimates of the logarithms of RR's. Similarly, with a quantitative variate representing the determinant, the coefficient multiplied by the distance (difference) in the variate corresponding to any particular contrast again represents the estimate of the logarithm of the corresponding RR. In this situation, the formulation of the logistic model, and the interpretation of the results, involves no novelty or subtlety beyond what was discussed in previous sections.

The use of a stratified sample of the base—formally stratified in the sense of matching, or nonrepresentative by virtue of the source of the sample (Section 4.3)—introduces problems. They derive from the need to explore the occurrence relation conditionally on the covariates, in terms of which the base sample is nonrepresentative (stratified), and the failure of the ordinary regression analysis to address this. The problem comes to focus when considering case-referent series individually matched for a continuous covariate such as age. The concern is to contrast the case-referent odds between the compared categories of the determinant, and this comparison is to be conditional on the matching characteristic. Inclusion of the covariate in the model as a single, continuous variate fails to assure that the analysis is conditional on that covariate; since the case-referent ratio is constant over the covariate, its coefficient in the fitted model is apt to be zero, which is tantamount to not controlling the matching characteristic.

If the empirical scale of the determinant is binary, with no study subject belonging to an extraneous ("other") category, the problem has the simple solution of shifting from an "outcome function" to a "determinant function," meaning that the roles of the outcome and the determinant are interchanged. The "dependent variate" Y now has to do with the determinant status, and the actual outcome now becomes one of its "determinant" (X_i), along with whatever covariates are to be controlled (Miettinen, 1976b; Prentice, 1976). The coefficient of the outcome variate in the determinant function has the role of the determinant variate's coefficient in an outcome function. It represents the logarithm of the case-referent OR and, thus, of the RR of interest, and conditionality on the covariates entered into the model is achieved even in the face of matching or other nonrepresentativeness of the study base.

When the determinant realizations among the subjects included in the analysis cover categories other than those involved in a single contrast, the use of an outcome function is necessary, and nonrepresentativeness of the base sample in terms of a matching or other selection-stratification characteristic must be dealt with by the use of the *conditional likelihood* methods described by Breslow and Day (1981).

18.5. IMPLEMENTATION OF REGRESSION ANALYSIS

In the previous sections, the concern has been with the formulation of the regression model in a priori terms. In point of fact, the ultimate model is generally chosen in such terms in part only; the other category of considerations is constituted by the data themselves—findings from preliminary data examinations in terms of mere distribution patterns and results from preliminary model fittings. Moreover, proper interpretation or other use of the fitted model may well be dependent on interim results.

18.5.1. Preliminaries to Regression Analysis

Scrutinies of the data before the analysis begins are critical to proper regression analysis.

The preliminaries commence with an examination of *univariate* distributions. The purposes are to identify:

1. Potential errors, indicated by outlier values.
2. The need for censoring the range of the determinant(s) and/or modifiers, indicated by sparse representation of categories.
3. Appropriate categorization for the use of indicator variates, guided by frequencies of representation.
4. Appropriate ways of dealing with missing data, considering their frequencies as a basis for choosing between subject deletion and the modeling approach.

An examination of *bivariate* distributions is commonly also necessary. Here the purposes are to identify:

1. Potential errors, indicated by outlier values.
2. The need for censoring the ranges of confounders, indicated by major imbalance (nonoverlap especially) of the confounder distributions between the compared categories of the determinant.
3. The need to use median instead of mean as the outcome parameter with a quantitative outcome measure, and in such a case, the appropriate transformation to be used—the criterion being the nature of outcome distribution conditional on the determinant.

After censoring is done, it is useful to examine the outcome-determinant relation, both unconditionally (in crude terms) and also conditionally on (with stratification by) major confounders. The results, perhaps in terms of such simple analyses as are presented in Sections 12.3, 13.3, and 14.3, serve as reference points to help assure the correctness of the regression analyses that follow.

18.5.2. Fitting of Causal Model

When the analysis addresses a problem of causation or prevention rather than a descriptive relation, the place to start actual regression analysis is replication, in regression terms, at the unconditional relation between the outcome and the determinant. This fitting should then be extended to regression replications of the stratified analyses carried out in the preliminary stage. In these "runs," the determinant is represented by indicator variates, and the main purpose is to assure that the regression approach is correct. The accent is on point estimation and, in these terms, the result of the preliminary crude relation should be replicated exactly, whereas the results of stratified analyses need to be replicated in approximate terms only (since the weighting schemes in the two types of analysis are not the same).

With this assurance that the regression approach is functioning (as to the definition of the variates conceptually and in programming terms), the actual analysis can commence.

In the context of an ordinal or a quantitative determinant, the first step is to fit a "full" model involving all potential confounders (and nonconfounding determinants of the outcome) together with the determinant, with the determinant represented by indicator variates. The model can be additive as to the confounders, and it should be free of any covariate-determinant product terms. The purpose of this fitting is to examine the nature of the outcome-determinant relation, conditional in all relevant regards, so as to provide an empirical basis for shifting from the indicator representation of the determinant categories to the use of quantitative representation.

With a simple representation of the determinant achieved, so that ready quantification of the occurrence relation is provided for, there is commonly a need to gain insight into the thoroughness of the attained control of confounding in the face of unsatisfactory empirical scales. To this end, it is useful to derive the empirical value of the relation parameter in two stages: with control of only well-measured confounders (age, gender, hospital, etc.), and then with added control of those confounders whose empirical scale is of dubious accuracy (socioeconomic status as measured by years of education or neighborhood, "medicalization" as measured by number of recent medical encounters, confounders with missing information, etc.). With these two estimates of the relation parameter (e.g., rate ratio) obtained, one may be able to judge *what the likely strength of the residual (conditional) relation would have been had all of the confounders been measured on a truly meaningful scale.*

With all the potential confounders represented in the model, covariate-determinant product terms may be introduced and retained in the model if "significant." (Throughout, everything else has been retained in the model regardless of statistical significance.)

This final model is then the basis for computing individual outcome scores, or outcome-parameter estimates, as a foundation for exploring modification by "background" level for the outcome parameter, and for presentation of the essential results in terms of stratified analysis.

18.5.3. Fitting of Descriptive Model

When the analysis is directed to the development of an occurrence relation that is to predict or estimate, the basic conceptualization of determinant vs. confounders and modifiers is not necessary. In fact, the goal is not understanding in any sense, but the development of a *well-performing function*.

In these analyses, the *statistical variates are grouped according to their respective sources* of information—history or physical examination, electrocardiography, radiography, biochemical assessments, and so on. In these terms, each regression analysis addresses a given type of situation as to what information is available.

With a given range of input information, the guiding principle in model formation is *thorough utilization of the information*. Thus the analysis commences with the fitting of a full model involving all the available items of information in terms of indicator variates and without product terms. The purpose is, again, to examine the nature of the individual relations, conditional on representation of all the other information items, as a basis for deriving simpler representation in terms of quantitative statistical variates.

Given a full additive model, with simple representation of the various potential determinants, the next concern is to *reduce* it. This should not be guided by "proportion of variance explained," because, for example, a rare but highly prognostic or diagnostic finding is of great medical import even if it "explains" only a very small proportion of the outcome variability. Instead, *statistical significance coupled with prior credibility* of relevance serves as the basis for retaining the variate(s) for a particular information item in the model; in its absence, the term(s) pertaining to a given information item is (are) deleted. The deletions are done in a "stepwise" fashion, one by one. Once no further reduction seems justifiable, it is often useful to reenter, separately, each of the items deleted before the last step, to see whether they seem to be informative in the context of the reduced model.

With the full additive model reduced, product terms may be entered on a trial basis, one by one, and they are retained predominantly on the basis of statistical significance.

It is useful to *apply the final model to the study subjects themselves*. Their individual estimates for the outcome parameter are derived, and the subjects are then stratified according to those estimates, and the empirical value of the outcome parameter is computed for each stratum. The purpose is to check that the empirical values are consonant with the stratum-specific values (ranges) of the estimates. This provides assurance that the regression analysis did not involve gross errors, but it does not assure that similar conformity between predictions or estimates and observations will be obtained in future applications of the empirical occurrence relation. Nor can the future performance be inferred on the basis of random splitting of the data base—fitting the model in one part and examining its performance in the other. The best statistical assurance for generalizability of the performance to future applications is in keeping the number of statistical variates in the full model down to a small fraction of the number of subjects in the data base.

APPENDIX 1

Rate Measures of Occurrence

A.1.1. PREVALENCE RATE

Prevalence is a phenomenon in populations only, not in individuals. It has to do with occurrence in the sense of the existence of individuals with some particular state (condition or trait). It is quantified in terms of a *prevalence rate*, which is the proportion of individuals (in the population at issue) who are in that state. Examples of prevalence rate thus include the proportions of people who have bloodtype AB, "hypertension," or a congenital malformation, respectively, and the proportion of patients with "hypertension" who have manifested complications of it. As a proportion, prevalence rate is a dimensionless quality, a "pure number."

In the context of a prevalent belief to the contrary, it may be helpful to note that a prevalence rate is not inherently momentary, any more than velocity is in physics. Of course, the prevalences of many conditions or traits are functions of time (age or other), as are incidence and velocity. When prevalence is a function of time, one may still address the average prevalence (expressly) or even ignore this dependence (along with many others, known and unknown).

There are also those who insist that "prevalence rate" is not a rate but a proportion, that is, that proportions such as the prevalence measure are not rates (see, e.g., Elandt-Johnson, 1975). The essence of the argument is

245

that a rate R is, by definition, of the form of a change in a dependent quantity ΔY divided by the corresponding change in a determinant of this quantity ΔX,

$$R = \frac{\Delta Y}{\Delta X},$$
(A.1.1)

and that "prevalence rate" is not of this form. It is the author's tenet that it is. One can think of prevalence as the occurrence of "cases" (individuals with the condition or trait) in the process, actual or hypothetical, of moving across a population (as in screening). If X denotes the number of individuals examined and Y the number of "cases" observed, the "local" prevalence rate is $\Delta Y/\Delta X$, and the overall (average) prevalence rate is Y/X, which is in full accord with the definition given above. More to the point, one need, and should, not insist on a latter-day mathematician's definition of "rate." The original Latin word takes direct manifestation in today's "unemployment rate," "tax rate," and so on.

A.1.2.   INCIDENCE RATES

Incidence is not as singularly a population phenomenon as prevalence, because it refers to changes *within* individuals (prevalence has to do with differences *among* them). Thus, an incidence rate could, in principle at least, characterize the intraindividual frequency of some recurrent event (seizure, arrhythmia, infection, intoxication, etc.). It is, however, characteristic of the epidemiologic outlook to make a sharp distinction between individual and population characterizations (cf. Examples 1.1–1.4), and in this spirit the recurrence pattern within individuals is viewed as an aspect of the condition itself, a basis for quantification of severity perhaps, and the incidence concept is confined to events that occur *among* individuals.

Because the concept of incidence is divorced from that of recurrence, it generally refers to *first* events only, but there is subtlety to this. The first event may be first only in the sense of *first new* event or *first recurrence* (of heart attack, for example). For individuals with one previous event, the first new event (first recurrence) is obviously the second event overall, and the occurrence of a possible third event would be ignored in the incidence rate. Similarly, for those who have already had two events, one considers the incidence of the third event, ignoring any potential subsequent recurrences. The point is that *no more than one event* (new) is properly tallied for any given individual toward an incidence measure for a population.

Although individuals who have had an event are candidates for a subsequent event, those who have had a first (kth) event are no longer candidates for a first (kth) event (ever). To say in the latter case that the incidence is zero is not to express knowledge about reality; it is, instead, a statement that involves an absurd mental construct. To avoid such problems, incidence is *defined* only for populations of *candidates* for the event—individuals who could experience the event in principle (as a matter of logic). Thus

1. Incidence of cervical cancer for those who have had this disease but do not have it any more *is* defined.
2. Incidence of cervical cancer for men and for women without a cervix *is* defined. (Indeed, even its magnitude is known a priori, not by mere logic but through substantive insight into the prerequisites for its occurrence.)
3. Incidence of cervical cancer for those who have this disease is *not* defined (as only noncases are logically candidates for it).
4. Incidence of cervical cancer is *not* defined for a mixture of cases and noncases (because it is undefined for the cases).
5. The incidence of death among the dead is *not* defined. (Only the living are logically candidates for death, by the very nature of the concept of death, that is, death is construed to occur among the living only.)

It should be noted that for incidence to be defined, that is, for a population to be one of candidates, the population need *not* be "*at risk*" in the sense of having a nonzero incidence (just as velocity need not be nonzero for it to be defined). Thus it is consonant with proper conceptualization of incidence to say that the incidence of cervical cancer in men is zero.

For a candidate population to manifest incidence (events) it must move over *time*. In this regard, there is a need to distinguish between two basic types of population experience over time:

1. *Cohort* experience (Section 3.2.1.1), in which an enumerable set of individuals, all candidates initially (at $T = t_0$), moves over the *risk period* (Section 3.3) at issue.
2. *Dynamic-population* experience (Section 3.2.1.2), in which a population of a given size but with turnover of membership moves over *calendar time*, with all members being candidates throughout (so that the event at issue is among the mechanisms of removal of individuals from the candidate population).

These two types of population experience may be viewed in terms of different types of incidence rate.

The availability of a cohort experience may suggest its direct characterization in terms of *cohort*, or *cumulative*, incidence rate. This type of incidence rate is a proportion, the proportion of the population of candidates, defined as of some zero time ($T = t_0$), who experience the event during the risk period at issue. It is an attractive direct measure of observed occurrence predominantly, though not exclusively, in situations in which each member of the cohort is followed up to the event at issue or to the end of the risk period, without attrition of the cohort due to loss to follow-up or extraneous mortality. This type of incidence rate is often of theoretical and practical interest as well.

The definition of the risk period to which a cohort (cumulative) incidence rate (an incidence proportion) refers is either substantive (and variable) or arbitrary (and fixed). Examples of the former type of incidence rate in epidemiology include the following:

1. "Hospital mortality" in myocardial infarction (proportion of patients entering a hospital who die before discharge).
2. "Fetal death rate" (proportion of youngest fetuses dying any time in the prenatal period).
3. "Life-time incidence" of breast cancer (proportion of young people who will ever develop breast cancer).
4. "Incidence" of postpartum depression (proportion of deliveries followed by maternal depression attributable to the delivery).
5. "Incidence" of venereal disease in subsequent contacts of active cases, or "secondary attack rate" (proportion of contacts who develop the disease from the contact).

The cohort-type incidence rate with an arbitrary, fixed risk period is exemplified by the following:

1. "Neonatal death rate" (proportion of live-born babies dying within 28 days).
2. "Five-year mortality" among survivors of first myocardial infarction (proportion of cases of first, nonfatal infarction dying within 5 years).

Cohort incidence rates of this latter type translate immediately to fractiles of the *precurrence period* (waiting time) to the event. For example, if 35- and 75-year incidence rates of death for a birth cohort are 5 and 50%, respectively, these ages represent the 5th and 50th centiles of the waiting time (at birth) to death, that is, of the duration of death's precurrence period (life).

Whereas the amount of experience in an empirical cohort incidence rate (for a given span of time) is characterized in terms of the size (S) of the cohort, dynamic-population experience is measured in terms of time (T) or more specifically *candidate time*, which is the integral of the size of the (dynamic) candidate population over the observation period.

For an experience of this latter type, with a certain number c of events occurring in it (cases "emitted" from it), the incidence rate is, naturally, that number divided by the candidate time, c/T. This rate is not a proportion, as the numerator is not a subset of the denominator. Rather, it is of the form of *density* measures in general. The dimensionality of this particular measure—*incidence density*—is inverse time. For example, if 15 cases arose from an experience of 5000 candidate years, the incidence density was $3/(10^3 \text{yr})$.

There is a direct relation between incidence density (*ID*) and cohort (cumulative) incidence (*CI*) of the second type. Specifically, incidence density determines for a cohort (defined at $T = t_0$) the proportion which *in the absence of attrition* experiences the event before some common, quantitatively (nonsubstantively) defined subsequent point in the time ($T = t_1$). With ID_t the *ID* at $T = t$, the *CI* for the interval t_0 to t_1 is (Chiang, 1968, Miettinen, 1976a)

$$CI_{t_0,t_1} = 1 - \exp\left[- \int_{t_0}^{t_1} (ID_t)\, dt \right]. \qquad (A.1.2)$$

If the incidence density is known for categories of time (e.g., age categories) in the interval at issue, the cohort (cumulative) incidence may be derived as follows:

$$CI_{t_0,t_1} = 1 - \exp\left[- \sum_i(ID_i)d_i \right], \qquad (A.1.3)$$

where the summation is over the categories in the interval (t_0 to t_1), and d_i is the duration of the *i*th interval.

It should be noted that this relation does not obtain between *ID* and *CI* referring to a substantively defined period of time. The latter depends not only on ID_t but also on the distribution of the risk period among individuals, that is, on the density of risk-time terminations for reasons unrelated to the event at issue.

A.1.3. RISK

The concept of *risk* is related to that of incidence proportion. It is the probability of a particular event, especially an untoward one, such as the inception of a particular illness. Thus, the risk of an (adverse) event is akin to its incidence in the sense that it has to do with its inception. As a probability, however, risk is inherently a *theoretical*, nonempirical entity, whereas incidence can be either theoretical or empirical. Moreover, it refers to *individuals* (of a given kind), whereas incidence characterizes populations. Thus, in a given kind of surgical situation, an empirical incidence of operative death among a series of patients serves as an estimate of the theoretical incidence among patients of that kind, operated on in that manner. By the same token, it serves as an estimate of the risk for a patient of that kind, not otherwise specified, to die after being operated on in that manner. The individual risk of operative death, a theoretical value, estimated from all the relevant experience, is not revealed by the actual, empirical outcome of the operation. Thus, if the risk was 5% before the operation, it remains 5% even in light of and regardless of the outcome.

Analogously with incidence, risk is not a singular parameter of nature. Its value depends on the specifications of the situation, on *determinants* of risk. In a further analogy, such a conditional risk remains quantitatively nebulous, because it depends on yet other, unspecified determinants.

A.1.4. PROPORTIONATE RATE

In the context of two or more mutually exclusive states or events, such as two subtypes of an illness, deaths from alternative causes, or care actions of various levels of quality, it may be of interest to consider their relative rates of occurrence in terms of a *proportionate rate*. Thus, information about the proportion that the prevalence of "secondary hypertension" represents of the prevalence of all "hypertension" is very helpful for the development of algorithms of care for newly diagnosed "hypertensives," the proportion that the incidence of "sudden cardiac death" represents of the incidence of all "acute coronary events" is helpful for planning the relative roles of prevention and treatment in the control of coronary heart disease; and the proportion of substandard care in a given clinical setting guides remedial administrative action.

However, proportionate rates do not always constitute reasonable substitutes for actual rates in scientific studies of occurrence relations, despite the commonality of their usage in situations in which the denominators of the compared rates cannot be quantified (in absolute terms). Instead of proportionate occurrence, *occurrence odds* should be considered in such situations, as is discussed in Section A.2.6.

It is of theoretical interest to note that, in the context of events (as with types of care action), the proportionate rates are neither prevalence nor incidence rates. They are not prevalence rates because they do not address (prevailing) states; and they are not incidence rates as they do not represent occurrence of events in units in the context of their motion over time.

APPENDIX 2

Measures of
Occurrence Relation

A.2.1. FUNDAMENTAL MEASURES OF
SUSCEPTIBILITY AND RESISTANCE

To say that a characteristic of individuals has an effect on some aspect of health means that there are *instances* in which the status of the characteristic makes a difference in the subsequent course of that aspect of health. For example, to say that a certain drug causes a particular type of adverse event means that there have been instances of that event among users of the drug that would not have occurred without it (everything else being equal), or that among nonusers there would have been such events had they used it.

Quantification of the effect of a particular (index) category of a characteristic relative to a chosen reference category of it is a matter of determining the frequency of such instances in some sense. Consider the effect of surgery on short-term survival in some type of life-threatening condition. There are instances of a patient being "saved" by the operation, and there are instances of death due to the operation. The survival effect of surgery (for that period) would be properly characterized in terms of the respective frequencies of each of these types of instance. The remainder of patients would have survived with or without surgery, or they would have died with or without it.

A complete characterization of a population's responsiveness to a particular index category $D = 1$ of a determinant D, relative to a particular reference category of it $D = 0$, can be based on the proportions of individuals of each of four types (cf. Miettinen, 1982a):

S_c = Proportion *causally susceptible* (event on $D = 1$, not on $D = 0$).

S_p = Proportion *preventively susceptible* (no event on $D = 1$, event on $D = 0$).

R_c = Proportion *causally resistant* (no event regardless of D).

R_p = Proportion *preventively resistant* (event regardless of D).

A.2.2. SUSCEPTIBILITY/RESISTANCE AND MEASURES OF RELATION

A.2.2.1. Rate Difference

In the terms introduced above, if everyone were in the index category, the rate (incidence proportion) would be

$$R_1^* = S_c + R_p \qquad (A.2.1)$$

(the asterisk denoting the conditional nature of the rate), and if everyone were in the reference state, it would be

$$R_0^* = S_p + R_p. \qquad (A.2.2)$$

Consequently, if everyone in the population were in the index category, the *effect* (absolute) that would result (relative to everyone in the reference category) would be the causal rate (theoretical) or risk *difference*,

$$RD^* = R_1^* - R_0^* \\ = S_c - S_p. \qquad (A.2.3)$$

In fact, this is the effect regardless of the population's status or distribution according to the determinant. For example, nuclear explosion has a deadly effect on any population, even if the population is spared of that effect through nonexposure.

A.2.2.2. Derivatives of Rate Ratio

One may wish to think of the magnitude of that effect—that rate difference—in *relative* terms. One possibility is the ratio of the magnitude of the effect relative to the "background" rate R_0^*. This relative measure is

$$
\begin{aligned}
\frac{RD^*}{R_0^*} &= \frac{R_1^*}{R_0^*} - 1 \\[2mm]
&= RR^* - 1 \\[2mm]
&= \frac{S_c + R_p}{S_p + R_p} - 1 \\[2mm]
&= \frac{S_c - S_p}{S_p + R_p},
\end{aligned}
\qquad (A.2.4)
$$

where RR^* stands for the *rate ratio* R_1^*/R_0^*.

Alternatively, with $RD^* > 0$, one may wish to express the effect as a proportion of the total rate conditional on the index category of the determinant:

$$
\begin{aligned}
\frac{RD^*}{R_1^*} &= \frac{RR^* - 1}{RR^*} \\[2mm]
&= \frac{S_c - S_p}{S_c + R_p}.
\end{aligned}
\qquad (A.2.5)
$$

Yet another possibility is to express the effect's magnitude as a proportion of the size of the domain of individuals who would be safe without the effect. This proportion is

$$
\begin{aligned}
\frac{RD^*}{1 - R_0^*} &= 1 - \frac{1 - R_1^*}{1 - R_0^*} \\[2mm]
&= 1 - SR^* \\[2mm]
&= 1 - \frac{S_p + R_c}{S_c + R_c} \\[2mm]
&= \frac{S_c - S_p}{S_c + R_c},
\end{aligned}
$$

where SR^* denotes the *safety ratio* (the ratio of the complements of rates or risks).

If $RD^* < 0$, there is interest in the absolute value of the effect relative to the "background" rate R_0^*:

$$
\begin{aligned}
\frac{-RD^*}{R_0^*} &= 1 - RR^* \\[2mm]
&= \frac{S_p - S_c}{S_p + R_p}.
\end{aligned}
\qquad (A.2.7)
$$

One may also wish to consider the relative enlargement of the safe domain, using the ratio

$$\frac{-RD^*}{1 - R_0^*} = SR^* - 1$$

$$= \frac{S_p + R_c}{S_c + R_c} - 1 \qquad (A.2.8)$$

$$= \frac{S_p - S_c}{S_c + R_c}.$$

A.2.3. DERIVATIVES OF OBSERVED AND EXPECTED NUMBERS OF CASES

Thus far, the effect of a particular (index) category of a determinant (relative to a chosen reference category) has been considered for a particular base in terms of the responsiveness of that *base at large*, regardless of the actual distribution of the determinant in that base. This outlook is appropriate for experimental research, wherein the determinant distribution is both arbitrary (set by the investigator) and unrelated to the susceptibilities in the base.

In nonexperimental contexts the effect of a particular category of the determinant tends to be of interest first and foremost in reference to *those actually in the index category*, that is, those who actually could have experienced the effect. This effect is embodied in the empirical rate r_1 for the index category, which involves the *observed* number of cases,

$$c_1 = O_1. \qquad (A.2.9)$$

The structure of the empirical rate in terms of the fundamental proportions is

$$r_1 = S_{c,1} + R_{p,1}, \qquad (A.2.10)$$

with the component proportions generally peculiar to the subpopulation in the index category (hence the subscripts).

If the index population had not experienced the effect, a certain *null expected* number (E_1) of exposed cases would have materialized in it, and the index rate would have been

$$\frac{E_1}{O_1} r_1 = S_{p,1} + R_{p,1}. \qquad (A.2.11)$$

Thus the absolute effect that the index population experienced was

$$r_1 - \frac{E_1}{O_1} r_1 = \frac{O_1 - E_1}{O_1} r_1$$

$$= S_{c,1} - S_{p,1}. \tag{A.2.12}$$

It is the difference between the crude rate for the index category and the reference rate adjusted to the structure of the index domain with respect to all confounders of the base (see Section 2.6 and Appendix 4).

If $O_1 > E_1$, the empirical *etiologic fraction* (*EF*) (Miettinen, 1974b) in the index population is

$$EF_1 = \frac{O_1 - E_1}{O_1}. \tag{A.2.13}$$

It is the proportion of the number of cases, in the experience of the population representing the index category, that is due to the cause at issue. It is also the proportion of the actual cases in the index domain that are caused by the cause at issue on the condition that in the population at issue there are no instances of preventive susceptibility (Section A.2.1). If such instances do exist, the proportion of the cases in the index domain that is attributable to the cause at issue is higher than the etiologic fraction (Equation A.2.13).

If $O_1 < E_1$, the *preventive fraction* (*PF*) (Miettinen, 1974b) in the index experience is

$$PF_1 = \frac{E_1 - O_1}{E_1}. \tag{A.2.14}$$

This is the proportion that was prevented by the index status within the case load that would have appeared in the absence of the effect.

In particularistic contexts there can also be interest in the *effect of the actual distribution* of the determinant relative to particular alternative distributions. The absolute effect of the actual distribution relative to everyone having been in the reference category is

$$\frac{\sum_i O_i - \sum_i E_i}{\sum_i O_i} r, \tag{A.2.15}$$

where the summations are over all categories of the determinant. (In the reference category, $O_i - E_i = O_0 - E_0 = 0$.)

If $\sum_i O_i > \sum_i E_i$, the *EF* for the actual distribution (relative to everyone's being in the reference category) is

$$EF = \frac{\sum_i O_i - \sum_i E_i}{\sum_i O_i}. \tag{A.2.16}$$

For example, if the determinant is *dichotomous*, with the index category a cause relative to the reference category, the *EF* for the distribution is

$$EF = \frac{O_1 - E_1}{O_0 + O_1}$$

$$= \frac{O_1 - E_1}{O_1} \quad \frac{O_1}{O_0 + O_1},$$

(A.2.17)

that is, the *EF* for those in the index domain (cf. Equation A.2.18) multiplied by the fraction of cases arising from that domain (Miettinen, 1974b).

If $\sum_i O_i < \sum_i E_i$, the *PF* that corresponds to the actual distribution (relative to everyone's being in the reference category) is

$$PF = \frac{\sum_i E_i - \sum_i O_i}{\sum E_i}.$$

(A.2.18)

In the context of a binary determinant this measure takes the form

$$PF = \frac{E_1 - O_1}{E_0 + E_1}$$

$$= \frac{E_1 - O_1}{E_1} \quad \frac{E_1}{O_0 + E_1},$$

(A.2.19)

that is, the *PF* in the index domain (Equation A.2.14) multiplied by the proportion of cases that would arise from this domain (of preventability) in the absence of the preventive effect (Miettinen, 1974b).

The remaining *preventable* fraction is the proportion of cases due to the actual distribution relative to everyone's being in the preventive index category. Thus, it is the etiologic fraction for the actual distribution, with everyone in the index category as the alternative. Its structure, therefore, involves the empirical number in the reference category together with its expected counterpart, based on the specific rates in the index domain and the structure of the reference domain.

A.2.4. ODDS RATIO

From the concepts discussed above it is evident, first, that the absolute effect is the rate difference RD^* contrasting the situation of everyone's being in the index category to its alternative of everyone being in the reference category. Second, all conceivable yet reasonable *relative* measures of the effect turn out to be functions of the corresponding *RR* or the safety ratio $SR = (1 - R_1)/(1 - R_0)$.

This leaves out the *OR*, one of the most popular relative measures of occurrence relation in epidemiology today. The odds conditional on the index category are $R_1/(1 - R_1)$, and conditional on the reference category they are $R_0/(1 - R_0)$. Consequently, the *OR* contrasting the two is

$$OR = \frac{R_1}{1 - R_1} \bigg/ \frac{R_0}{1 - R_0}. \qquad (A.2.20)$$

This measure of relation is an amalgamation of *RR* and *SR*:

$$OR = \frac{RR}{SR}, \qquad (A.2.21)$$

where $SR = (1 - R_1)/(1 - R_0)$. In terms of the fundamental proportions in the context of causal inference its structure is

$$OR^* = \frac{(S_c + R_p)(S_c + R_c)}{(S_p + R_p)(S_p + R_c)}. \qquad (A.2.22)$$

It is quite apparent that the *OR* parameter has not gained its epidemiologic popularity on the basis of intelligibility. Instead, its reason for being, such as it is, is none other than mathematical convenience (e.g., in logistic regression). Even less intelligible is the *logit difference* (*LD*), another popular parameter in modern analysis of epidemiologic data. Its structure is

$$LD = \log \frac{R_1}{1 - R_1} - \log \frac{R_0}{1 - R_0}$$
$$= \log(OR). \qquad (A.2.23)$$

Despite the unattractiveness of *OR* with reference to proportion-type rates for the outcome under study, the ratio of *case-base odds*, contrasting the index and reference categories of the determinant as always, is of express interest as an estimate of *RR* in the context of the case-base (case-referent) sampling strategy (Section 4.1, Chapter 17, and Section A.2.6).

A.2.5. CORRELATION AND REGRESSION COEFFICIENTS

Correlation between a subject characteristic and a measure of health outcome reflects linear association between the two. Thus, a coefficient of either simple or partial correlation may be entertained as a measure of occurrence relation.

As a measure of relation, the coefficient of correlation has two drawbacks. One is *unintelligibility*. Interpretation is commonly attempted for its square, which is viewed as the proportion of the variance of the outcome measure "explained" by the determinant. One can attach ready meaning to "proportion" and to "explained," but "variance" can pose an insurmountable intellectual challenge. Defined as the average squared deviation from the mean, its visualization in the context of a distance measure as an area is possible, but it strains the intellect to think of area as a measure of the variability of a linear measure. Even the visualization of variance poses a problem when dealing with various other types of quantity. Consider pressure as an example. The dimensionality of variance is the square of that of pressure (which is force per area), with units such as square Pascal or (mm Hg)^2. When variance cannot be visualized, a proportion of it can scarcely be explained in terms of a determinant.

The other drawback of the correlation coefficient as a parameter for scientific purposes is its *lack of invariance* with respect to arbitrary features of study design. A correlation coefficient does not characterize nature per se (as a scientific parameter should), but it represents a mixture of inputs from nature (the occurrence relation under study) and the study plan. In the latter category of inputs the elements are the variability of the determinant in the study base (Section 3.2.2) and that of the empirical measure of outcome (Section 5.7).

These drawbacks of the correlation coefficient are not shared by the coefficient of *regression*. A regression model expresses a parameter as a function of its determinant(s). Thus, it serves as a formal expression for the occurrence relation under study.

Intelligibility of regression coefficient(s), even for quantitative purposes, can be preserved by a modicum of care in the construction of the model. The first condition is that the dependent parameter represents the occurrence parameter of interest without any obfuscating transformations. When studying cohort (cumulative) incidence (see Appendix 1), the parameter might have to be that proportion itself rather than its logit, for example (see Section A.2.4). Similarly, when the concern is with a quantitative aspect of health, such as serum triglyceride level, the dependent parameter should be a meaningful descriptor of its distribution, such as the logarithm of its median. Statistical convenience or elegance are not cogent reasons for any willful disfiguration of the very object of scientific inquiry, the parameter whose magnitude is being studied in relation to certain determinants of this magnitude. Even less tenable as a reason is assurance that the model-implied value for the parameter remains within its theoretical bounds regardless of how absurd the values entertained for the determinant(s) may be. A model addresses a particular range of a determinant only. Thus it is no liability of the model if outside this range a thoughtless observer calculates an inadmissible value for the parameter, a negative risk for a coronary event at zero blood pressure, for example. (The "intercept" of the model can be interpreted as the value of the dependent parameter corresponding to all the determinant values being zero only insofar as this case is indeed intended to belong in the domain that the model addresses.)

The other condition for intelligibility is that the relation of the parameter to any given determinant must have a reasonably *simple* representation in the function. After all, when simplicity has been lost, the function is not a model—a formal and simplified representation of its object.

When these conditions for an intelligible regression function are met, with the determinant at issue represented by a single term, and with all confounders properly accounted for, the coefficient of this term can be the effect of a unit increment in the determinant. For example, if the dependent parameter is cumulative incidence (risk) and an all-or-none exposure is represented by an indicator of the exposure ($X = 1$ for exposed, $X = 0$ for unexposed, with a separate indicator for "other") in a linear, additive model, the coefficient of the exposure indicator is the *RD* in the causal/preventive sense. Similarly, if the dependent parameter is mean blood pressure, the coefficient of the exposure indicator in such a model is the mean effect of the exposure, -10 mm Hg, for example.

Quite commonly, though, even on the conditions stated, a regression coefficient is not the effect of a unit increment. This is the case when the determinant is not a "pure number" (dimensionless), but is dimensioned. For example, if B is the coefficient of the rate of sodium intake in a regression model for mean blood pressure, B is not the effect of a unit increment in the rate of sodium intake; it does not have even the dimensionality of pressure. It is *the ratio of the effect of a unit increment of the determinant to that increment,* for example, $B = 0.5$ mm Hg/(g/day). The effect itself of a unit change in the determinant is B times that change, in this example [0.5 mm Hg/(g/day)] (g/day) = 0.5 mm Hg. This ratio structure is characteristic of linear regression coefficients in general, and the situation considered in the paragraph above is a special case.

This interpretation of a regression coefficient applies to the occurrence parameter that the linear compound of the B's, together with the "intercept" A, represents—in logistic regression, the logit of rate R, that is, $\log[R/(1 - R)]$. When, as in logistic regression, the dependent parameter is not of interest per se, the actual measure of effect must be derived as a more complicated metameter of the regression coefficient. For example, when the incidence of neonatal RDS in relation to GA and maternal glucocorticoid use is studied by the use of an additive logistic model (Example 18.2), the coefficient of the indicator of exposure B_2 represents effect in the sense of *LD* (Section A.2.4). This is unintelligible. Its antilog, the *OR* is also unattractive (Section A.2.4). By contrast, real interest centers on the shift in the location of the incidence curve over GA, which is characterized for the unexposed by the "intercept" A and the coefficient of GA, B_1. The shift of interest is $-B_2/B_1$ (Example 18.2).

A.2.6. PROPORTIONATE MORTALITY RATIO

In occupational mortality analysis, which is concerned with the effects of particular occupations on mortality from particular causes, it is commonplace to employ the so called *Proportional Mortality Ratio* or *Proportionate Mortality Ratio,* the *PMR,* as the parameter of effect.

Suppose that in the occupational category of interest, the index occupation, there were, in a particular time interval, c_1 deaths from the cause of interest and b_1 deaths from other causes, either all other causes or a selected subset. Suppose, too, that the corresponding numbers were c_0 and b_0 for a reference experience, for either the nation at large or a select, more comparable occupational group (see Section 2.3). The corresponding Proportionate Mortality Rates are $c_1/(c_1 + b_1)$ and $c_0/(c_0 + b_0)$. The *PMR* is then

$$PMR = \frac{c_1/(c_1 + b_1)}{c_0/(c_0 + b_0)}. \tag{A.2.24}$$

This parameter addresses the effect at issue only insofar as the rate of occurrence of death from the "other" cause(s) is identical between the index and reference experiences. On this condition, the ratio of the numbers of deaths from those other causes is the ratio of the respective rate denominators, usually in terms of population time (Appendix 1). Thus, the *RR* of interest, the rate in the index occupation divided by that in the reference experience, is

$$RR = \frac{c_1/c_0}{b_1/b_0}. \tag{A.2.25}$$

This parameter is identical to the mortality-odds ratio (*MOR*), contrasting the two experiences (Miettinen and Wang, 1981):

$$MOR = \frac{c_1/b_1}{c_0/b_0}. \tag{A.2.26}$$

It is evident that the *PMR* is *redundant* as a parameter. Moreover, it has the drawback of *lack of invariance* with respect to the arbitrary design decision as to the size of the domain of the "other" causes of death—a problem that is not shared by the alternative *MOR* formulation.

In point of fact, the type of situation represented by occupational mortality analyses does not justify the invocation of any ad hoc parameter. Instead, these studies should be thought of as case-referent studies in the ordinary sense. The case series is the deaths from the cause of interest, distributed between the index and reference domains, and the reference series consists of the deaths from the "other" causes, similarly distributed (cf. Example 5.3, and Wang and Miettinen, 1982).

A.2.7. DEATHS PREVENTED (LIVES SAVED)

The merits of intervention programs are sometimes viewed in terms of the annual number of "deaths prevented" or "lives saved." Thus, in the context of a randomized trial being launched in the area of preventive cardiology, the principal investigator was reported to have said that "a positive result . . . would have an enormous impact. 'A mere 10-percent reduction in mortality . . . could, in theory, prevent 60,000 premature deaths a year, while a 20-percent reduction could prevent 120,000 such deaths annually,' . . ." (*Boston Globe*, 3/16/82).

The concept of the number of deaths ("premature," "mature," or "postmature") prevented in unit time suggests that with the prevention there would be fewer deaths in unit time. This is akin to the concept that preventive medicine, to the extent that it is efficacious, reduces the annual number of hospitalizations. In point of fact, deaths cannot be prevented but only postponed, so that, in a stable state, the annual number of deaths equals the annual number of births, regardless of the success of death-postponing programs. Thus, instead of the "annual number of deaths prevented" one should think of a program's impact in the duration of life (Miettinen, 1983a), which is a corollary of its effect in terms of the cumulative incidence of death (Appendix 1). By the same token, it is a case of specious logic to think that preventive medicine would reduce the costs of therapeutic medicine (Miettinen, 1979).

APPENDIX 3

Causal and Preventive Interdependence (Synergism and Antagonism)

A.3.1. DEFINITIONS

Synergism has to do with cooperation, antagonism with opposition; both therefore represent *interdependence* in coaction. This concept is not properly referred to as "*interation*" (which refers to mutual or reciprocal action), even though the distinction is not always made.

The definitions of causal and preventive interdependencies, or synergism and antagonism, must be in conformity with those of "causation" and "prevention" themselves. "Causation" may be said to mean the existence of instances in which the "cause" is critical for the development of the event (meaning that conditionally on the alternative, reference category of the determinant, it would not develop). "Prevention" may be defined analogously, in terms of nondevelopment. It seems desirable, however, to distinguish between two types of prevention: noncausation and blockage. In the former sense, the alternative to a cause (its absence, the reference category) is a preventive. The latter type of preventive acts on an otherwise sufficient cause, frustrating it, blocking its effect. This is the meaning of prevention in the context of immunization, contraception, and so on; it is defensive and downstream, in the nature of goaltending.

In these terms, *synergism* of action between two causes or preventives may be defined as the existence of instances such that their joint action (coation) has the effect (production or blockage) whereas solo actions do not (Miettinen, 1982a). Thus, for agents A and B, with complements $\bar{A}$ and $\bar{B}$, respectively, synergism means that all three of the following obtain:

1. $A\bar{B}$ has *no* effect.
2. $\bar{A}B$ has *no* effect.
3. AB has effect.

Evidently, synergism between two factors is inherently a *mutual* interdependence of effect.

Analogously, *antagonism* of action between two causes or preventives may be said to mean the existence of instances in which one of them blocks the effect of the other. Antagonism may be *mutual*, so that all three of the following obtain:

1. $A\bar{B}$ has effect.
2. $\bar{A}B$ has effect.
3. AB has no effect.

In contrast to the inherent symmetry of synergism, there are also *one-way* antagonisms. One possibility is the following triad:

1. $A\bar{B}$ has effect.
2. $\bar{A}B$ has *no* effect.
3. AB has *no* effect.

The other possibility is the combination of the following:

1. $A\bar{B}$ has *no* effect.
2. $\bar{A}B$ has effect.
3. AB has *no* effect.

The coaction of two factors may involve synergy in some instances and antagonism in others. When this is the case (or a possibility), the concepts can be applied with reference to the dominant form of coaction.

Independence of the effects of two factors may be defined as the absence of both synergism and antagonism, that is, of instances in which the effect of one of the factors depends on the presence of the other, or to balance between synergism and antagonism (Miettinen, 1982a).

A.3.2. RATE CRITERIA

Whereas causal and preventive interdependence or independence are defined (see Section A.3.1) with reference to individual instances, there arises the question of what *rate criteria* may be used for their detection. Let

$RD_{10}^* =$ Effect of $A\bar{B}$ relative to $\bar{A}\bar{B}$.
$RD_{01}^* =$ Effect of $\bar{A}B$ relative to $\bar{A}\bar{B}$.
$RD_{11}^* =$ Effect of AB relative to $\bar{A}\bar{B}$.

The problem is the relation of RD_{11}^* to RD_{10}^* and RD_{01}^* under independence of actions. Consider two examples.

EXAMPLE A.3.1.   Suppose that the susceptibility patterns of five subjects are as follows (with " + " and " − " denoting susceptibility and lack of it for the factor constellation at issue):

	1	2	3	4	5
$A\bar{B}$	+	+	−	−	−
$\bar{A}B$	+	+	+	−	−
AB	+	+	+	−	−

Here, $RD_{10}^* = \frac{2}{5}$, $RD_{01}^* = \frac{3}{5}$, and $RD_{11}^* = \frac{3}{5} = \max (RD_{10}^*, RD_{01}^*)$.

EXAMPLE A.3.2.   Now suppose that another five subjects have as their susceptibility patterns the following:

	1	2	3	4	5
$A\bar{B}$	+	+	−	−	−
$\bar{A}B$	−	−	+	+	+
AB	+	+	+	+	+

Here, $RD_{11}^* = RD_{10}^* + RD_{01}^*$.

These examples indicate that the rate criterion for independence of action must account for possible *correlatedness of susceptibilities* to the two factors, respectively (Wahrendorf and Brown, 1980). Moreover, it is evident from the examples that, in the context of *causal* agents and under independence of the actions, RD_{11}^* is bounded as follows:

$$\max(RD_{10}^*, RD_{01}^*) \leq RD_{11}^*$$
$$\leq \min(RD_{10}^* + RD_{01}^*, 1 - R_{00}^*). \qquad (A.3.1)$$

(Koopman, 1981; Miettinen, 1982a). With high positive correlation of the susceptibilities, RD_{11}^* is close to its lower bound, while the upper bound corresponds to extreme *negative* correlation. The analogous interval in the case of two preventives is (Miettinen, 1982a)

$$\max(\,|\,RD^*_{10}\,|,\,|\,RD^*_{01}\,|\,) \leq RD^*_{11}$$
$$\leq \min(\,|\,RD^*_{10}\,|\,+\,|\,RD^*_{01}\,|,\,|\,R^*_{00}\,|\,).$$

(A.3.2)

APPENDIX 4

Crude, Adjusted, and Standardized Rates

Rates characterize populations (cf. Appendix 1), and populations generally are quite inhomogeneous as to the commonality of any given phenomenon. Thus there is a need for rate concepts according to how the *overall* (unconditional) rate is constituted in the context of variation among *specific* (conditional) rates that characterize subdomains of the population.

A.4.1. CRUDE RATE AS A WEIGHTED AVERAGE OF SPECIFIC RATES

With reference to any particular population experience, or study base to be specific, the *actual* (empirical) overall rate r is referred to as the crude rate. Thus, a crude rate (CR) is simply

$$CR = \frac{c}{B}, \qquad (A.4.1.)$$

where c is the total empirical number of cases and B is the size of the base (number of subjects S or amount of population time T).

EXAMPLE A.4.1. Consider the mortality data for male agricultural workers in Table A.4.1. In the age range considered therein, 14,000 deaths occurred

TABLE A.4.1.

Mortality data, actual and hypothetical, for males in England, 1951[a]

Age (yr)	Agricultural Workers			Hypothetical Occupational Group			National Rate in $(10^3y)^{-1}$
	Deaths in 1949–1953	Population in 1951	Rate in $(10^3y)^{-1}$	Deaths in 1949–1953	Population in 1951	Rate in $(10^3y)^{-1}$	
20–24	540	83,400	1.3	65	10,000	1.3	1.4
25–34	960	133,300	1.4	144	20,000	1.4	1.6
35–44	1,500	131,600	2.3	57	5,000	2.3	2.9
45–54	3,420	117,200	5.8	58	2,000	5.8	8.2
55–64	7,530	90,600	16.6	83	1,000	16.6	23.0
20–64	14,000	556,100		407	38,000		

[a] Cf. Schilling, 1973

267

in a dynamic population of (average) size 556,100 followed for the 5-year period of 1949–1953. Thus, the crude death rate (incidence density of death) was 14,000 cases in a 556,100(5 y) space of population time (candidate time T), that is, $CR = 14,000/[556,100(5y)] = 5.0/(10^3 y)$.

A CR has the structure of being a *weighted average* of the constituent specific rates, with weights equal (or proprotional) to the sizes of the respective subdomains of the actual base:

$$CR = \frac{\sum_j W_j(c_j/B_j)}{\sum_j W_j},$$ (A.4.2)

where

$$W_j = \frac{B_j}{B}.$$

This relation, which is fundamental to all understanding of rates, is a mere algebraic truism.

EXAMPLE A.4.2.   Recall Example A.4.1, where $CR = 5.0/(10^3 y)$. From the specific rates in Table A.4.1 this crude value may be summarized as follows: $\{[83.4(1.3) + 133.3(1.4) + 131.6(2.3) + 117.2(5.8) + 90.6(16.6)]/ (83.4 + 133.3 + 131.6 + 117.2 + 90.6)\}/(10^3 y) = 5.0/(10^3 y)$.

A CR thus reflects not only the specific rates of the various subdomains but also the relative sizes of the latter, through latent weights of a totally ad hoc nature. This makes such rates ill-suited for many purposes, particularistic as well as scientific.

A.4.2. ADJUSTMENT AND STANDARDIZATION: THE IDEAS

There is a need to separate the two elements in a CR—the set of specific *rates* on one hand and the set of their corresponding *weights* on the other.

The most elementary, yet thorough, way of coping with this need is to consider the set of specific rates, as in Table A.4.1. The drawback with this is complexity, difficulty with assimilation in the context of excess detail. Hence there *is* a need for overall rates, but with deliberately chosen weights, the "native" weights of the CR being but one among the options.

In an *adjusted* rate, the native weights (proportional to the base experiences themselves) are replaced by some other, external set of weights. This transforms the CR, the actual overall rate, into its equivalent in the context of a *hypothetical* structure of the base. The adjusted rate expresses what the overall *CR* would have been, had the base had the alternative structure and had the specific rates remained unchanged.

EXAMPLE A.4.3.   Recall the two examples presented above, with the crude overall death rate of $5.0/(10^3 y)$ for male agricultural workers. One might ask—perhaps ill-advisedly (Wang and Miettinen, 1982)—how this rate compares with the male mortality in the nation at large. One would not wish this comparison to be clouded by the difference in age structure between the two populations; rather, the comparison ought to address, in an overall sense, the relative magnitudes of age-specific rates between the compared populations. To this end, one option is to adjust the national *CR* to the age structure of the agricultural workers. This means replacing the weights inherent in the national *CR* by ones proportional to the age-specific base sizes in the agricultural experience, that is, to the numbers of person years of observation by age in that hypothetical structure for the national experience. This adjusted national rate is $\{[83.4(1.4) + 133.3(1.6) + 131.6(2.9) + 117.2(8.2) + 90.6(23.0)]/556.1\}/(10^3 y) = 6.8/(10^3 y)$. The difference between this adjusted rate for the nation and the *CR* for the agricultural occupation is no longer attributable to the difference in age structure between the two.

When two or more rates involve a common set of weights, whatever this set may be, they are said to be *standardized*—meaning *mutually* standardized. This does not mean that the rates involved are all adjusted; a *CR* may be a member of a mutually standardized set of rates, as in Example A.4.3. The point is merely that the weights are the same, so that any difference(s) between (among) the rates is (are) not attributable to difference(s) in structure (weights), but must be a reflection of differences in the specific rates. (Lack of difference, however, does not mean that the values of the specific rates are the same for each of the compared populations.)

A.4.3.   THE NOTION OF "INDIRECT" STANDARDIZATION

There are those who believe that there are two types of mutually standardized rate pairs or rate sets, *"directly"* and *"indirectly"* standardized. This is a misapprehension. As noted, the issue is singular, modification of weights, and the role of the "standard" is to supply those weights.

The notion of a duality of standardizations arises from the consideration of *observed* and *expected* numbers of cases in some base of interest. The observed number ($c_1 = O_1$) is the actual number, the numerator of the *CR* for this *index* experience. The "expected" number ($\hat{E}_1$) is hypothetical, the number that would have materialized in the index base had the specific rates of a *reference* population, such as those of the nation at large, obtained in the index experience. The ratio $O_1/\hat{E}_1$ characterizes the relative magnitudes of the rates in the index and reference experiences, indicating the relative size of the index rate in comparison with the reference rate, upon standardization for age or whatever. Thus, one may use the comparison

$$\frac{O_1}{\hat{E}_1} (CR_0) \text{ vs. } CR_0 \qquad \text{(A.4.3.)}$$

with the assurance inherent in standardization, namely that any difference is indicative of nonidentity of the set of specific rates between the index and reference experiences. It is $(O_1/\hat{E}_1)(CR_0)$ that is thought of as the "indirectly standardized" rate, with the "indirectness" meaning that the specific rates of the index experience never need to be considered. The observed number is the numerator of the CR, and the "expected" number involves only the structure of the index experience with the empirical rate elements derived from the reference experience:

$$\hat{E}_1 = \sum_j B_{1j} r_{0j}. \qquad \text{(A.4.4.)}$$

Not only is this calculation thought to represent a special form of standardization, but it is also thought to be preferable to "direct" standardization when the index experience is small relative to the reference experience. After all, it focuses directly on the total number cases in the scarce index experience.

To gain insight into these notions, consider the structure of the comparison shown in Equation A.4.3 in terms of the elements that are relevant to standardization—the specific rates in the index experience, $\{r_{1j}\}$, those in the reference experience, $\{r_{0j}\}$, and the common set of weights, $\{W_j\}$. The essence of the formulation is the contrast between the observed and "expected" numbers, and it can be recast as

$$\frac{O_1}{B_1} \text{ vs. } \frac{\hat{E}_1}{B_1}. \qquad \text{(A.4.5.)}$$

The left-hand element is, evidently, the CR for the index experience and, recalling the structure of E_1 (Equation A.4.4), the right-hand element evidently is the reference rate standardized to the structure of the index experience. There is nothing "direct" or "indirect" about this standardization; it is just standardization, of the one and only kind. A point of note is, however, that the common *weights derive from the index experience*.

A.4.4. THE STANDARDIZED MORTALITY (MORBIDITY) RATIO

In the context of dynamic-population mortality (incidence density of death), the ratio of two rates standardized by the use of weights from the index experience is commonly termed *the standardized mortality ratio, the SMR*.

Sometimes the acronym is applied to morbidity density as well, with the same implication of uniqueness. Either way,

$$SMR = \frac{O_1}{\hat{E}_1}$$

$$= \frac{O_1/B_1}{\hat{E}_1/B_1} \qquad\qquad (A.4.6.)$$

$$= \frac{\sum_j B_{1j} r_{1j}}{\sum_j B_{1j} r_{0j}}.$$

EXAMPLE A.4.4.   Recall Example A.4.3. For the agricultural workers (the domain of express interest, the index domain), the observed number of deaths was 14,000. The corresponding expected number, had the age-specific national rates applied to the agricultural subpopulation as well, would have been $83{,}000(5y)$ $[1.4/(10^3 y)]$ + $133{,}300(5y)$ $[1.6/(10^3 y)]$ + . . . = 18,800. Thus, the observed-to-expected ratio for the agricultural workers, with the national population as the referent, was $14{,}000/18{,}800 = 0.74$. This is also the ratio of the respective mortality rates, mutually standardized, with the index experience (that of agricultural workers) providing the common weights. Hence, the ratio involves the CR for agricultural workers, $5.0/(10^3 y)$ (cf. Example A.4.1), and the reference rate adjusted to the structure of the agricultural population, $6.8/(10^3 y)$ (cf. Example A.4.3). The ratio is $5.0/6.8 = 0.74$, the $O/\hat{E}$ ratio.

Since the weights in an $O/\hat{E}$ ratio derive from the index experience, they are specific to each index category in the context of two or more ratios. Thus, even though each $O/\hat{E}$ ratio is *internally* standardized, a set of such ratios is *not mutually* standardized (Miettinen, 1972b). In other words, a difference between two $O/\hat{E}$ ratios does not indicate that there must be a difference between the respective sets of specific rates.

EXAMPLE A.4.5.   Consider again the data in Table A.4.1. The agricultural and the hypothetical occupational categories are characterized by identical age-specific rates. Thus, any comparable, mutually standardized, overall measures for those two experiences are identical. The $O/\hat{E}$ ratio for the agricultural experience is 0.74 (cf. Example A.4.4). For the hypothetical population it is $407/\{10{,}000(5y)$ $[1.4/(10^3 y)]$ + $20{,}000(5y)$ $[1.6/(10^3 y)]$ + . . .} = 0.81. This value differs from the 0.74 for the agricultural experience, reflecting the incomparability of a set of $O/\hat{E}$ ratios rather than differences between the respective sets of specific rates.

Comparability among the values in a set of rate ratios presupposes the employment of a common set of internal standards for each. One possibility is to use the referent as the common standard as well. This means using the specific rates of the ith index category to compute the respective "expected" number in the reference category, $\hat{E}_{0i}$. The rate ratios, internally and mutually standardized, for the various compared categories are then $\{\hat{E}_{0i}/O_0\}$ (Miettinen, 1973).

A.4.5.   PRECISION-MAXIMIZING WEIGHTS

When one attempts to maximize the *precision* of a single contrast of rates, a reasonable choice of the weights of the internal standard is to draw them from one of the compared experiences, the one in which the experience is more *sparse* (Miettinen, 1972a)—often the index experience. It is even better to employ a standard in which the weights are proportional to the respective amounts of comparative information among the subcategories (cf. Section 11.1.2). This means taking the weights as

$$W_j = \left(\frac{1}{B_{1j}} + \frac{1}{B_{0j}}\right)^{-1}, \quad j = 1, \ldots \quad \text{(A.4.7)}$$

When several categories of a determinant of the magnitude of the rate at issue are being compared, the choice of precision-maximizing weights for internal and mutual standardization involves consideration of relative importance among the contrasts. Where such distinctions do not exist, the choice of weights should again reflect the amount of comparative information alone. Such weights, as an extension of those given above, are

$$W_j = \left[\sum_i \left(\frac{1}{B_{ij}}\right)\right]^{-1}, \quad j = 1, \ldots \quad \text{(A.4.8)}$$

Census vs. Case-Referent Approach

Relative Informativeness

Suppose that the study base embodies the rates

$$r_i = \frac{c_i}{B_i}, \qquad i = 1, \ldots \qquad \text{(A.5.1)}$$

for different categories of a determinant of interest (with c denoting the empirical number of cases and B the size of the corresponding base; cf. Section 4.1). Potential interest in these rates, with the base itself as the technical referent (Section 1.6), is mainly of two types:

1. It may be particularistic to the point where the actual realizations r_i are of interest per se.
2. The base experience may be viewed as a (simple random) sample of an infinite amount of experience of its kind, actual or hypothetical, and the

interest is in the parameters of that larger reality—the "superpopula-tion" (cf. Section 9.1).

These two types of potential interest in the base experience have different implications for the thoroughness with which the case-referent strategy har-vests the information in the base. (The census approach provides all the available information in either case.)

Consider first the assessment of the *realizations* themselves (a question of potential particularistic, but not really of scientific, interest). All the cases (*c* in number) are identified and classified according to the determinant, and a simple random sample (of size *b*) of the base (of size *B*) is also drawn and its members are similarly classified. The resulting point estimates of the $\{r_i\}$ are

$$\hat{r}_i = \frac{c_i}{Bb_i/b}, \qquad i = 1, \ldots \tag{A.5.2}$$

(cf. Section 4.1). In this estimate the number of cases is a constant, and the statistical uncertainty arises solely from the use of b_i/b as an estimate of B_i/B, that is, sampling variability in the reference series is the only source of uncertainty. In these terms, the variance of $\hat{r}_i$ is

$$V_{\hat{r}_i} = \left(\frac{c_i}{B}\right)^2 V_{b/b_i}. \tag{A.5.3}$$

By the use of a first-order Taylor-series approximation, thus,

$$V_{\hat{r}_i} = (r_i)^2 \left(1 - \frac{b}{B}\right) \left(\frac{1}{E_{b_i}} - \frac{1}{b}\right). \tag{A.5.4}$$

This procedure can have the alternative of focusing on the *noncases* in the base sample, that is, of supplementing the case census by a sample of the noncases. This is an alternative only when dealing with prevalence or cohort (cumulative) incidence (incidence proportion; see Appendix 1), whereas in the context of a dynamic-population base the distinction is moot (Miettinen, 1976a). If the number of noncases is *n* out of a total of $N = B - c$, and if n_i of them fall in the *i*th category of the determinant, the coun-terpart of the estimate in Equation A.5.2 is

$$\hat{r}_i = \frac{c_i}{c_i + Nn_i/n}. \tag{A.5.5}$$

For this estimate the variance arising from mere sampling of the noncases is

$$\hat{V}_{\hat{r}_i} = [r_i(1 - r_i)]^2 \left(1 - \frac{n}{N}\right) \left(\frac{1}{E_{n_i}} - \frac{1}{n}\right). \qquad (A.5.6)$$

Evidently, even though the noncases are only a subset of the base sample, with

$$E_n = b \left(1 - \frac{c}{B}\right), \qquad (A.5.7)$$

the latter analysis, involving only the noncases in the base sample, is more informative than that without the exclusions.

The variance of the relative error ($\hat{r}/r - 1$), owing to mere sampling of the base/noncases, that is, $V_{\hat{r}_i/r_i} = V_{\hat{r}_i}/(r_i)^2$, is attractively small, even for the rarest category of the determinant, if for this category the *expected* number of noncases is one hundred or more (which makes the standard deviation of the relative error 10% or less).

When the interest is in *expected* rates in the context of regarding the base as a sample of abstract reality (the usual scientific view; cf. Section 9.1), the point estimators are the same as those given above (Equations A.5.2 and A.5.5). However, r_i is now construed as a sampling realization, an estimate of some unknown rate R_i, and hence the variance becomes larger. Consider estimation based on noncases in the base sample. Taking the hypothetical sampling behind the base and the random sampling of the base to be independent, and applying again the first-order Taylor-series approximation, the variance may be written as

$$V_{\hat{r}_i} = [R_i(1 - R_i)]^2 \left[\frac{1 - R_i}{R_i B_i}\right.$$
$$\left. + \left(1 - \frac{n}{N}\right) \left(\frac{1}{E_{n_i}} - \frac{1}{n}\right)\right]. \qquad (A.5.8)$$

This variance has an implication very different from that derived in the previous case. Now the imprecision that is due to mere sampling of the base/noncases (in lieu of a census) is not the sole component of imprecision; and the other component is inherent in the base, influencing the informativeness of a census as well. Thus, the design concern is only with the *relative* contribution of the case-referent approach to the total imprecision of the rate estimates.

It is evident from Equation A.5.8 that resorting to the case-referent strategy increases the standard deviation of the relative error by a factor of

$$\left[1 + \frac{(1 - n/N)(1/E_{n_i} - 1/n)B_i R_i}{1 - R_i}\right]^{1/2}. \qquad (A.5.9)$$

In the usual context of low rates, and for the most critical (rarest) categories of the determinant, this factor is seen to depend on the *size of the base sample relative to the total number of cases*, through $B_i R_i / E_{n_i} = E_{c_i} / E_{n_i}$. In particular, the case-base strategy of information acquisition is an excellent substitute for the census approach, even in the context of a low sampling fraction and an infrequent category of the determinant, if the base sample is at least fivefold relative to the number of cases (in which case the error standard deviation is increased by less than 10% relative to the census result).

APPENDIX 6

Case-Referent Approach

Sample of Base (Referent) vs. Sample of Noncase Subdomain of Base

The prevailing concept of the case-referent ("case-control") approach is that it "involves the comparison of patients (cases) with a group of controls that consists of persons who are free of the disease under study" (Schlesselman, 1982, p. vii).

In this text the outlook is somewhat different. Regardless of whether the case-referent approach is employed, the conceptual focus of research is taken to be an occurrence relation (Section 1.3). Thus, concerns for comparisons are confined to those between/among categories of *determinants* of parameters of occurrence for the outcome phenomenon (Sections 4.1 and 17.1). With the outcome of interest an all-or-none state or event, the concern is to compare its rate of occurrence between/among categories of the determinant(s) of interest. The comparison, which is empirical, is done directly in the realm of the study base, and this, then, is the direct *referent* of the empirical relation from the study (Section 1.6 and Chapter 3).

With the cases in the study base identified and information on them obtained, one is in a position to know the numerators of the compared rates in the study base. The remaining concern is not that of comparing these cases with noncases, but that of learning about the denominators of the empirical rates (Sections 4.1 and 17.1).

Fundamentally, the case series is not *compared* with anything, but is *supplemented* with information about the study base. The obvious approach would be to sample the study base (the direct referent of the study result) per se. However, the prevailing notion of "comparing" the cases with noncases suggests sampling of the noncase subdomain of the study base. This raises the question of the relative merits of these two approaches to sampling the study base.

When, in an incidence study, the base is a dynamic-population experience (Section 3.2.2, Appendix 1) the distinction between the two types of base sampling is moot, because the entire base has to do with an experience of noncases. In this situation the reference series can be thought of as a sample of the population time of the study base. It thus provides for learning about the relative magnitudes of the denominators of the compared rates and, thereby, for the estimation of rate (incidence density) ratios (Miettinen, 1976a).

The choice is substantive in instances in which the base is a cohort experience or a population cross section; at the end of a follow-up, or at the time of "cross sectioning" (of a cohort or a dynamic population), there can be cases as well as noncases in the base. If a sample of the base at large is employed, the case-referent data provide for the estimation of *RR* values without any "rare-disease assumption" (Miettinen, 1982b and Section 17.2). Moreover, such a sample can be the basis for estimating the compared rates themselves from case-referent data, even if only the noncases in the sample have bearing on significance testing of the differences between/among the compared categories of the determinant (Miettinen 1982b).

As a sample of the base at large thus tends to be more informative than a sample of its noncase subdomain, the question is whether the former is appreciably less practical than the latter. It is not. Double ascertainment of the cases is inconsequential, and sampling frames for the base at large are generally more, not less, readily available than lists of the noncase subdomain of the base.

For these reasons, it seems that the notion of case-noncase comparison as the essence of case-referent studies should give way to one of sampling, because the experience of the study base is captured by ascertaining and examining the cases that occur (occurred) in it, and by obtaining a *sample of the base itself* (Miettinen, 1985). To insist that the sample is to be drawn from the noncase subdomain of the base (cohort or cross-sectional) is to obfuscate the basic concept that for the comparison of rates one needs information on their numerators—from a case series—and on their denominators—from a sample of the base (and direct referent) of the study (Sections 4.1 and 17.1). Such insistence also obfuscates the realization that sampling of the base itself is an option in these studies that makes preoccupation with the "rare-disease assumption" (Cornfield, 1951) unnecessary (Miettinen, 1976; 1982b).

APPENDIX 7

Relative Sizes of Compared Series

Suppose that, after the set-up costs of a study, a total amount of C can be expended, and that the unit costs for the index and reference subjects are C_1 and C_0, respectively. Then the sizes S_1 and S_0 of the index and reference series, respectively, must satisfy the condition

$$C = S_1 C_1 + S_0 C_0 \qquad \text{(A.7.1)}$$
$$= S_1 (C_1 + R C_0),$$

where $R = S_0/S_1$.

As for the information yield of this investment, suppose that the individual observations have, uniformly, variance V. Then the variance of the difference between the index and reference series in the case of no covariates is $V(1/S_1 + 1/S_2)$, so that the information about the difference is

$$I = \left[V \left(\frac{1}{S_1} + \frac{1}{S_0} \right) \right]^{-1} \qquad \text{(A.7.2)}$$
$$= \left[\frac{V}{S_1} (1 + R^{-1}) \right]^{-1}$$

The relative sizes of the index and reference series, when subjects for each are readily available at those unit costs, are then chosen with a view

280

to maximizing I conditionally on C. Solving Equation A.7.1 for S_1 and substituting this to Equation A.7.2, differentiating with respect to R, setting the derivate equal to zero, and solving for R yields

$$R = \frac{S_0}{S_1} = \left(\frac{C_1}{C_0}\right)^{1/2}. \tag{A.7.3}$$

Thus, in the simple situation in which no covariates are being considered, *the optimal size ratio is the square root of the inverse of the unit cost ratio.*

This result is readily seen to apply also to the case of stratified data with a constant size ratio over the strata, that is, to the case of *matched* series (Miettinen, 1969).

Consider next the case of two strata, indexed by $j = 1, 2$. The cost constraint is that

$$
\begin{aligned}
C &= \sum_j S_{1,j}(C_1 + R_j C_0) \\
&= S_{1,1}(1 + Q)(C_1 + RC_0),
\end{aligned}
\tag{A.7.4}
$$

where

$$
\begin{aligned}
R &= \frac{\sum_j S_{0,j}}{\sum_j S_{1,j}} \\
&= \frac{R_1 + R_2 Q}{1 + Q},
\end{aligned}
\tag{A.7.5}
$$

$$Q = \frac{S_{1,2}}{S_{1,1}}.$$

The information is

$$
\begin{aligned}
I &= \sum_k I_k \\
&= \sum_k \left(\frac{V}{S_{1,k}}\right)(1 + R_k^{-1})^{-1} \\
&= \left(\frac{V}{S_{1,1}}\right)^{-1} \left\{ \left[1 + \frac{R^{-1}(1 + QT)}{1 + Q}\right]^{-1} \right. \\
&\quad \left. + S^{-1}\left[1 + \frac{R^{-1}(1 + QT)}{(1 + Q)T}\right]^{-1} \right\},
\end{aligned}
\tag{A.7.6}
$$

where

$$T = \frac{R_2}{R_1}. \tag{A.7.7}$$

Substituting $S_{1,1}$ from Equation A.7.4 to Equation A.7.6, differentiating with respect to R, and setting the derivate equal to zero leads to an awkward equation that has no closed solution for R. It is possible, however, to infer that when $T \neq 1$, the optimal R-value is larger than $(C_1/C_0)^{1/2}$ when the latter is larger than one $(C_0 < C_1)$. Similarly, if $C_0 > C_1$, the optimal S_0/S_1 ratio is smaller than $(C_1/C_0)^{1/2}$.

Either way, the prospect of stratification in the analysis, in the absence of matching in subject selection, calls for a more extreme departure from equal allocation than is implied by Equation A.7.3 (cf. Section 4.3).

APPENDIX 8

Review of Study Design

A.8.1. QUESTIONS OF VALIDITY IN THE DESIGN STAGE

A. Conceptualization of phenomenon: Is it truly consonant with the essence of the research problem, the motive for the study? (Section 2.1.)

B. Empirical scales of outcome, determinant, and modifiers: Are they of optimal dimensionality (unidimensional if at all possible) and in optimal correspondence with the respective conceptual scales? (Section 2.1.)

C. Time relation: Is the difference (lag) between the time referents of outcome and determinant informations optimal in the sense of providing the best possible reflection of the relation in terms of the presumed actual lag (induction period)? (Sections 2.4 and 5.2.)

D. Contrast(s) on determinant(s): Does it (do they) assure comparability (of extraneous effects, populations, and information) conditionally on what covariates can be controlled in the analysis? (Section 2.3.)

E. Confounders: Is information on *all* potential confounders, left for analytic control in the context of the empirical contrast (item A above), to be recorded on sufficiently valid scales? (Sections 2.6 and 2.7.)

F. Study base: Is its selection independent of what that particular base is likely to show? (Sections 3.4.2 and 3.4.3.)

G. Termination of follow-up (given a cohort base): Is it independent of the outcome? (Section 3.4.4.)

H. Case series vis-à-vis base sample (given a case-referent strategy): Do they represent the same population experience? In the context of a base secondary to case selection, specifically, is the base series *representative* of the base experience implied by the case selection? (Section 4.4.2.)

I. Index series vis-à-vis reference series: Is the accuracy of information *comparable*? (Sections 2.3.3, 5.2, and 5.6.)

A.8.2. QUESTIONS OF EFFICIENCY IN THE DESIGN STAGE

A. Domain of study: Is its definition optimal with a view to the relation under study being most readily apparent (in qualitative research)? (Section 2.8.)

B. Distribution matrix: Is it optimal? (Sections 3.2.2 and 3.3.)

C. Place and time: Is the base optimal in these terms? (Section 3.2.1.5.)

D. Sampling: Is advantage going to be taken of the possibility of the case-referent strategy as an alternative to the census approach; and if so, is stratification going to be used to best advantage, and is the size of the base sample optimal relative to that of the case series? (Chapter 4.)

E. Information: Is all of it on each subject justifiable? (Sections 5.3 and 5.4.)

F. Information: Is its accuracy optimal? (Section 5.7.)

A.8.3. QUESTIONS IN THE REVIEW OF "POSITIVE" STUDIES

A. To what extent is the empirical relation explicable in terms of the overall bias based on the following:

1. Incomparability of the extraneous effects of the index and reference categories of the determinant. (Section 2.3.1.)

2. Incomparability of the compared populations conditionally on what confounders were "controlled." (Sections 1.5, 2.3.2, and 2.6.)

3. Inadequacy of the empirical scales of the "controlled" confounders. (Section 2.7.)

4. Inadequacy of the procedures of control in the analysis (applied to the "controlled" confounders).

5. Given a primary base, incomparability of outcome information (Sections 2.3.3, 4.4.1, and 5.6.); or, given a base secondary to available cases, lack of representativeness (as to sampling) and/or comparability (as to information) of the reference series. (Sections 4.4.2, 5.2, and 5.6.)

6. Biasedness of the study base. (Section 3.4.)

B. To the extent that an empirical relation remains upon allowance (informal) for the overall bias, how strong would the residual relation be upon allowance for the overall "dilution" from the following:

1. Inaccuracy of the empirical scale of the determinant. (Section 5.7.)
2. Misclassification of the outcomes (nominal). (Section 5.7.)
3. The empirical relation being unduly cross-sectional or unduly longitudinal. (Section 2.4.)

C. Given the strength of the relation after "adjustments" for bias (of the "malignant" sort) and "dilution," what are the relative merits of the hypothesis, quantitatively specified in terms of a prior distribution, and its denial, in explaining that relation? (Section 9.7.2.)

A.8.4. QUESTIONS IN THE REVIEW OF "NEGATIVE" STUDIES

A. Is the study truly "negative" or is it only inconclusive? That is, are the data, on the surface, inconsistent with the hypothesized relation, or are they simply consistent with the denial of the hypothesis, and with the hypothesis as well? (Section 9.3.2.)

B. Insofar as it is "negative" in the proper sense of the word, to what extent is this explicable, under the hypothesis at issue, in terms of the biases and "dilution" mechanisms considered for "positive" studies in Section A.8.3?

APPENDIX 9

Distribution of *P*-Value and Interpretation of Test Results

Insofar as the *P*-value for the "null hypothesis" is used as the summary of evidence in hypothesis testing, it is essential to understand its distribution not only on the "null hypothesis" but also on the hypothesis itself. The null distribution is simple and singular; it is uniform in the range from zero to one. By contrast, the distribution under the hypothesis depends on the amount of information in the study, in addition to the value of the parameter under study.

It is the purpose here to illustrate the latter distributions. It will serve to justify the principles of informal *P*-value interpretation presented in Section 9.3.2. It will also give insight into the proposition that, if the distributions of the *P*-value are examined formally for various values of the parameter, the result is the *LR* function as a summary of the evidence in the data. Thus the larger purpose here is to give further insight into the proposition that the ultimate summary of evidence in the data (apart from issues of validity) is the *LR* function, not only for hypothesis testing but for estimation as well (cf. Section 9.7.2).

It will suffice to consider a single, simple situation and model. Suppose the hypothesis is that the mean M_1 of the outcome criterion in the index category $D = 1$ of the determinant is higher than the mean M_0 in the reference

TABLE A.9.1.

Probability density of the distribution of a *P*-value in selected intervals of its realizations, listed separately for selected values of the "noncentrality parameter" for the test statistic, E_X (the deviation from the null value divided by the standard deviation of its estimate)[a]

P-Value Range	E_X			
	0.00	1.00	3.00	5.00
0.000–0.001	1.0	18	460	970
0.001–0.010	1.0	8.2	32	2.7
0.010–0.050	1.0	4.2	4.1	0.084
0.050–0.100	1.0	2.6	0.90	0.0059
0.200–0.300	1.0	1.2	0.088	
0.400–0.500	1.0	0.69	0.017	
0.800–0.900	1.0	0.22		

[a] Cf. Figure A.9.1.

category $D = 0$; and consider a model on which the outcome variate is Gaussian with mean M_i and variance V, with V known and unrelated to M. Let m_1 and m_0 denote the empirical means, and S_1 and S_0 the numbers of subjects, corresponding to $D = 1$ and $D = 0$, respectively. With these specifications, the test statistic may be taken as

$$X = \frac{m_1 - m_0}{[V(1/S_1 + 1/S_0)]^{1/2}} . \qquad (A.9.1)$$

The appropriate *P*-value is the "upper-tail" value P_{ut}—the probability with which a standard Gaussian variate exceeds X. Thus,

$$P = P_{ut} \qquad (A.9.2)$$
$$= 1 - F_g(X),$$

where $F_g(X)$ is the cumulative probability of the standard Gaussian distribution at the realization of the test statistic. For example, if the test statistic X takes on the value 1.96, $F_g(X) = 0.975$ (Appendix 11) and $P = 0.025$; when $X = -1.96$, $F_g(X) = 0.025$ and $P = 0.975$.

If $M_1 = M_0$ ("null hypothesis"), the test statistic X is a standard Gaussian variate. It follows that $F_g(X)$ has a uniform distribution in the 0–1 range, that is, that $\Pr[F_g(X) < \alpha] = \alpha$ for any α in that range; and as a consequence, $\Pr(P < \alpha) = \alpha$ for $0 \leq \alpha \leq 1$. For example, $\Pr[F_g(X) < 0.975] = \Pr(X < 1.96) = 0.975$, so that $\Pr(P < 0.025) = 1 - \Pr[F_g(X) < 0.975] = 0.025$. Thus, the null probability for any interval of *P*-values equals the width of that interval. For example, the null probability of $0.05 \leq P \leq 0.10 = \Pr(P$

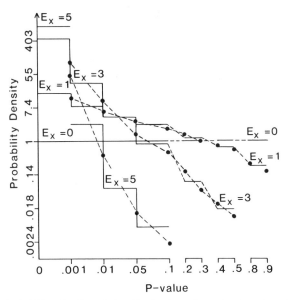

Figure A.9.1. Probability density of the distribution of *P*-value in selected intervals of its realizations, separately for selected values of the "noncentrality parameter" for the test statistic E_X (the deviation from the null value divided by the standard deviation of its estimate) (cf. Table A.9.1). Values of the *LR* function (Equation A.9.7) at the boundary points of the intervals for the *P*-value (cf. Table A.9.2) are also shown.

TABLE A.9.2.

Relation between "upper-tail" *P*-value, *X* statistic (Equation A.9.1), and *LR* (Equation A.9.7), listed separately for selected values of the "noncentrality parameter" for the test statistic, E_X (the deviation from the null value divided by the standard error of the estimator).

P_{ut}	X	$LR = \exp\{E_X[X - \frac{1}{2}E_X]\}$			
		$E_X = 0$	$E_X = 1$	$E_X = 3$	$E_X = 5$
0.001	3.09	1	13	120	19
0.01	2.33	1	6.2	12	0.43
0.05	1.64	1	3.1	1.5	0.014
0.1	1.28	1	2.2	0.52	0.0022
0.2	0.84	1	1.4	0.14	
0.3	0.52	1	1.0	0.053	
0.4	0.25	1	0.8	0.024	
0.5	0.00	1	0.6	0.011	
0.8	−0.84	1	0.26	0.001	
0.9	−1.28	1	0.17		

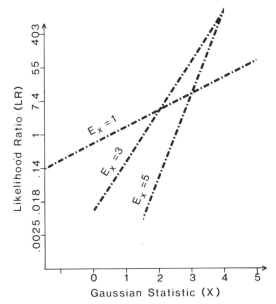

Figure A.9.2. Relation between Gaussian test statistic X (Equation A.9.1) and likelihood ratio LR (Equation A.9.7), for selected values of E_X = (theoretical mean difference)/(standard error of empirical mean difference), assuming, as before, that variance is independent of the mean (cf. Table A.9.3).

< 0.10) $-$ Pr($P < 0.05$) $= 0.10 - 0.05 = 0.05$. By the same token, the probability density of the P-value in any given interval between zero and one (the probability divided by the width of the interval) is one. For example, for the range from $P = 0.05$ to $P = 0.10$, the probability is 0.05, so that the probability density is $0.05/(0.10 - 0.05) = 1$.

If the hypothesis $M_1 > M_0$ is correct, the test statistic is Gaussian with mean

$$E_X = \frac{M_1 - M_0}{[V(1/S_1 + 1/S_0)]^{1/2}} \tag{A.9.3}$$

and variance $V_X = 1$. It is evident that the distribution of the test statistic in the general, nonnull case does indeed depend on the degree of the parameter's deviation ($M_1 - M_0$) from the null value (zero) together with the amount of information in the study, with the latter manifest in (the inverse of the square of) the standard deviation of the estimate of the parameter.

Under this general model for the distribution of the test statistic, for any α in the 0–1 range,

$$\text{Pr}(P < \alpha) = 1 - F_g(g_\alpha - E_X) > \alpha, \tag{A.9.4}$$

with g_α the $100(1 - \alpha)$ centile of the standard Gaussian distribution. For

TABLE A.9.3.

Relation between a Gaussian test statistic X (Equation A.9.1) and LR (Equation A.9.7), for selected values of E_X = (theoretical mean difference)/(standard error of empirical mean difference), assuming that variance is independent of the mean[a]

X	$E_X = 1$		$E_X = 3$		$E_X = 5$	
	Log (LR)	LR	Log (LR)	LR	Log (LR)	LR
−1.5	−2	0.14				
0.0	−0.5	0.61	−4.5	0.01		
1.0	0.5	1.6	−1.5	0.22		
1.5	1.0	2.7	0.0	1.00	−5.0	0.007
2.0	1.5	4.5	1.5	4.5	−2.5	0.082
2.5	2.0	7.4	3.0	20	0.0	1.00
3.0	2.5	12	4.5	90	2.5	12
4.0	3.5	33	7.5	1800	7.5	1800
5.0	4.5	90				

[a] Cf. Figure A.9.2.

example, if the deviation from the null state equals one standard deviation of the estimate ($E_X = 1$), $\Pr(P < 0.025) = 1 - F_g(1.96 - 1) = 1 - F_g(0.96) = 1 - 0.83 = 0.17$. By the same token,

$$\Pr(\alpha_1 < P < \alpha_2) = \Pr(P < \alpha_2) - \Pr(P < \alpha_1) \qquad (A.9.5)$$
$$= F_g(g_{\alpha_1} - E_X) - F_g(g_{\alpha_2} - E_X),$$

and the probability density of the distribution of the P-value, averaged for this interval, is

$$\frac{F_g(g_{\alpha_1} - E_X) - F_g(g_{\alpha_2} - E_X)}{\alpha_2 - \alpha_1}. \qquad (A.9.6)$$

Thus, for the interval $0.05 \leq P \leq 0.10$, the P-value density is $[F_g (1.645 - E_X) - F_g(1.282 - E_X)/(0.10 - 0.05)$, so that with $E_X = 0$ it is $(0.95 - 0.90)/0.05 = 1$, and with $E_X = 1$ it is $[F_g(0.645) - F_g(0.282)]/0.05 = (0.74 - 0.61)/0.05 = 2.6$.

These average densities of the P-value for various intervals of its realizations are given in Table A.9.1, separately for selected values of the "noncentrality parameter" E_X. These densities are also shown in histogram form in Figure A.9.1.

It is seen, once again, that on the "null hypothesis" ($E_X = 0$) the distribution of the P-value is uniform in the 0–1 range, meaning that the probability density is unity for all intervals in that range, that is, that $\Pr(P < \alpha) = \alpha$ for any α in that range (cf. Section 9.3.1).

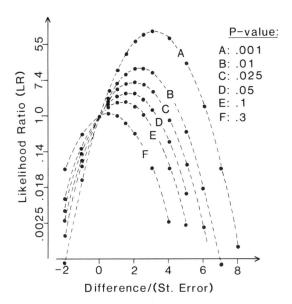

Figure A.9.3.   Translation of *P*-value to *LR* as a function of the parameter divided by its standard error for the situation in which the variance of the estimator is unrelated to the parameter itself (cf. Table A.10.4).

It is evident that if the imprecision of the study is appreciable relative to the parameter's hypothesized deviation from the null value, then the *P*-value (or any other statistic) is not a good discriminator between the hypothesis and its denial. Thus, when the standard error of the estimate of the parameter of interest equals the parameter's hypothesized deviation from the null value ($E_X = 1$), *P*-values that are "significant" ($P < 0.05$), but not "highly significant" ($P < 0.01$), are only 4.2 times as common on the hypothesis as on its denial. Even "very highly significant" values ($P < 0.001$) are only 18 times as common on the hypothesis as on its denial (cf. Table A.9.1). Thus, if the prior probability (P') of the hypothesis is 1%, a "highly significant" *P*-value, unspecified as to detail, means that the posterior credibility (P''), conditional on total validity of the study, is only $1/[1 + (0.99/0.01)/18] = 15\%$ (cf. Section 9.7.2). It is worthy of careful note also that with $E_X = 1$ a "nonsignificant" *P*-value in the 0.05–0.10 range is more common (2.6 times) on the hypothesis than on its denial. Hence, such a *P*-value, insofar as it does serve as evidence, supports the hypothesis rather than detracts from it. The *P*-value that is "neutral" between the hypothesis and its denial, given $E_X = 1$, is $P = 0.31$ (cf. Figure A.9.1); and a value in the 0.8–0.9 range is 22% as common on the hypothesis as when its denial obtains.

If imprecision is small relative to the hypothesized deviation from the null state, small *P*-values can be so common that even a "significant" result may detract from, rather than support, the hypothesis. Thus, if $E_X = 5$, a *P*-

TABLE A.9.4.

Translation of P-value and the value of a Gaussian test statistic to LR [and log (LR)] as a function of E_X (Equation A.9.7), given that variance is unrelated to the mean[a]

E_X	P: 0.001 / X: 3.09	0.01 / 2.33	0.025 / 1.96	0.05 / 1.64	0.1 / 1.28	0.3 / 0.52
−2.0	0.003 (−8.2)	0.001 (−6.7)	0.003 (−5.9)	0.005 (−5.3)	0.01 (−4.6)	0.048 (−3.0)
−1.0	0.028 (−3.6)	0.059 (−2.8)	0.085 (−2.5)	0.12 (−2.1)	0.17 (−1.8)	0.36 (−1.0)
0.0	1.0 (0.0)	1.0 (0.0)	1.0 (0.0)	1.0 (0.0)	1.0 (0.0)	1.0 (0.0)
0.5	4.1 (1.4)	2.8 (1.00)	2.4 (0.86)	2.0 (0.70)	1.7 (0.52)	1.1 (0.14)
1.0	13 (2.6)	6.2 (1.8)	4.3 (1.5)	3.1 (1.1)	2.2 (0.78)	1.0 (0.02)
1.5	33 (3.5)	11 (2.4)	6.1 (1.8)	3.8 (1.3)	2.2 (0.80)	0.71 (−0.35)
2.0	65 (4.2)	14 (2.7)	6.8 (1.9)	3.6 (1.3)	1.8 (0.56)	0.38 (0.96)
2.5	99 (4.6)	15 (2.7)	5.9 (1.8)	2.7 (0.98)	1.1 (0.08)	0.19 (−1.7)
3.0	120 (4.8)	12 (2.5)	4.0 (1.4)	1.5 (0.42)	0.52 (−0.66)	0.0053 (−2.9)
4.0	78 (4.4)	3.7 (1.3)	0.85 (−0.16)	0.24 (−1.4)	0.056 (−2.9)	0.0027 (−5.9)
5.0	19 (3.0)	0.43 (−0.85)	0.067 (−2.7)	0.014 (−4.3)	0.0022 (−6.1)	
6.0	1.7 (0.54)	0.018 (−4.0)	0.0019 (−6.2)			
7.0	0.057 (−2.9)	0.003 (−8.2)				
8.0	0.0007 (−7.3)					

[a] Cf. Figure A.9.3.

value in the 0.05–0.10 range is only 0.6% as common on the hypothesis as on its denial, so that with a prior probability of $P' = 0.50$, for example, the corresponding posterior probability is $P'' = 0.006$. The "neutral" outcome is that which corresponds to $X^2 = (X - 5)^2$, that is, to $X = 2.5$ and, thus, to $P = 0.006$—a "highly significant" value in terms of ordinary language and thought in epidemiology.

It is evident that mechanistic translation of P-values to "significance" and inference, with no regard for the precision of the study, is absurd. For any given realization of the P-value statistic one should compare the null density of unity with the density on particular deviations from the null state under the hypothesis. Since the null density is one, the nonnull density is the likelihood ratio LR. This density equals the Gaussian density ratio at the realization X for the test statistic. The numerator, the nonnull density, is standard Gaussian density at $X - E_X$, and its corresponding denominator, the null density, is the standard Gaussian density of X. Thus the LR, or the nonnull density of the P-value at its realization, is

$$LR = \exp\{-\tfrac{1}{2}[(X - E_X)^2 - X^2]\}$$
$$= \exp\{E_X[X - \tfrac{1}{2}E_X]\}.$$

(A.9.7)

This alternative to the P-value metameter of X, for selected values of E_X, is depicted in Figure A.9.1 and tabulated in Table A.9.2. The corresponding functions of X itself are shown in Figure A.9.2 and given numerically in Table A.9.3. The ultimate interest is in LR as a function of E_X conditional on the X-value (and its associated P-value) actually obtained. These relations, for selected values of X, are shown in Figure A.9.3 and Table A.9.4. Their interpretation is discussed in Section 9.7.2.

APPENDIX 10

Some Probability Models

A.10.1. BINOMIAL DISTRIBUTIONS

Consider a set of N independent "trials," with the same probability P of "success" in each. The total number of "successes" X is a *binomial* random variate. Specifically,

$$X \sim B(P, N), \tag{A.10.1}$$

where B denotes "binomial" (and the parameters of the particular binomial distribution are specified in the parentheses).

Evidently, the range of possible values for the variate is

$$0 \leq X \leq N. \tag{A.10.2}$$

The probability of any particular realization $X = x$ within that range is

$$\Pr(X = x) = C_{N,x} P^x (1 - P)^{N-x}, \tag{A.10.3}$$

where

$$C_{N,x} = \frac{N!}{[x!(N - x)!]}. \tag{A.10.4}$$

The expectation (mean) and variance of this distribution are

$$E = NP \tag{A.10.5}$$

and

$$V = NP(1 - P), \tag{A.10.6}$$

respectively.

A.10.2. POISSON DISTRIBUTIONS

A special case of the binomial family of models that is commonly of interest in epidemiology is the Poisson family of distributions. It is the limiting case when N approaches infinity and P approaches zero, with $NP = E$ remaining finite and nonzero.

In the Poisson case, the range of possible values for the random variate is the entirety of nonnegative integers:

$$0 \le X \le \infty. \tag{A.10.7}$$

In this limiting case, the binomial probability model assumes the form

$$\begin{aligned} \Pr(X = x) &= \frac{e^{-E}E^x}{x!} \\ &= \frac{[\exp(-E)]E^x}{x!}, \end{aligned} \tag{A.10.8}$$

where e is the base of natural logarithms and, as before, E is the expected number of events.

In the Poisson case of binomial distributions, $NP = NP(1 - P)$, so that variance equals expectation,

$$V = E. \tag{A.10.9}$$

A.10.3. HYPERGEOMETRIC DISTRIBUTIONS

Consider two independent binomial variates with identical probabilities of "success,"

$$\begin{aligned} X_1 &\sim B(P, N_1) \\ X_2 &\sim B(P, N_2). \end{aligned} \tag{A.10.10}$$

The distribution of one of these binomial variates conditional on the sum of the two has a hypergeometric distribution. Thus,

$$(X_1 \mid X_1 + X_2 = M_1) \sim H(M_1, N_1, T), \qquad (A.10.11)$$

where $T = N_1 + N_2$. Similarly,

$$(X_2 \mid X_1 + X_2 = M_1) \sim H(M_1, N_2, T). \qquad (A.10.12)$$

The range of possible values for X_1 is

$$\max(0, M_1 - N_2) \le X_1 \le \min(M_1, N_1). \qquad (A.10.13)$$

The probability of $X_1 = x_1$ within that range is

$$\Pr(X_1 = x_1) = \frac{C_{N_1, x_1} C_{N_2, x_2}}{C_{T, M_1}}. \qquad (A.10.14)$$

where $x_2 = M_1 - x_1$, and the expectation and variance for X_1 are

$$E = \frac{M_1 N_1}{T}$$

$$V = \frac{M_1 M_2 N_1 N_2}{[T^2(T - 1)]}, \qquad (A.10.15)$$

respectively, with $M_2 = T - M_1$ and $N_2 = T - N_1$.

The hypergeometric distribution of X_1 has binomial distributions as limiting cases. For example,

$$\frac{M_1}{T} \to 0$$

$$\Rightarrow H(M_1, N_1, T) \to B\left(\frac{N_1}{T}, M_1\right) \qquad (A.10.16)$$

where $N_1/T = P$ and $M_1 = N$ in terms of the notation in Section A.9.1. Similarly,

$$\frac{N_1}{T} \to 0$$

$$\Rightarrow H(M_1, N_1, T) \to B\left(\frac{M_1}{T}, N_1\right) \qquad (A.10.17)$$

When both of these conditions obtain, the limit is a Poisson distribution:

$$\frac{M_1}{T} \to 0, \qquad \frac{N_1}{T} \to 0$$

$$\Rightarrow H(M_1, N_1, T) \to P\left(\frac{M_1 N_1}{T}\right). \tag{A.10.18}$$

The computation of hypergeometric probabilities is facilitated by the use of recursion formulas. Thus,

$$\Pr(X_1 = x_1 + 1) = \Pr(X_1 = x_1) \frac{(x_1 + 1)(N_1 - x_1)}{x_2(N_2 - x_2 + 1)} \tag{A.10.19}$$

and

$$\Pr(X_1 = x_1 - 1) = \Pr(X_1 = x_1) \frac{(x_2 + 1)(N_2 - x_2)}{x_1(N_1 - x_1 + 1)}, \tag{A.10.20}$$

where $x_2 = M_1 - x_1$.

A.10.4. NONCENTRAL HYPERGEOMETRIC DISTRIBUTIONS

In the hypergeometric distribution, the two underlying independent binomial distributions have, as was noted, identical probabilities for the event, that is, $P_1 = P_2$. In this way, the hypergeometric distributions are subsumed under the more general case of $P_1 \neq P_2$. For this generalization, the *non-central hypergeometric* distributions, the probability of $X_1 = x_1$ is

$$\Pr(X_1 = x_1) = \frac{C_{N_1, x_1} C_{N_2, x_2} (OR)^{x_1}}{\sum_i C_{N_1, i} C_{N_2 M_1 - i,} (OR)^{i}}, \tag{A.10.21}$$

where OR represents the odds ratio, that is,

$$OR = \frac{P_1/(1 - P_1)}{P_2/(1 - P_2)}, \tag{A.10.22}$$

and the summation ranges over the range of possible realizations for X_1 (Equation A.10.13).

The OR and expectation E of X_1 have the asymptotic relation

$$OR = \frac{E(T - M_1 - N_1 + E)}{(M_1 - E)(N_1 - E)}. \tag{A.10.23}$$

Given that the expectation of X_1 is E, the corresponding asymptotic variance (first-order Taylor-series approximation) is

$$V = \left[\frac{1}{E} + \frac{1}{M_1 - E} + \frac{1}{N_1 - E}\right.$$
$$\left. + \frac{1}{T - M_1 - N_1 + E}\right]^{-1}. \qquad (A.10.24)$$

A.10.5. GAUSSIAN DISTRIBUTIONS

All of the probability models above deal with discrete distributions, ones in which the random variate takes on integer values only.

Among statistical models for *continuous* distributions, the most important one, by far, for epidemiologic purposes is the *Gaussian*, or *normal*, distribution model. The basis for this is not that health-outcome characteristics or their determinants tend to have Gaussian distributions among individuals; they do not. Instead, various evidence-summarizing *statistics* have approximately Gaussian *sampling distributions*, and the more closely Gaussian the greater the amount of information in the data.

A Gaussian variate has a range that covers all possible values on the real-number axis:

$$-\infty \le X \le \infty. \qquad (A.10.25)$$

Since the distribution is continuous, any given realization has a probability of zero. For this reason, the probability model specifies only the *probability density* for various values of the random variate. This density function is

$$f(X = x) = (2\pi V)^{-1/2}\exp\left[-\frac{1}{2}\frac{(x - E)^2}{V}\right], \qquad (A.10.26)$$

where, as before, E and V denote the expectation and variance of the distribution (and "exp" means "antilog base e").

The probability for any given range of the distribution is derived, in principle, by integrating the density function over that range. Alternatively, such a probability is the difference between the cumulative probabilities at the upper and lower bounds of the range.

For reading such probabilities, it suffices to have access to a tabulation of the cumulative probabilities for the *standard Gaussian distribution*, characterized by $E = 0$ and $V = 1$. The basis for this is the relation of

$$\Pr[G(E, V) < x] = \Pr\left[G(0, 1) < \frac{x - E}{V^{1/2}}\right]. \qquad (A.10.27)$$

The complement of the cumulative probabilities for various values of a standard Gaussian variate are tabulated in Appendix 11.

APPENDIX 11

P-Value from Standard Gaussian Statistic

The table presented below lists various positive realizations g for a standard Gaussian test statistic G. Next to each realization is given the corresponding exceedance probability $\Pr(G > g)$, which is the "upper-tail" P-value P_{ut}. The corresponding "lower-tail" P-value is $1 - P_{ut}$. For any realization $g < 0$, the corresponding "lower-tail" P-value equals the P_{ut} for $|g|$, and the "upper-tail" value is again its complement.

g	P_{ut}	g	P_{ut}	g	P_{ut}	g	P_{ut}
0.00	0.50	1.00	0.16	2.00	0.023	3.00	0.0014
0.05	0.48	1.05	0.15	2.05	0.020	3.10	0.00097
0.10	0.46	1.10	0.14	2.10	0.018	3.20	0.00069
0.15	0.44	1.15	0.13	2.15	0.016	3.30	0.00048
0.20	0.42	1.20	0.12	2.20	0.014	3.40	0.00034
0.25	0.40	1.25	0.11	2.25	0.012	3.50	0.00023
0.30	0.38	1.30	0.10	2.30	0.011	3.60	0.00016
0.35	0.36	1.35	0.089	2.35	0.0094	3.70	0.00011
0.40	0.34	1.40	0.081	2.40	0.0082	3.80	0.000072
0.45	0.33	1.45	0.074	2.45	0.0071	3.90	0.000048
0.50	0.31	1.50	0.067	2.50	0.0062	4.00	0.000032
0.55	0.29	1.55	0.061	2.55	0.0054	4.10	0.000021
0.60	0.27	1.60	0.055	2.60	0.0047	4.20	0.000013
0.65	0.26	1.65	0.049	2.65	0.0040	4.30	0.000009
0.70	0.24	1.70	0.045	2.70	0.0035	4.40	0.000005
0.75	0.23	1.75	0.040	2.75	0.0030	4.50	0.000003
0.80	0.21	1.80	0.036	2.80	0.0026	4.60	0.000002
0.85	0.20	1.85	0.032	2.85	0.0022	4.70	0.000001
0.90	0.18	1.90	0.029	2.90	0.0019	4.80	0.000001
0.95	0.17	1.95	0.026	2.95	0.0016	4.90	0.000000

APPENDIX 12

P-Value from Chi Square Statistic

The table presented below lists various realizations X^2 for a chi square statistic (1 df). Next to each realization is given the corresponding exceedance probability $\Pr(\chi^2 > X^2)$, which is the "two-tailed" P-value P_{tt}. The corresponding "upper-tail" P-value is either $P_{ut} = (\frac{1}{2})P_{tt}$ or $P_{ut} = 1 - (\frac{1}{2})P_{tt}$, according to whether empirical association is positive or negative, and $P_{1t} = 1 - P_{ut}$ (cf. Equations 10.8 and 10.9).

X^2	P_{tt}	X^2	P_{tt}	X^2	P_{tt}	X^2	P_{tt}
0.0	1.00	2.5	0.11	5.0	0.025	7.5	0.0062
0.1	0.75	2.6	0.11	5.1	0.024	7.6	0.0058
0.2	0.66	2.7	0.10	5.2	0.023	7.7	0.0055
0.3	0.58	2.8	0.094	5.3	0.021	7.8	0.0052
0.4	0.53	2.9	0.089	5.4	0.020	7.9	0.0049
0.5	0.48	3.0	0.083	5.5	0.019	8.0	0.0047
0.6	0.44	3.1	0.078	5.6	0.018	8.2	0.0042
0.7	0.40	3.2	0.074	5.7	0.017	8.4	0.0037
0.8	0.37	3.3	0.069	5.8	0.016	8.6	0.0034
0.9	0.34	3.4	0.065	5.9	0.015	8.8	0.0030
1.0	0.32	3.5	0.061	6.0	0.014	9.0	0.0027
1.1	0.29	3.6	0.058	6.1	0.014	9.2	0.0024
1.2	0.27	3.7	0.054	6.2	0.013	9.4	0.0022
1.3	0.25	3.8	0.051	6.3	0.012	9.6	0.0019
1.4	0.24	3.9	0.048	6.4	0.011	9.8	0.0017
1.5	0.22	4.0	0.046	6.5	0.011	10.0	0.0016
1.6	0.21	4.1	0.043	6.6	0.010	10.5	0.0012
1.7	0.19	4.2	0.040	6.7	0.0096	11.0	0.00091
1.8	0.18	4.3	0.038	6.8	0.0091	11.5	0.00070
1.9	0.17	4.4	0.036	6.9	0.0086	12.0	0.00053
2.0	0.16	4.5	0.034	7.0	0.0082	12.5	0.00041
2.1	0.15	4.6	0.032	7.1	0.0077	13.0	0.00031
2.2	0.14	4.7	0.030	7.2	0.0073	13.5	0.00024
2.3	0.13	4.8	0.028	7.3	0.0069	14.0	0.00018
2.4	0.12	4.9	0.027	7.4	0.0065	14.5	0.00014

APPENDIX 13

Analysis of Matched Series:

Variance Estimates for X^2 Functions of Rate Difference and Rate Ratio

A.13.1. RATE DIFFERENCE (EQUATION 12.20)

R	RD	u	v	$\bar{R}_0$	$\bar{V}_{RD}$
1	-.5	1	1	1.000	0.500
		1	0	0.750	0.750
		0	1	0.750	0.750
		0	0	0.500	0.500
	-.4	1	1	1.000	0.480
		1	0	0.700	0.840
		0	1	0.700	0.840
		0	0	0.400	0.480
	-.3	1	1	1.000	0.420
		1	0	0.650	0.910
		0	1	0.650	0.910
		0	0	0.300	0.420
	-.2	1	1	1.000	0.320
		1	0	0.600	0.960
		0	1	0.600	0.960
		0	0	0.200	0.320
	-.1	1	1	1.000	0.180
		1	0	0.550	0.990
		0	1	0.550	0.990
		0	0	0.100	0.180
	.0	1	1	1.000	0.000
		1	0	0.500	1.000
		0	1	0.500	1.000
		0	0	0.000	0.000
	.1	1	1	0.900	0.180
		1	0	0.450	0.990
		0	1	0.450	0.990
		0	0	0.000	0.180
	.2	1	1	0.800	0.320
		1	0	0.400	0.960
		0	1	0.400	0.960
		0	0	0.000	0.320
	.3	1	1	0.700	0.420
		1	0	0.350	0.910
		0	1	0.350	0.910
		0	0	0.000	0.420
	.4	1	1	0.600	0.480
		1	0	0.300	0.840
		0	1	0.300	0.840
		0	0	0.000	0.480
	.5	1	1	0.500	0.500
		1	0	0.250	0.750
		0	1	0.250	0.750
		0	0	0.000	0.500

R	RD	u	v	$\bar{R}_0$	$\bar{V}_{RD}$
2	-.5	1	2	1.000	0.375
		1	1	0.788	0.433
		1	0	0.666	0.374
		0	2	1.000	0.375
		0	1	0.500	0.188
		0	0	0.500	0.188
	-.4	1	2	1.000	0.360
		1	1	0.757	0.482
		1	0	0.600	0.420
		0	2	0.933	0.420
		0	1	0.400	0.180
		0	0	0.400	0.180
	-.3	1	2	1.000	0.315
		1	1	0.729	0.516
		1	0	0.533	0.455
		0	2	0.866	0.455
		0	1	0.373	0.277
		0	0	0.300	0.158
	-.2	1	2	1.000	0.240
		1	1	0.705	0.531
		1	0	0.466	0.479
		0	2	0.800	0.480
		0	1	0.362	0.377
		0	0	0.200	0.120
	-.1	1	2	1.000	0.135
		1	1	0.684	0.527
		1	0	0.399	0.494
		0	2	0.733	0.495
		0	1	0.348	0.450
		0	0	0.100	0.068
	.0	1	2	1.000	0.000
		1	1	0.666	0.500
		1	0	0.333	0.500
		0	2	0.666	0.500
		0	1	0.333	0.500
		0	0	0.000	0.000
	.1	1	2	0.900	0.068
		1	1	0.651	0.451
		1	0	0.266	0.494
		0	2	0.600	0.495
		0	1	0.315	0.526
		0	0	0.000	0.135
	.2	1	2	0.800	0.120
		1	1	0.637	0.378
		1	0	0.200	0.480
		0	2	0.533	0.480
		0	1	0.294	0.531
		0	0	0.000	0.240
	.3	1	2	0.700	0.158
		1	1	0.626	0.278
		1	0	0.133	0.455
		0	2	0.466	0.455
		0	1	0.270	0.515
		0	0	0.000	0.315
	.4	1	2	0.600	0.180
		1	1	0.600	0.180
		1	0	0.066	0.419
		0	2	0.400	0.420
		0	1	0.242	0.482
		0	0	0.000	0.360
	.5	1	2	0.500	0.188
		1	1	0.500	0.188
		1	0	0.000	0.375
		0	2	0.333	0.375
		0	1	0.211	0.433
		0	0	0.000	0.375

R	RD	u	v	$\tilde{R}_0$	$\tilde{V}_{RD}$	RD	u	v	$\tilde{R}_0$	$\tilde{V}_{RD}$
3	-.5	1	3	1.000	0.333	.1	1	3	0.900	0.040
		1	2	0.820	0.356		1	2	0.742	0.262
		1	1	0.695	0.304		1	1	0.477	0.436
		1	0	0.625	0.250		1	0	0.175	0.330
		0	3	1.000	0.333		0	3	0.675	0.330
		0	2	0.578	0.204		0	2	0.472	0.437
		0	1	0.500	0.111		0	1	0.240	0.380
		0	0	0.500	0.111		0	0	0.000	0.120
	-.4	1	3	1.000	0.320	.2	1	3	0.800	0.071
		1	2	0.800	0.391		1	2	0.735	0.168
		1	1	0.644	0.348		1	1	0.458	0.410
		1	0	0.549	0.279		1	0	0.100	0.320
		0	3	1.000	0.320		0	3	0.600	0.320
		0	2	0.568	0.295		0	2	0.439	0.417
		0	1	0.400	0.107		0	1	0.229	0.405
		0	0	0.400	0.107		0	0	0.000	0.213
	-.3	1	3	1.000	0.280	.3	1	3	0.700	0.093
		1	2	0.783	0.408		1	2	0.700	0.093
		1	1	0.600	0.387		1	1	0.443	0.364
		1	0	0.475	0.303		1	0	0.025	0.303
		0	3	0.975	0.303		0	3	0.525	0.303
		0	2	0.566	0.370		0	2	0.399	0.387
		0	1	0.300	0.093		0	1	0.216	0.408
		0	0	0.300	0.093		0	0	0.000	0.280
	-.2	1	3	1.000	0.213	.4	1	3	0.600	0.107
		1	2	0.770	0.406		1	2	0.600	0.107
		1	1	0.560	0.417		1	1	0.431	0.296
		1	0	0.400	0.320		1	0	0.000	0.320
		0	3	0.900	0.320		0	3	0.450	0.280
		0	2	0.541	0.410		0	2	0.355	0.348
		0	1	0.264	0.166		0	1	0.200	0.391
		0	0	0.200	0.071		0	0	0.000	0.320
	-.1	1	3	1.000	0.120	.5	1	3	0.500	0.111
		1	2	0.759	0.381		1	2	0.500	0.111
		1	1	0.527	0.437		1	1	0.421	0.205
		1	0	0.325	0.330		1	0	0.000	0.333
		0	3	0.825	0.330		0	3	0.375	0.250
		0	2	0.522	0.436		0	2	0.304	0.304
		0	1	0.257	0.261		0	1	0.179	0.356
		0	0	0.100	0.040		0	0	0.000	0.333
	.0	1	3	1.000	0.000					
		1	2	0.750	0.333					
		1	1	0.500	0.444					
		1	0	0.250	0.333					
		0	3	0.750	0.333					
		0	2	0.500	0.444					
		0	1	0.250	0.333					
		0	0	0.000	0.000					

(*continued*)

A.13.1. (continued)

R	RD	u	v	$\tilde{R}_0$	$\tilde{V}_{RD}$	RD	u	v	$\tilde{R}_0$	$\tilde{V}_{RD}$
4	-.5	1	4	1.000	0.313	.1	1	4	0.900	0.028
		1	3	0.844	0.323		1	3	0.795	0.168
		1	2	0.723	0.279		1	2	0.588	0.344
		1	1	0.644	0.226		1	1	0.373	0.385
		1	0	0.600	0.188		1	0	0.120	0.248
		0	4	1.000	0.313		0	4	0.720	0.248
		0	3	0.683	0.255		0	3	0.566	0.355
		0	2	0.500	0.078		0	2	0.385	0.386
		0	1	0.500	0.078		0	1	0.194	0.308
		0	0	0.500	0.078		0	0	0.000	0.113
	-.4	1	4	1.000	0.300	.2	1	4	0.800	0.050
		1	3	0.831	0.350		1	3	0.791	0.063
		1	2	0.687	0.323		1	2	0.578	0.292
		1	1	0.582	0.262		1	1	0.353	0.380
		1	0	0.520	0.210		1	0	0.040	0.240
		0	4	1.000	0.300		0	4	0.640	0.240
		0	3	0.674	0.317		0	3	0.524	0.328
		0	2	0.436	0.120		0	2	0.366	0.380
		0	1	0.400	0.075		0	1	0.187	0.344
		0	0	0.400	0.075		0	0	0.000	0.200
	-.3	1	4	1.000	0.263	.3	1	4	0.700	0.066
		1	3	0.820	0.358		1	3	0.700	0.066
		1	2	0.657	0.357		1	2	0.570	0.218
		1	1	0.525	0.296		1	1	0.337	0.359
		1	0	0.440	0.228		1	0	0.000	0.263
		0	4	1.000	0.263		0	4	0.560	0.228
		0	3	0.662	0.359		0	3	0.474	0.297
		0	2	0.429	0.217		0	2	0.342	0.358
		0	1	0.300	0.066		0	1	0.179	0.358
		0	0	0.300	0.066		0	0	0.000	0.263
	-.2	1	4	1.000	0.200	.4	1	4	0.600	0.075
		1	3	0.812	0.345		1	3	0.600	0.075
		1	2	0.633	0.379		1	2	0.563	0.121
		1	1	0.475	0.327		1	1	0.325	0.318
		1	0	0.360	0.240		1	0	0.000	0.300
		0	4	0.959	0.241		0	4	0.480	0.210
		0	3	0.646	0.380		0	3	0.417	0.263
		0	2	0.421	0.291		0	2	0.312	0.323
		0	1	0.208	0.061		0	1	0.168	0.350
		0	0	0.200	0.050		0	0	0.000	0.300
	-.1	1	4	1.000	0.113	.5	1	4	0.500	0.078
		1	3	0.805	0.309		1	3	0.500	0.078
		1	2	0.614	0.386		1	2	0.500	0.078
		1	1	0.433	0.354		1	1	0.316	0.255
		1	0	0.279	0.247		1	0	0.000	0.313
		0	4	0.879	0.248		0	4	0.400	0.188
		0	3	0.626	0.385		0	3	0.355	0.227
		0	2	0.411	0.343		0	2	0.276	0.280
		0	1	0.204	0.167		0	1	0.155	0.323
		0	0	0.100	0.028		0	0	0.000	0.313
	.0	1	4	1.000	0.000					
		1	3	0.800	0.250					
		1	2	0.600	0.375					
		1	1	0.400	0.375					
		1	0	0.200	0.250					
		0	4	0.799	0.251					
		0	3	0.600	0.375					
		0	2	0.400	0.375					
		0	1	0.200	0.250					
		0	0	0.000	0.000					

R	RD	u	v	$\bar{R}_0$	$\bar{V}_{RD}$	RD	u	v	$\bar{R}_0$	$\bar{V}_{RD}$
5	-.5	1	5	1.000	0.300	.0	0	5	0.833	0.200
		1	4	0.864	0.306		0	4	0.666	0.320
		1	3	0.750	0.270		0	3	0.500	0.360
		1	2	0.666	0.220		0	2	0.333	0.320
		1	1	0.614	0.178		0	1	0.166	0.199
		1	0	0.583	0.150		0	0	0.000	0.000
		0	5	1.000	0.300	.1	1	5	0.900	0.022
		0	4	0.749	0.270		1	4	0.830	0.112
		0	3	0.547	0.113		1	3	0.659	0.273
		0	2	0.500	0.060		1	2	0.485	0.351
		0	1	0.500	0.060		1	1	0.304	0.340
		0	0	0.500	0.060		1	0	0.083	0.198
	-.4	1	5	1.000	0.288		0	5	0.749	0.199
		1	4	0.854	0.327		0	4	0.628	0.294
		1	3	0.723	0.310		0	3	0.480	0.352
		1	2	0.617	0.261		0	2	0.323	0.345
		1	1	0.544	0.207		0	1	0.162	0.265
		1	0	0.500	0.168		0	0	0.000	0.108
		0	5	1.000	0.288	.2	1	5	0.800	0.038
		0	4	0.741	0.316		1	4	0.800	0.038
		0	3	0.542	0.206		1	3	0.653	0.205
		0	2	0.400	0.058		1	2	0.473	0.324
		0	1	0.400	0.058		1	1	0.284	0.348
		0	0	0.400	0.058		1	0	0.000	0.192
	-.3	1	5	1.000	0.252		0	5	0.666	0.193
		1	4	0.847	0.328		0	4	0.579	0.265
		1	3	0.703	0.339		0	3	0.455	0.331
		1	2	0.576	0.298		0	2	0.312	0.351
		1	1	0.478	0.235		0	1	0.158	0.308
		1	0	0.416	0.181		0	0	0.000	0.192
		0	5	1.000	0.252	.3	1	5	0.700	0.050
		0	4	0.730	0.341		1	4	0.700	0.050
		0	3	0.534	0.275		1	3	0.648	0.114
		0	2	0.351	0.113		1	2	0.465	0.275
		0	1	0.300	0.050		1	1	0.269	0.341
		0	0	0.300	0.050		1	0	0.000	0.252
	-.2	1	5	1.000	0.192		0	5	0.583	0.182
		1	4	0.841	0.308		0	4	0.521	0.236
		1	3	0.687	0.351		0	3	0.423	0.299
		1	2	0.544	0.330		0	2	0.296	0.339
		1	1	0.420	0.264		0	1	0.152	0.328
		1	0	0.333	0.192		0	0	0.000	0.252
		0	5	1.000	0.192	.4	1	5	0.600	0.058
		0	4	0.715	0.349		1	4	0.600	0.058
		0	3	0.526	0.324		1	3	0.600	0.058
		0	2	0.346	0.204		1	2	0.457	0.207
		0	1	0.200	0.038		1	1	0.258	0.316
		0	0	0.200	0.038		1	0	0.000	0.288
	-.1	1	5	1.000	0.108		0	5	0.500	0.168
		1	4	0.837	0.265		0	4	0.455	0.208
		1	3	0.676	0.346		0	3	0.382	0.261
		1	2	0.519	0.352		0	2	0.276	0.311
		1	1	0.371	0.293		0	1	0.145	0.327
		1	0	0.249	0.197		0	0	0.000	0.288
		0	5	0.916	0.199	.5	1	5	0.500	0.060
		0	4	0.695	0.340		1	4	0.500	0.060
		0	3	0.514	0.351		1	3	0.500	0.060
		0	2	0.340	0.273		1	2	0.452	0.114
		0	1	0.169	0.111		1	1	0.250	0.270
		0	0	0.100	0.022		1	0	0.000	0.300
	.0	1	5	1.000	0.000		0	5	0.416	0.151
		1	4	0.833	0.200		0	4	0.385	0.179
		1	3	0.666	0.320		0	3	0.333	0.220
		1	2	0.500	0.360		0	2	0.250	0.270
		1	1	0.333	0.320		0	1	0.135	0.306
		1	0	0.166	0.199		0	0	0.000	0.300

A.13.2. RATE RATIO (EQUATION 13.19)

R	RR	u	v	$\tilde{R}_0$	$\tilde{V}_{r_1-(RR)r_0}$	R	RR	u	v	$\tilde{R}_0$	$\tilde{V}_{r_1-(RR)r_0}$
1	0.2	1	1	1.000	0.320	2	0.2	1	2	1.000	0.240
		1	0	0.500	0.200			1	1	0.667	0.180
		0	1	1.000	0.320			1	0	0.333	0.100
		0	0	0.000	0.000			0	2	1.000	0.240
								0	1	0.472	0.136
								0	0	0.000	0.000
	0.4	1	1	1.000	0.480		0.4	1	2	1.000	0.360
		1	0	0.500	0.400			1	1	0.667	0.320
		0	1	1.000	0.480			1	0	0.333	0.200
		0	0	0.000	0.000			0	2	1.000	0.360
								0	1	0.440	0.247
								0	0	0.000	0.000
	0.6	1	1	1.000	0.480		0.6	1	2	1.000	0.360
		1	0	0.500	0.600			1	1	0.667	0.420
		0	1	0.833	0.600			1	0	0.333	0.300
		0	0	0.000	0.000			0	2	1.000	0.360
								0	1	0.405	0.341
								0	0	0.000	0.000
	0.8	1	1	1.000	0.320		0.8	1	2	1.000	0.240
		1	0	0.500	0.800			1	1	0.667	0.480
		0	1	0.625	0.800			1	0	0.333	0.400
		0	0	0.000	0.000			0	2	0.833	0.400
								0	1	0.368	0.423
								0	0	0.000	0.000
	1.0	1	1	1.000	0.000		1.0	1	2	1.000	0.000
		1	0	0.500	1.000			1	1	0.667	0.500
		0	1	0.500	1.000			1	0	0.333	0.500
		0	0	0.000	0.000			0	2	0.667	0.500
								0	1	0.333	0.500
								0	0	0.000	0.000
	1.5	1	1	0.667	1.000		1.5	1	2	0.667	0.375
		1	0	0.500	1.500			1	1	0.667	0.375
		0	1	0.333	1.500			1	0	0.333	0.750
		0	0	0.000	0.000			0	2	0.444	0.750
								0	1	0.262	0.684
								0	0	0.000	0.000
	2.0	1	1	0.500	2.000		2.0	1	2	0.500	0.750
		1	0	0.500	2.000			1	1	0.500	0.750
		0	1	0.250	2.000			1	0	0.333	1.000
		0	0	0.000	0.000			0	2	0.333	1.000
								0	1	0.211	0.866
								0	0	0.000	0.000
	2.5	1	1	0.400	3.000		2.5	1	2	0.400	1.125
		1	0	0.400	3.000			1	1	0.400	1.125
		0	1	0.200	2.500			1	0	0.333	1.250
		0	0	0.000	0.000			0	2	0.267	1.250
								0	1	0.176	1.050
								0	0	0.000	0.000
	3.0	1	1	0.333	4.000		3.0	1	2	0.333	1.500
		1	0	0.333	4.000			1	1	0.333	1.500
		0	1	0.167	3.000			1	0	0.333	1.500
		0	0	0.000	0.000			0	2	0.222	1.500
								0	1	0.150	1.234
								0	0	0.000	0.000
	4.0	1	1	0.250	6.000		4.0	1	2	0.250	2.250
		1	0	0.250	6.000			1	1	0.250	2.250
		0	1	0.125	4.000			1	0	0.250	2.250
		0	0	0.000	0.000			0	2	0.167	2.000
								0	1	0.116	1.606
								0	0	0.000	0.000
	5.0	1	1	0.200	8.000		5.0	1	2	0.200	3.000
		1	0	0.200	8.000			1	1	0.200	3.000
		0	1	0.100	5.000			1	0	0.200	3.000
		0	0	0.000	0.000			0	2	0.133	2.500
								0	1	0.094	1.978
								0	0	0.000	0.000

R	RR	u	v	$\bar{R}_0$	$\bar{V}_{r_1-(RR)r_0}$	RR	u	v	$\bar{R}_0$	$\bar{V}_{r_1-(RR)r_0}$
3	0.2	1	3	1.000	0.213	2.0	1	3	0.500	0.444
		1	2	0.750	0.173		1	2	0.500	0.444
		1	1	0.500	0.124		1	1	0.500	0.444
		1	0	0.250	0.067		1	0	0.250	0.667
		0	3	1.000	0.213		0	3	0.375	0.667
		0	2	0.649	0.155		0	2	0.305	0.694
		0	1	0.318	0.083		0	1	0.180	0.569
		0	0	0.000	0.000		0	0	0.000	0.000
	0.4	1	3	1.000	0.320	2.5	1	3	0.400	0.667
		1	2	0.750	0.293		1	2	0.400	0.667
		1	1	0.500	0.231		1	1	0.400	0.667
		1	0	0.250	0.133		1	0	0.250	0.833
		0	3	1.000	0.320		0	3	0.300	0.833
		0	2	0.625	0.267		0	2	0.250	0.833
		0	1	0.301	0.156		0	1	0.155	0.680
		0	0	0.000	0.000		0	0	0.000	0.000
	0.6	1	3	1.000	0.320	3.0	1	3	0.333	0.889
		1	2	0.750	0.360		1	2	0.333	0.889
		1	1	0.500	0.320		1	1	0.333	0.889
		1	0	0.250	0.200		1	0	0.250	1.000
		0	3	1.000	0.320		0	3	0.250	1.000
		0	2	0.592	0.344		0	2	0.211	0.976
		0	1	0.284	0.221		0	1	0.136	0.791
		0	0	0.000	0.000		0	0	0.000	0.000
	0.8	1	3	1.000	0.213	4.0	1	3	0.250	1.333
		1	2	0.750	0.373		1	2	0.250	1.333
		1	1	0.500	0.391		1	1	0.250	1.333
		1	0	0.250	0.267		1	0	0.250	1.333
		0	3	0.938	0.267		0	3	0.188	1.333
		0	2	0.549	0.399		0	2	0.161	1.266
		0	1	0.267	0.280		0	1	0.108	1.011
		0	0	0.000	0.000		0	0	0.000	0.000
	1.0	1	3	1.000	0.000	5.0	1	3	0.200	1.778
		1	2	0.750	0.333		1	2	0.200	1.778
		1	1	0.500	0.444		1	1	0.200	1.778
		1	0	0.250	0.333		1	0	0.200	1.778
		0	3	0.750	0.333		0	3	0.150	1.667
		0	2	0.500	0.444		0	2	0.130	1.559
		0	1	0.250	0.333		0	1	0.089	1.232
		0	0	0.000	0.000		0	0	0.000	0.000
	1.5	1	3	0.667	0.222					
		1	2	0.667	0.222					
		1	1	0.500	0.500					
		1	0	0.250	0.500					
		0	3	0.500	0.500					
		0	2	0.386	0.562					
		0	1	0.211	0.455					
		0	0	0.000	0.000					

(*continued*)

A.13.2. (continued)

R	RR	u	v	$\bar{R}_0$	$\bar{V}_{r_1-(RR)r_0}$	RR	u	v	$\bar{R}_0$	$\bar{V}_{r_1-(RR)r_0}$
4	0.2	1	4	1.000	0.200	2.0	1	4	0.500	0.313
		1	3	0.800	0.170		1	3	0.500	0.313
		1	2	0.600	0.135		1	2	0.500	0.313
		1	1	0.400	0.095		1	1	0.400	0.500
		1	0	0.200	0.050		1	0	0.200	0.500
		0	4	1.000	0.200		0	4	0.400	0.500
		0	3	0.739	0.160		0	3	0.355	0.544
		0	2	0.486	0.113		0	2	0.276	0.559
		0	1	0.240	0.059		0	1	0.155	0.431
		0	0	0.000	0.000		0	0	0.000	0.000
	0.4	1	4	1.000	0.300	2.5	1	4	0.400	0.469
		1	3	0.800	0.280		1	3	0.400	0.469
		1	2	0.600	0.240		1	2	0.400	0.469
		1	1	0.400	0.180		1	1	0.400	0.469
		1	0	0.200	0.100		1	0	0.200	0.625
		0	4	1.000	0.300		0	4	0.320	0.625
		0	3	0.722	0.267		0	3	0.289	0.652
		0	2	0.469	0.203		0	2	0.233	0.653
		0	1	0.230	0.113		0	1	0.137	0.513
		0	0	0.000	0.000		0	0	0.000	0.000
	0.6	1	4	1.000	0.300	3.0	1	4	0.333	0.625
		1	3	0.800	0.330		1	3	0.333	0.625
		1	2	0.600	0.315		1	2	0.333	0.625
		1	1	0.400	0.255		1	1	0.333	0.625
		1	0	0.200	0.150		1	0	0.200	0.750
		0	4	1.000	0.300		0	4	0.267	0.750
		0	3	0.695	0.328		0	3	0.243	0.764
		0	2	0.449	0.274		0	2	0.200	0.750
		0	1	0.220	0.163		0	1	0.123	0.593
		0	0	0.000	0.000		0	0	0.000	0.000
	0.8	1	4	1.000	0.200	4.0	1	4	0.250	0.938
		1	3	0.800	0.320		1	3	0.250	0.938
		1	2	0.600	0.360		1	2	0.250	0.938
		1	1	0.400	0.320		1	1	0.250	0.938
		1	0	0.200	0.200		1	0	0.200	1.000
		0	4	1.000	0.200		0	4	0.200	1.000
		0	3	0.655	0.357		0	3	0.184	0.993
		0	2	0.426	0.330		0	2	0.155	0.949
		0	1	0.210	0.208		0	1	0.100	0.750
		0	0	0.000	0.000		0	0	0.000	0.000
	1.0	1	4	1.000	0.000	5.0	1	4	0.200	1.250
		1	3	0.800	0.250		1	3	0.200	1.250
		1	2	0.600	0.375		1	2	0.200	1.250
		1	1	0.400	0.375		1	1	0.200	1.250
		1	0	0.200	0.250		1	0	0.200	1.250
		0	4	0.800	0.250		0	4	0.160	1.250
		0	3	0.600	0.375		0	3	0.148	1.225
		0	2	0.400	0.375		0	2	0.126	1.153
		0	1	0.200	0.250		0	1	0.084	0.906
		0	0	0.000	0.000		0	0	0.000	0.000
	1.5	1	4	0.667	0.156					
		1	3	0.667	0.156					
		1	2	0.600	0.281					
		1	1	0.400	0.469					
		1	0	0.200	0.375					
		0	4	0.533	0.375					
		0	3	0.456	0.445					
		0	2	0.333	0.469					
		0	1	0.176	0.345					
		0	0	0.000	0.000					

R	RR	u	v	$\bar{R}_0$	$\dot{V}_{r_1-(RR)_{r_0}}$	RR	u	v	$\bar{R}_0$	$\dot{V}_{r_1-(RR)_{r_0}}$
5	0.2	1	5	1.000	0.192	1.5	0	5	0.556	0.300
		1	4	0.833	0.168		0	4	0.500	0.360
		1	3	0.667	0.141		0	3	0.411	0.414
		1	2	0.500	0.110		0	2	0.290	0.406
		1	1	0.333	0.077		0	1	0.150	0.279
		1	0	0.167	0.040		0	0	0.000	0.000
		0	5	1.000	0.192	2.0	1	5	0.500	0.240
		0	4	0.792	0.162		1	4	0.500	0.240
		0	3	0.589	0.127		1	3	0.500	0.240
		0	2	0.390	0.089		1	2	0.500	0.240
		0	1	0.194	0.046		1	1	0.333	0.480
		0	0	0.000	0.000		1	0	0.167	0.400
	0.4	1	5	1.000	0.288		0	5	0.417	0.400
		1	4	0.833	0.272		0	4	0.386	0.439
		1	3	0.667	0.243		0	3	0.333	0.480
		1	2	0.500	0.202		0	2	0.250	0.480
		1	1	0.333	0.147		0	1	0.136	0.350
		1	0	0.167	0.080		0	0	0.000	0.000
		0	5	1.000	0.288	2.5	1	5	0.400	0.360
		0	4	0.780	0.264		1	4	0.400	0.360
		0	3	0.575	0.222		1	3	0.400	0.360
		0	2	0.378	0.163		1	2	0.400	0.360
		0	1	0.187	0.089		1	1	0.333	0.500
		0	0	0.000	0.000		1	0	0.167	0.500
	0.6	1	5	1.000	0.288		0	5	0.333	0.500
		1	4	0.833	0.312		0	4	0.312	0.528
		1	3	0.667	0.307		0	3	0.276	0.556
		1	2	0.500	0.274		0	2	0.216	0.552
		1	1	0.333	0.211		0	1	0.123	0.416
		1	0	0.167	0.120		0	0	0.000	0.000
		0	5	1.000	0.288	3.0	1	5	0.333	0.480
		0	4	0.760	0.313		1	4	0.333	0.480
		0	3	0.556	0.288		1	3	0.333	0.480
		0	2	0.364	0.225		1	2	0.333	0.480
		0	1	0.180	0.128		1	1	0.333	0.480
		0	0	0.000	0.000		1	0	0.167	0.600
	0.8	1	5	1.000	0.192		0	5	0.278	0.600
		1	4	0.833	0.288		0	4	0.262	0.620
		1	3	0.667	0.333		0	3	0.235	0.638
		1	2	0.500	0.326		0	2	0.189	0.625
		1	1	0.333	0.269		0	1	0.111	0.480
		1	0	0.167	0.160		0	0	0.000	0.000
		0	5	1.000	0.192	4.0	1	5	0.250	0.720
		0	4	0.724	0.323		1	4	0.250	0.720
		0	3	0.531	0.331		1	3	0.250	0.720
		0	2	0.350	0.277		1	2	0.250	0.720
		0	1	0.173	0.165		1	1	0.250	0.720
		0	0	0.000	0.000		1	0	0.167	0.800
	1.0	1	5	1.000	0.000		0	5	0.208	0.800
		1	4	0.833	0.200		0	4	0.197	0.808
		1	3	0.667	0.320		0	3	0.180	0.809
		1	2	0.500	0.360		0	2	0.149	0.776
		1	1	0.333	0.320		0	1	0.093	0.604
		1	0	0.167	0.200		0	0	0.000	0.000
		0	5	0.833	0.200	5.0	1	5	0.200	0.960
		0	4	0.667	0.320		1	4	0.200	0.960
		0	3	0.500	0.360		1	3	0.200	0.960
		0	2	0.333	0.320		1	2	0.200	0.960
		0	1	0.167	0.200		1	1	0.200	0.960
		0	0	0.000	0.000		1	0	0.167	1.000
	1.5	1	5	0.667	0.120		0	5	0.167	1.000
		1	4	0.667	0.120		0	4	0.158	0.998
		1	3	0.667	0.120		0	3	0.145	0.984
		1	2	0.500	0.360		0	2	0.123	0.930
		1	1	0.333	0.420		0	1	0.079	0.725
		1	0	0.167	0.300		0	0	0.000	0.000

APPENDIX 14

Analysis of
Matched Series

X^2 Function of Odds Ratio:
Elements for Equation 14.16

R	OR	u	v	g	h	R	OR	u	v	g	h
1	0.2	1	0	0.691	0.214	2	0.2	1	1	0.575	0.212
		0	1	-0.309	0.214			1	0	0.867	0.140
								0	2	-0.425	0.212
								0	1	-0.133	0.140
	0.4	1	0	0.613	0.237		0.4	1	1	0.472	0.228
		0	1	-0.387	0.237			1	0	0.792	0.184
								0	2	-0.528	0.228
								0	1	-0.208	0.184
	0.6	1	0	0.564	0.246		0.6	1	1	0.411	0.229
		0	1	-0.436	0.246			1	0	0.740	0.204
								0	2	-0.589	0.229
								0	1	-0.260	0.204
	0.8	1	0	0.528	0.249		0.8	1	1	0.367	0.227
		0	1	-0.472	0.249			1	0	0.699	0.216
								0	2	-0.633	0.227
								0	1	-0.301	0.216
	1.1	1	0	0.488	0.250		1.1	1	1	0.319	0.220
		0	1	-0.512	0.250			1	0	0.652	0.224
								0	2	-0.681	0.220
								0	1	-0.348	0.224
	1.5	1	0	0.449	0.247		1.5	1	1	0.275	0.209
		0	1	-0.551	0.247			1	0	0.606	0.229
								0	2	-0.725	0.209
								0	1	-0.394	0.229
	2.0	1	0	0.414	0.243		2.0	1	1	0.236	0.196
		0	1	-0.586	0.243			1	0	0.562	0.229
								0	2	-0.764	0.196
								0	1	-0.438	0.229
	2.5	1	0	0.387	0.237		2.5	1	1	0.208	0.184
		0	1	-0.613	0.237			1	0	0.528	0.228
								0	2	-0.792	0.184
								0	1	-0.472	0.228
	3.0	1	0	0.366	0.232		3.0	1	1	0.186	0.173
		0	1	-0.634	0.232			1	0	0.500	0.225
								0	2	-0.814	0.173
								0	1	-0.500	0.225
	4.0	1	0	0.333	0.222		4.0	1	1	0.155	0.155
		0	1	-0.667	0.222			1	0	0.457	0.219
								0	2	-0.845	0.155
								0	1	-0.543	0.219
	5.0	1	0	0.309	0.214		5.0	1	1	0.133	0.140
		0	1	-0.691	0.214			1	0	0.425	0.212
								0	2	-0.867	0.140
								0	1	-0.575	0.212

(*continued*)

313

R	OR	u	v	g	h	OR	u	v	g	h
3	0.2	1	2	0.500	0.208	2.0	1	2	0.162	0.148
		1	1	0.775	0.187		1	1	0.372	0.237
		1	0	0.919	0.089		1	0	0.646	0.210
		0	3	-0.500	0.208		0	3	-0.838	0.148
		0	2	-0.225	0.187		0	2	-0.628	0.237
		0	1	-0.081	0.089		0	1	-0.354	0.210
	0.4	1	2	0.390	0.213	2.5	1	2	0.139	0.133
		1	1	0.667	0.228		1	1	0.333	0.228
		1	0	0.861	0.133		1	0	0.610	0.213
		0	3	-0.610	0.213		0	3	-0.861	0.133
		0	2	-0.333	0.228		0	2	-0.667	0.228
		0	1	-0.139	0.133		0	1	-0.390	0.213
	0.6	1	2	0.326	0.206	3.0	1	2	0.121	0.121
		1	1	0.595	0.243		1	1	0.303	0.219
		1	0	0.817	0.159		1	0	0.581	0.214
		0	3	-0.674	0.206		0	3	-0.879	0.121
		0	2	-0.405	0.243		0	2	-0.697	0.219
		0	1	-0.183	0.159		0	1	-0.419	0.214
	0.8	1	2	0.282	0.197	4.0	1	2	0.097	0.103
		1	1	0.542	0.249		1	1	0.257	0.202
		1	0	0.780	0.176		1	0	0.535	0.212
		0	3	-0.718	0.197		0	3	-0.903	0.103
		0	2	-0.458	0.249		0	2	-0.743	0.202
		0	1	-0.220	0.176		0	1	-0.465	0.212
	1.1	1	2	0.237	0.183	5.0	1	2	0.081	0.089
		1	1	0.482	0.250		1	1	0.225	0.187
		1	0	0.736	0.192		1	0	0.500	0.208
		0	3	-0.763	0.183		0	3	-0.919	0.089
		0	2	-0.518	0.250		0	2	-0.775	0.187
		0	1	-0.264	0.192		0	1	-0.500	0.208
	1.5	1	2	0.196	0.166					
		1	1	0.424	0.246					
		1	0	0.690	0.203					
		0	3	-0.804	0.166					
		0	2	-0.576	0.246					
		0	1	-0.310	0.203					

R	OR	u	v	g	h	OR	u	v	g	h
4	0.2	1	3	0.446	0.204	2.0	1	3	0.123	0.117
		1	2	0.705	0.210		1	2	0.275	0.207
		1	1	0.853	0.139		1	1	0.464	0.245
		1	0	0.942	0.064		1	0	0.702	0.192
		0	4	-0.554	0.204		0	4	-0.877	0.117
		0	3	-0.295	0.210		0	3	-0.725	0.207
		0	2	-0.147	0.139		0	2	-0.536	0.245
		0	1	-0.058	0.064		0	1	-0.298	0.192
	0.4	1	3	0.333	0.198	2.5	1	3	0.104	0.102
		1	2	0.579	0.241		1	2	0.239	0.192
		1	1	0.761	0.192		1	1	0.421	0.241
		1	0	0.896	0.102		1	0	0.667	0.198
		0	4	-0.667	0.198		0	4	-0.896	0.102
		0	3	-0.421	0.241		0	3	-0.761	0.192
		0	2	-0.239	0.192		0	2	-0.579	0.241
		0	1	-0.104	0.102		0	1	-0.333	0.198
	0.6	1	3	0.271	0.185	3.0	1	3	0.089	0.091
		1	2	0.500	0.247		1	2	0.212	0.179
		1	1	0.694	0.218		1	1	0.386	0.235
		1	0	0.859	0.128		1	0	0.637	0.202
		0	4	-0.729	0.185		0	4	-0.911	0.091
		0	3	-0.500	0.247		0	3	-0.788	0.179
		0	2	-0.306	0.218		0	2	-0.614	0.235
		0	1	-0.141	0.128		0	1	-0.363	0.202
	0.8	1	3	0.230	0.172	4.0	1	3	0.070	0.075
		1	2	0.443	0.245		1	2	0.174	0.157
		1	1	0.642	0.232		1	1	0.333	0.222
		1	0	0.827	0.147		1	0	0.591	0.204
		0	4	-0.770	0.172		0	4	-0.930	0.075
		0	3	-0.557	0.245		0	3	-0.826	0.157
		0	2	-0.358	0.232		0	2	-0.667	0.222
		0	1	-0.173	0.147		0	1	-0.409	0.204
	1.1	1	3	0.188	0.154	5.0	1	3	0.058	0.064
		1	2	0.382	0.237		1	2	0.147	0.139
		1	1	0.582	0.242		1	1	0.295	0.210
		1	0	0.788	0.165		1	0	0.554	0.204
		0	4	-0.812	0.154		0	4	-0.942	0.064
		0	3	-0.618	0.237		0	3	-0.853	0.139
		0	2	-0.418	0.242		0	2	-0.705	0.210
		0	1	-0.212	0.165		0	1	-0.446	0.204
	1.5	1	3	0.152	0.135					
		1	2	0.325	0.224					
		1	1	0.521	0.247					
		1	0	0.745	0.181					
		0	4	-0.848	0.135					
		0	3	-0.675	0.224					
		0	2	-0.479	0.247					
		0	1	-0.255	0.181					

(continued)

315

R	OR	u	v	g	h	OR	u	v	g	h
5	0.2	1	4	0.404	0.198	2.0	1	4	0.099	0.096
		1	3	0.649	0.222		1	3	0.217	0.178
		1	2	0.797	0.171		1	2	0.359	0.233
		1	1	0.892	0.107		1	1	0.531	0.242
		1	0	0.955	0.049		1	0	0.742	0.176
		0	5	-0.596	0.198		0	5	-0.901	0.096
		0	4	-0.351	0.222		0	4	-0.783	0.178
		0	3	-0.203	0.171		0	3	-0.641	0.233
		0	2	-0.108	0.107		0	2	-0.469	0.242
		0	1	-0.045	0.049		0	1	-0.258	0.176
	0.4	1	4	0.292	0.185	2.5	1	4	0.082	0.082
		1	3	0.514	0.242		1	3	0.186	0.160
		1	2	0.683	0.221		1	2	0.317	0.221
		1	1	0.814	0.160		1	1	0.486	0.242
		1	0	0.918	0.082		1	0	0.708	0.185
		0	5	-0.708	0.185		0	5	-0.918	0.082
		0	4	-0.486	0.242		0	4	-0.814	0.160
		0	3	-0.317	0.221		0	3	-0.683	0.221
		0	2	-0.186	0.160		0	2	-0.514	0.242
		0	1	-0.082	0.082		0	1	-0.292	0.185
	0.6	1	4	0.232	0.168	3.0	1	4	0.071	0.073
		1	3	0.432	0.240		1	3	0.162	0.146
		1	2	0.605	0.241		1	2	0.284	0.210
		1	1	0.755	0.191		1	1	0.449	0.239
		1	0	0.886	0.107		1	0	0.679	0.191
		0	5	-0.768	0.168		0	5	-0.929	0.073
		0	4	-0.568	0.240		0	4	-0.838	0.146
		0	3	-0.395	0.241		0	3	-0.716	0.210
		0	2	-0.245	0.191		0	2	-0.551	0.239
		0	1	-0.114	0.107		0	1	-0.321	0.191
	0.8	1	4	0.194	0.152	4.0	1	4	0.055	0.058
		1	3	0.376	0.232		1	3	0.130	0.124
		1	2	0.546	0.248		1	2	0.236	0.189
		1	1	0.707	0.210		1	1	0.393	0.231
		1	0	0.858	0.125		1	0	0.633	0.196
		0	5	-0.806	0.152		0	5	-0.945	0.058
		0	4	-0.624	0.232		0	4	-0.870	0.124
		0	3	-0.454	0.248		0	3	-0.764	0.189
		0	2	-0.293	0.210		0	2	-0.607	0.231
		0	1	-0.142	0.125		0	1	-0.367	0.196
	1.1	1	4	0.156	0.133	5.0	1	4	0.045	0.049
		1	3	0.316	0.217		1	3	0.108	0.107
		1	2	0.480	0.250		1	2	0.203	0.171
		1	1	0.649	0.227		1	1	0.351	0.222
		1	0	0.822	0.145		1	0	0.596	0.198
		0	5	-0.844	0.133		0	5	-0.955	0.049
		0	4	-0.684	0.217		0	4	-0.892	0.107
		0	3	-0.520	0.250		0	3	-0.797	0.171
		0	2	-0.351	0.227		0	2	-0.649	0.222
		0	1	-0.178	0.145		0	1	-0.404	0.198
	1.5	1	4	0.124	0.113					
		1	3	0.262	0.198					
		1	2	0.416	0.244					
		1	1	0.589	0.238					
		1	0	0.782	0.162					
		0	5	-0.876	0.113					
		0	4	-0.738	0.198					
		0	3	-0.584	0.244					
		0	2	-0.411	0.238					
		0	1	-0.218	0.162					

Glossary

ABSTRACT   Theoretical (q.v.).

ABSTRACT-GENERAL   Theoretical (q.v.)

ACCURACY   Degree of lack of error (cf. PRECISION and VALIDITY).

ACQUIRED   Postnatal in origin (as opposed to congenital).

ACUTE
1. Of short duration.
2. Of sudden onset.

ADDITIVE MODEL   A regression model without any term whose X is a product of two other X's in the model representing separate items of information.

ADJUSTED MEASURE OF RELATION   (e.g., adjusted rate difference) A measure based on conditional comparative information (cf. CRUDE and STANDARDIZED).

ADJUSTED RATE   The projection of a crude rate to another (possibly hypothetical) population structure; that is, a weighted average of specific (conditional) rates, with the weights proportional to the sizes of the corresponding experiences in another population (cf. CRUDE and STANDARDIZED).

ADMINISTRATIVE   Having to do with actual delivery of health care in a particularistic setting (as opposed to its scientific premises).

ADMISSIBILITY (into the study base)   The property of satisfying the criteria of membership (potential or actual) in the population whose experience constitutes the study base.

ALTERNATIVE HYPOTHESIS

1.   In science—a hypothesis entertained as a "competitor" for the hypothesis at issue.
2.   In statistics—the range of parameter values corresponding to the hypothesis at issue (as opposed to the null value or "null hypothesis").

ANALYSIS OF DATA   The process of summarizing, under a statistical model, the evidence in the data with reference to the object of research.

ANALYTIC EPIDEMIOLOGY   Misnomer for epidemiologic hypothesis testing (whose logic is synthetic, not analytic). In terms of a classical misapprehension, "analytic epidemiology" is viewed as the alternative to descriptive epidemiology (q.v.).

ANTAGONISM   One factor's inhibition of the effect of another.

APPLIED HEALTH SCIENCE   Scientific research with direct implications for health care (i.e., assessment of relative merits of alternative algorithms of care) (cf. BASIC HEALTH SCIENCE).

ASSESSMENT   Classification according to a scale of quantity (cf. EVALUATION).

ASSOCIATION   Occurrence relation (q.v.).

AT RISK   Not known to have zero risk (cf. CANDIDATE).

ATTACK RATE   In communicable-disease epidemiology, the proportion of candidates who come down with the illness in a particular (usually short) period of time, as in "secondary attack rate" (the proportion of the "contacts" of cases that comes down with the disease, presumably as a consequence of contact with a case).

ATTRIBUTABLE RISK   Misnomer for rate difference (q.v.).

BACKGROUND LEVEL (of a parameter of occurrence)   Level determined by characteristics other than that under study.

BASE   See STUDY BASE.

BASE POPULATION   The population whose experience (in a defined segment of time) constitutes the study base (q.v.).

BASELINE   The starting point of the risk period under study, or of follow-up.

BASIC HEALTH SCIENCE   Science (q.v.) motivated by intent to provide new theoretical foundations for innovations in health care (cf. APPLIED HEALTH SCIENCE).

BAYESIAN STATISTICS   Statistics concerned with the use of data in the modification of the probabilities (credibilities) of various values of the parameter of interest (cf. FREQUENTIST STATISTICS.)

BIAS
1. MEAN BIAS   Mean error, that is, difference between the *mean* of empirical values (over a large number of hypothetical replications) and the theoretical value.
2. MEDIAN BIAS   Median error, that is, difference between the *median* of empirical values (over a large number of hypothetical replications) and the theoretical value.
3. Tendency for error on the mean or median.

BIASED BASE   A study base formed conditionally on what it shows, or with membership that is outcome-selective (conducive to biased result).

BIASED RESULT   A result (empirical value) from a biased study or procedure, that is, a result with *median* bias.

BIASED SAMPLING   Sampling in which the sampling probability depends in an unknown way on a determinant of the observation

BIASED STUDY   A study with invalidity of design (conducive to a biased result).

BINARY   Consisting of (or viewed as if consisting of) two categories.

BIOMETRY   The discipline of how to study statistical problems in biology and medicine.

BIOSTATISTICS   Biometry (q.v.).

BLINDED STUDY   Study characterized by arrangements designed to assure the observers' and/or the subjects' lack of awareness of whether the subject is a member of the index or the reference series.

BLOCKING   Restriction of randomization; that is, the use of separate randomizations within categories of a covariate, with the aim of assuring similarity of the distribution of the covariate between the index and reference series (in the study base).

CANDIDATE   An individual who, by virtue of not having the state (illness) at issue, could logically experience its inception (even if, in light of substantive facts, the risk is known to be zero).

CANDIDATE TIME   The amount of candidate experience (in terms of the integral of the size of the candidate population over the period of observation).

CASE
1. In medicine—episode of illness, as in "a case of gonorrhea."
2. In epidemiology—a person representing a case (in the medical sense) of some state or event, as in "the interviews of cases."

CASE-CONTROL STUDY   Case-referent (case-base) study (q.v.).

CASE-REFERENT STUDY   A study involving the sampling design of enrolling all of the cases in the study base (in the direct referent of the empirical result) and, separately, a sample (not census) of the study base itself (or of its noncase segment).

CAUSAL RELATION   Occurrence relation reflecting a causal connection between the determinant and the outcome phenomenon (as opposed to confounding by extraneous determinants of the outcome parameter).

CAUSE   A category of a determinant, in relation to a particular reference category, capable of completing a sufficient cause in some instances in which the reference category is incapable of such completion. When, in this sense, a category (relative to a particular reference category) can be both a cause (in some instances) and a preventive (in some others), it is commonplace to mean by "cause" that causal instances are more common than preventive ones.

CENSUS   100% sampling, or 100% sample.

CENTILE   A fractile expressed in terms of a scale from 0 to 100% for the fraction involved, as in "the median is the 50th centile, or the 0.5 fractile."

CHARACTERISTIC (of person)
1. A dimension in which persons (units of observation) may be characterized, such as any risk indicator.
2. A realization in a dimension in which persons are characterized, such as any risk indication (q.v.).

CHI SQUARE   The square of a standard Gaussian variate (χ^2 with 1 df) or a statistic whose distribution conforms to that of the sum of two or more independent χ^2 1 df variates (χ^2 with 2 or more df).

CHRONIC   Long-lasting or long-term.

CHRONIC-DISEASE EPIDEMIOLOGY   Misnomer for epidemiology of noninfectious diseases.

CLINICAL   Having to do with patient care in a direct way (originally bedside).

COACTION (of factors)   Joint action.

COEFFICIENT OF CORRELATION   See CORRELATION COEFFICIENT.

COEFFICIENT OF REGRESSION   See REGRESSION COEFFICIENT.

COEFFICIENT OF VARIATION   Standard deviation divided by mean.

COHORT   A closed population (from Latin, *cohors*, enclosure); that is, a population whose membership is defined on the basis of some event, for ever after; that is, a population with fixed membership (cf. DYNAMIC POPULATION).

COHORT INCIDENCE   Proportion-type incidence (cf. incidence density)

COHORT STUDY   A study (of incidence or change) whose base is the experience of a cohort over time (as opposed to a dynamic-population study or a cross-sectional study).

COMMUNICABLE   Subject to transmission from one person to another, that is, contagious.

COMORBIDITY   Presence of associated illness.

COMPARABILITY OF EFFECTS   Identity of extraneous effects of the compared empirical categories of the determinant, as in "the treatment under study and the 'placebo' treatment have comparable effects (in studying the drug effect) if the extraneous (nondrug) aspects of the two treatments have identical effects, and if, in addition, the 'placebo' has no effect."

COMPARABILITY OF INFORMATION
1. Absence of differential errors in the outcome information between the compared populations (in the study base).
2. In case-referent studies, also absence of differential errors in the determinant information between the case series and the base sample.

COMPARABILITY OF POPULATIONS   Balanced distributions between populations representing the compared categories of the determinant, specifically distributions with respect to extraneous determinants of the outcome parameter (i.e., the property that randomization and "blocking" are designed to achieve in experiments).

COMPARATIVE STUDY   A study involving separate representations of the compared categories of the determinant (as opposed to a before-after study).

CONDITIONAL STATISTIC (estimate or test statistic)   Statistic derived with a restriction as to either the realization for an ancillary statistic (e.g., total number of cases), parameter space (e.g., all stratum-specific values of comparative parameter equal to a given theoretical value), or covariate.

CONFIDENCE INTERVAL   See ESTIMATE.

CONFOUNDER   An extraneous determinant of the outcome parameter in terms of which there is lack of comparability (q.v.) of effects and/or populations; sometimes the term is used also for an extraneous factor explanatory of lack of comparability of information.

CONFOUNDING FACTOR   Confounder (q.v.).

CONGENITAL   Present at birth already (as opposed to acquired).

CONSTITUTIONAL   Having to do with inherent susceptibility characteristics (inherited, other congenital, or acquired) of persons (as opposed to behavioral or environmental ones).

CONTAGIOUS   Communicable (q.v.).

CONTRAINDICATION   A situation in which a particular type of action is to be avoided, as in "propensity for bleeding as a contraindication for aspirin use" and "the potential matching factor's association with the determinant but not with the outcome as a contraindication for matching the base sample to the case series."

CONTROL   A member of that segment of the base population (q.v.) which represents the reference category of the determinant. Also used (as a misnomer) for a member of a base sample in a case-referent study (q.v.).

CONTROL GROUP/POPULATION   Reference group/population (q.v.).

CONTROL OF A COVARIATE   Any arrangement (restriction of study domain, balancing in the formation of the determinant contrast, "blocking" or matching of the study base, or conditioning of the analysis) that provides for examining the relation under study conditionally on the covariate.

CORRELATION   Association, dependence.

CORRELATION COEFFICIENT   Covariance (q.v.) divided by the product of the respective standard deviations (q.v.).

COST (of study)   The aggregate of investments into a study (monetary and other).

COST-EFFICIENCY (of study)   See EFFICIENCY.

COVARIANCE   Average of the product of two variates' deviations from their respective means.

COVARIATE   An extraneous variate that may have to be taken into account to avoid distortion or inefficiency in the study of the relation at issue (inherently conditional on the covariate).

CREDIBILITY   Probability (subjective) of the correctness of a proposition.

CROSS-SECTIONAL POPULATION   Misnomer for population cross-section; that is, the status of a population (cohort or dynamic) as of a particular point in time (individual or calendar).

CROSS-SECTIONAL RELATION (between outcome parameter and its determinant)   A relation in which the time referent of the information on the determinant coincides more with that on the outcome parameter than with the etiologic period.

CROSS-SECTIONAL STUDY   A study whose base is a population cross-section (as opposed to a population's experience over time).

CRUDE MEASURE OF RELATION (e.g., crude rate difference)   A measure based on unconditional comparative information (e.g., the difference of two crude rates).

CRUDE RATE   A directly empirical rate; that is, an unadjusted empirical rate; that is, a weighted average of empirical specific (conditional) rates, with weights proportional to the actual sizes of the experiences providing those specific rates (cf. ADJUSTED and STANDARDIZED).

CUMULATIVE INCIDENCE   The proportion of a cohort (of candidates) experiencing the event at issue over a particular risk period (fixed/arbitrary or individual/substantive), if time-specific incidence density (q.v.) is considered to operate over that period.

CURATIVE   Having to do with curing of cases of illness (cf. THERAPEUTIC).

DATA   Representations, especially recorded ones, of particularistic facts.

DATA ANALYSIS   See ANALYSIS OF DATA.

DECILE
1.   A centile for which the cumulative proportion is a multiple of 10%, as in "the median is the 5th decile of a distribution."
2.   Misnomer for interdecile range.

DEFECT   A stable state of illness, as in "congenital defect" (in Latin, *vitium*; cf. DISEASE).

DENIAL PROPOSITION/VALUE   Null (q.v.) "hypothesis"/value.

DEPENDENT VARIATE   A statistical variate representing the outcome in a regression analysis.

DEPENDENT PARAMETER   The parameter of the distribution of the dependent variate that is expressed as a function of its determinant(s) in a regression model.

DESCRIPTIVE   Without implication as to causality or noncausality. (Descriptive epidemiology need not involve populations as units of observation, contrary to classical insistence; and its alternative is not "analytic epidemiology" (q.v.) but causality-oriented epidemiology.)

DESIGN   See STUDY DESIGN.

DESIGN MATRIX   Distribution matrix (q.v.).

DETERMINANT (of occurrence)   A characteristic of individuals (constitutional, behavioral, or environmental) on which a parameter (q.v.) of occurrence depends (causally or noncausally).

DIAGNOSIS
1. The inferred (rather than necessarily the actual) state of, or event in, a person (or an object).
2. The process of arriving at an inference as to the state of, or event in, a person (or an object).

DICHOTOMOUS   Divided in two categories (cf. POLYTOMOUS and TRICHOTOMOUS).

DIFFERENTIAL (selection, errors, etc.)   Operating differently between/among the compared categories or series.

DIRECTLY STANDARDIZED   Misnomer for standardized (q.v.). (Cf. INDIRECTLY STANDARDIZED)

DISCIPLINE   Field learning and practice.

DISEASE   A process of illness, as in "neoplastic disease " (in Latin, *morbus*; cf. DEFECT and ILLNESS)

DISTRIBUTION MATRIX   The distribution of the base experience according to the determinant(s), modifiers, and confounders in the occurrence relation.

DOMAIN OF STUDY   The type of situation in which the object of the study (occurrence relation) will be (was) explored, as in "the effects of Indomethacin in the domain of the premature neonate with patent ductus arteriosus."

DOSE-RESPONSE
1. Dependence between the level of a determinant (causal or preventive) and the magnitude of effect, as in "there was evidence of dose-response."
2. The relation between the level of a determinant and the magnitude of the effect, as in "linear dose-response."

DOUBLE BLINDED   Blinded with respect to both the observer(s) and the subjects.

DYNAMIC POPULATION   An open population; that is, a population whose membership is defined on the basis of some state, for the duration of that state; that is, a population with turnover of membership (cf. COHORT).

DYNAMIC-POPULATION STUDY   A study (of incidence) whose base is the experience of a dynamic population (of candidates) over time [as opposed to a cohort study (q.v.) or a cross-sectional study (q.v.)].

EFFECT
1. In science—the change in the outcome parameter brought about by a particular cause or preventive.
2. In statistics—the value of a parameter of relation, as in "the main effect of X_i."

EFFECTIVENESS   Efficacy (q.v.)

EFFICACY (of intervention)   Ability to bring about the intended change in the outcome or outcome parameter.

EFFICIENCY (of study)
1. Informativeness with a given cost (cost-efficiency).
2. Informativeness with a given size (size-efficiency).

EMPIRICAL
1. Operational (as opposed to conceptual), as in "empirical scale."
2. Based directly on experience, as in "empirical rate."

END POINT   An event that terminates follow-up, especially the event whose occurrence is under study.

ENDEMIC OCCURRENCE   The usual rate of occurrence (cf. EPIDEMIC).

ENTRY COHORT   A cohort defined as of the beginning of the risk period under study (i.e., at "baseline").

ENVIRONMENTAL   Having to do with the settings in which individuals (units of observation) exist [as opposed to constitutional (q.v.) or behavioral].

EPIDEMIC   An episode, or relating to an episode, of unusually common occurrence.

EPIDEMIOLOGY
1. That aspect of a medical science or discipline which deals with the (frequency of the) occurrence of phenomena of interest in that field, as in "the epidemiology of oncology" (neoplastic or cancer epidemiology), or "health care epidemiology."
2. The (frequency of) occurrence aspect of a phenomenon, as in "the epidemiology of sudden death."
3. Research into the occurrence (epidemiologic) aspect of a phenomenon, as in "practice of epidemiology."

EPISTEMOLOGIC   Having to do with theoretical (rather than procedural) aspects of how to learn about the objects of research, that is, with theory of methodology (cf. ONTOLOGIC).

ESTIMATE

1. INTERVAL ESTIMATE (confidence interval) An interval (for a parameter) constructed (from a particular set of data) in a way designed to assure that in a specified proportion of such applications (out of a large number of them) it covers the actual value of the parameter.

2. POINT ESTIMATE   A 0% two-sided confidence interval; that is, a 50% one-sided confidence bound; that is, a value (for a parameter) computed (from a particular set of data) in a way designed to assure that in 50% of such applications (out of a large number of them) it exceeds, and in the other 50% it falls short of, the actual value of the parameter (cf. BIAS).

ESTIMATOR   A function of data, designed to provide estimates; that is, a way (conceptual) of computing an estimate (q.v.) from data.

ETIOLOGIC FRACTION   Of the actual total rate of occurrence (total load of cases), the proportion that is attributable to the cause at issue. It equals the proportion of actual cases that is attributable to the cause if there are no instances of preventive susceptibility (cf. PREVENTIVE FRACTION.)

ETIOLOGY   Causal origin, or causal explanation.

EVALUATION   Classification according to a scale of quality or preference (cf. OUTCOME EVALUATION, PRACTICE EVALUATION, PREMISE EVALUATION, and PROCESS EVALUATION). Also used (as a misnomer) for mere assessment (q.v.).

EVENT

1. An episode.

2. The transition (rapid) from one state to another.

EXACT MODEL/DISTRIBUTION   A model/distribution that represents exactly the sampling distribution of data on the premise that the study experience represents a probability sample of the abstract reality ("superpopulation") under study.

EXPECTATION   See EXPECTED VALUE

EXPECTED VALUE   Mean of sampling distribution (q.v.), often, implicitly, on the "null hypotheses" (q.v.).

EXPERIMENT   A study in which a determinant is intentionally perturbed for reasons none other than the goals of the study itself.

EXPLANATORY STUDY (of exposure or intervention)   Study that addresses the effect of a particular agent in the exposure or intervention (cf. PRAGMATIC STUDY).

EXPOSURE

1. A particular (index) category of a (potential) environmental (as opposed to constitutional or behavioral) determinant, entertained as a cause or preventive for the phenomenon of interest, relative to a particular other (reference) category.

2. Experiencing the index (exposure) category of an environmental determinant (potential) of the outcome.

3. Environmental determinant.

4. Misnomer for any determinant (i.e., constitutional or behavioral as well as environmental), or its index category.

EXPOSURE ODDS   In a case-referent study, the theoretical proportion of cases or members of the reference series representing the index category of an environmental determinant divided by the proportion representing the reference category.

EXPOSURE-ODDS RATIO   In a case-referent study, the exposure odds of cases divided by that of reference subjects.

EXTERNAL VALIDITY   Generalizability beyond the experience of the study (cf. INTERNAL VALIDITY).

EXTRANEOUS CHARACTERISTIC/FACTOR   A characteristic/factor that is not part of the object of research (occurrence relation) per se, but that may have to be considered in the interest of validity or efficiency (as a conditioning factor); that is, a characteristic/factor that a covariate (q.v.) represents.

FACTOR

1. A cause or a preventive (e.g., a category of blood pressure relative to another).

2. A causal or preventive determinant (e.g., blood pressure).

3. Misnomer for determinant (q.v.) or a category of it.

FALSE NEGATIVE RATE   The complement of sensitivity; that is, one minus sensitivity (q.v.).

FALSE POSITIVE RATE   The complement of specificity; that is, one minus specificity (q.v.).

FRACTILE   The value of a characteristic that corresponds to a given cumulative fraction (proportion) of its realizations, as in "the median is the 0.5 fractile of a distribution."

FREQUENTIST STATISTICS   Statistics concerned with the frequency behavior (sampling distribution) of quantities (statistics) derived from data, without addressing the probabilities (credibilities) of various values of the parameter of interest (cf. BAYESIAN STATISTICS).

FUNCTION   Relation between a dependent quantity and its determinant(s).

GENERAL EPIDEMIOLOGY   Theoretical epidemiology (q.v.).

GENERAL POPULATION   A broadly defined (and thus ill-defined) population (and a concept of inherently no value in science).

GENERALIZATION
1. In science—inference (inductive) from the empirical (particularistic) to the theoretical (abstract-general).
2. In statistics—inference (usually "frequentist"-mechanistic) from a sample to a population (particularistic).

GENETIC   Having to do with the genome (chromosomes).

HEALTH   The state of being, or the extent to which one is, as functional and symptom-free as is commonly attainable at the age at issue, and freedom from unusual (for age) constitutional indications of future disability, symptoms or death; in other words, freedom from illness (q.v.) or the extent to which one is free from illness.

HEALTH CARE   Any activity or arrangement aimed at the maintenance or improvement of health (whether education, regulation, or service; whether preventive or therapeutic) or adaptation to illness (rehabilitative).

HEALTH-CARE RESEARCH   Research into the realities (as opposed to premises) of health care (cf. HEALTH SCIENCE).

HEALTH SCIENCE   Science (q.v.), either basic (q.v.) or applied (q.v.), relevant to health care (its premises).

HEALTHY WORKER EFFECT   Tendency of occupationally defined populations to show lower mortality than "the general population," conditionally on controllable covariates (usually age, gender, race, and calendar time).

HOMOSCEDASTICITY   Constancy of the variance (theoretical) of the outcome measure over the determinants at issue.

HYPOTHESIS   A tentative piece of scientific (theoretical) knowledge; that is, a scientific idea (cf. ALTERNATIVE HYPOTHESIS and NULL HYPOTHESIS).

ILLNESS   Ill-health; that is, disease (q.v.) or defect (q.v.).

IMPRECISION   Lack of total precision (q.v.).

INCIDENCE   The appearance of events (q.v.) of a particular kind in a population (of candidates over time) (cf. PREVALENCE).

INCIDENCE DENSITY   The ratio of the number of events to the corresponding population time (candidate time).

INCIDENCE PROPORTION   See COHORT INCIDENCE and CUMULATIVE INCIDENCE.

INCIDENT CASES   Cases that appear (as against those that exist or prevail).

INCONCLUSIVE STUDY   A study whose result is reasonably consistent with both the hypothesis at issue and its denial (cf. NEGATIVE STUDY and POSITIVE STUDY).

INDEPENDENCE   Lack of association (relation) or of synergism and antagonism.

INDEPENDENT VARIATE   A variate (statistical) representing a determinant of the dependent parameter in a regression model.

INDEX   A measure that provides for ranking.

INDEX CATEGORY (of a determinant)   A category that is of express interest, for example, a particular new treatment under study (as opposed to the reference category of the "standard" treatment or, alternatively, no treatment).

INDEX EXPERIENCE/GROUP/POPULATION/SERIES
1. The experience/group/population/series representing an index category (in the study base).
2. The experience/group/population/series around which a study base is built (as is commonplace in case-referent studies, for example).

INDICATION
1. Realization of an indicator, indicative of the state or event at issue, as in "symptomatic improvement as an indication of therapeutic efficacy," or "test positivity as an indication of disease."
2. Situation that prompts a particular type of action, as in "the small size of the index series as an indication for matching."

INDICATOR   A characteristic (variate) whose realization, or a test whose outcome, conveys information about the presence or future occurrence of the phenomenon at issue.

INDICATOR VARIATE   Statistical variate representing a binary characteristic, usually with values 1 and 0 corresponding to the two categories, respectively.

INDIRECTLY STANDARDIZED   Misnomer for standardized according to the distribution of the index experience. (This means standardization between any given index rate and the reference rate, but not among two or more index rates.)

INDUCTION PERIOD   The time lag from the beginning of the causal process to the manifestation of the effect.

INFECTIOUS   Due to a microorganism.

INFERENCE (in statistical science)   The movement, presumptive, from the results of data analysis toward new knowledge (q.v.) about the object of study; that is, interpretation of statistics.

INFORMATION
1. In statistics—with reference to a particular parameter, the inverse of the sum of variance and the square of mean bias of its point estimator; that is, the inverse of the average of squared deviations of point estimates from the parameter value itself.
2. In statistical science—data and statistics serving as evidence for the advancement of knowledge about the object of study.

INFORMATIVENESS (of study)   The degree of evidence from a study (as determined by validity, efficiency, and size).

INTERACTION   Mutual influence between two factors (the factors' influence on each other). Also used, as a misnomer, for interdependence (q.v.) of coaction and the modification (q.v.) of relation (need for product term in regression analysis).

INTERCEPT   The value (actual or hypothetical) of the dependent parameter in a regression function that corresponds to all the independent variates in the function equaling zero.

INTERDEPENDENCE (of coaction)   Dependence of the effects of two factors on each other; that is, synergism (q.v.) or antagonism (q.v.).

INTERNAL VALIDITY   Validity with reference to the study base itself (the direct referent of the study result; cf. EXTERNAL VALIDITY).

INTERVAL ESTIMATE   See ESTIMATE.

INTERVENTION   Willful perturbation of a determinant, aimed at influencing the outcome.

KNOWLEDGE (scientific)   Strong expert belief, especially a consensus belief, about a scientific proposition.

LATENCY PERIOD   The span of time for which a state remains inapparent.

LEVEL OF TEST   An a priori "critical" level (α) for a P-value, such that $P < \alpha$ is deemed "significant" (at level α), and $P > \alpha$ is considered "nonsignificant," in the sense of calling for "acceptance" and "rejection" of the hypothesis, respectively.

LINK   Lay locution for causal connection.

LINKED   Lay locution for causally connected.

LOGIT   Logarithm (natural) of odds (q.v.).

LONGITUDINAL RELATION (between outcome parameter and its determinant)   A relation in which the time referent of the information on the determinant is antecedent to that on the outcome parameter by an amount consonant with the nature of the theoretical relation under study (e.g., length of the induction period) (cf. CROSS-SECTIONAL).

LONGITUDINAL STUDY   A study whose base is a population's experience over time (as opposed to a population cross-section).

MAIN EFFECT   Regression coefficient of a nonproduct term.

MALFORMATION   An anatomic defect of developmental origin.

MATCHING
   1. Selection of the base sample in such a way that its distribution according to a covariate becomes more similar to that of the case series than would tend to be the case if it were selected independently of the case series.
   2. Selection of the comparison group for the study base in such a way that its distribution according to a covariate becomes more similar to that of the other group than would tend to be the case if it were selected independently.

MATCHING RATIO   The ratio of the size of a matched base sample (case-referent matching) or matched comparison group (base matching) to that of the index series/group.

MEDIAN BIAS   See BIAS

MEDIAN UNBIASED ESTIMATOR   Estimator whose sampling distribution has the actual parameter value as its median (cf. BIAS).

MEDICAL
   1. Having to do with medicine, that is, with the prevention, diagnosis, or treatment of, or rehabilitation for, illness.
   2. Having to do with medicinal (as opposed to surgical) therapy.

MEDICINE
   1. The health field, as in "preventive medicine."
   2. The field of diagnosis and medicinal treatment of internal, somatic illness.

METAMETER (of a measure)   A transform of a measure.

METHOD   A planned means of achieving a preset end (as opposed to serendipity) (cf. PRINCIPLE).

METHODOLOGY   The body of methods in a discipline (cf. EPISTEMOLOGIC).

MODEL   A formal, simplified representation of, or the terms in which to consider, the object of study.

MODIFICATION   Inconstancy of a parameter of occurrence relation over another subject characteristic.

MODIFIER (of a relation)   A characteristic (of individuals) on which a parameter of occurrence relation depends.

MOR   See MORTALITY ODDS RATIO.

MORBIDITY   The occurrence of illness.

MORTALITY   The occurrence of death.

MORTALITY ODDS   Occurrence odds (q.v.) for a given cause of death relative to another (or a series of others).

MORTALITY ODDS RATIO   Ratio of mortality odds between two categories of a determinant.

NEGATIVE CONFOUNDING   Confounding that reduces, or even reverts, the empirical relation (relative to the theoretical one).

NEGATIVE STUDY   A study that detracts from the hypothesis at issue (cf. INCONCLUSIVE STUDY and POSITIVE STUDY).

NOMINAL P-VALUE   A P-value that is not subject to the usual interpretation.

NOMINAL SCALE   A scale without any quantitative implications (not even those of ranking) (cf. ORDINAL SCALE and QUANTITATIVE SCALE).

NONEXPERIMENTAL STUDY   A study that is not experimental (q.v.).

NOSOCOMIAL   Having to do with hospitals.

NUISANCE PARAMETER   An extraneous parameter that needs to be estimated (in assessing a parameter of express interest).

NULL DISTRIBUTION   The distribution that corresponds to the null hypothesis (q.v.).

NULL EXPECTATION   The mean of null distribution (q.v.).

NULL HYPOTHESIS   The denial, parsimonious, of a hypothesis (e.g., the proposition of no relation between an outcome parameter and its potential determinant, given a hypothesis of such a relation).

NULL VALUE   Parameter value corresponding to null hypothesis

NULL X^2 Statistic designed to have chi square (q.v.) distribution on the null hypothesis (q.v.).

OBJECT OF STUDY   That which is under study (in epidemiology, an occurrence relation).

OBJECTIVE OF STUDY   That which is to be achieved by a study (i.e., advancement of knowledge about the object of study).

OBJECTIVITY   The quality of being subject to agreement by independent qualified examiners.

OBLIQUE COHORT   A cohort whose zero time is distributed across the risk period under study (cf. ENTRY COHORT).

OBSERVATIONAL STUDY   Misnomer for nonexperimental study (q.v.). All empirical studies, experimental as well as nonexperimental, are observational (i.e., based on observation).

OCCURRENCE
1. A particular instance of a phenomenon, as in "this occurrence of complication."
2. The frequency (statistical) aspect of a phenomenon, as in "the occurrence of complications."

OCCURRENCE FUNCTION   Occurrence relation (q.v.).

OCCURRENCE ODDS
1. For a single theoretical rate of the form of a proportion (and for risk), the ratio of that rate (risk) to its complement (i.e., to one minus that rate or risk).
2. For two theoretical rates, having to do with alternative types of state or event in the same base, the ratio of the rate for one type to that for the other.

OCCURRENCE RELATION   The relation of a parameter of occurrence (e.g., incidence rate) to one or more characteristics of persons (or other units of observation).

ODDS   Ratio of probability (P) to its complement $(1 - P)$ [i.e., $P/(1 - P)$]. (See EXPOSURE ODDS and OCCURRENCE ODDS).

ODDS RATIO   The ratio of two odds (q.v.).

O/E RATIO   Observed-to-expected ratio (as to number of cases; for expected number, see NULL NUMBER).

ONTOLOGIC   Having to do with theoretical aspects of how to view nature and formulate the objects of research (cf. EPISTEMOLOGIC).

OR   Odds ratio (q.v.).

ORDINAL (QUASI-QUANTITATIVE) SCALE   A scale with implications for ranking, but not for absolute quantification of differences or ratios (cf. NOMINAL SCALE and QUANTITATIVE SCALE).

OUTCOME   The end stage of a process, as in "the health outcome following treatment" (distinct from the effect of treatment).

OUTCOME EVALUATION (of health care)   Premise evaluation (q.v.), or indirect process evaluation (q.v.).

OVERMATCHING   Matching that reduces the amount of information per subject; that is, matching of base sample to case series on a covariate that will not be controlled as a confounder nor explored as a potential modifier but is a correlate of the determinant in the study base.

P-VALUE   A statistic so derived that its sampling distribution is on the "null hypothesis" uniform in the zero-to-one range, with a shift to the left in this range on the hypothesis itself.

PARAMETER
1.   In medicine—a characteristic of interest in individual patients, as in "diagnostic parameter."
2.   In mathematics—a constant (as opposed to a variable).
3.   In mathematical statistics—a constant in a statistical (distribution) model.
4.   In epidemiology—a population measure of occurrence, or occurrence relation, empirical or theoretical.

PARSIMONIOUS   Conforming to the principle of parsimony.

PARSIMONY (principle of)
1.   Regarding concepts—one is to restrict the invocation of concepts to the minimum sufficient.
2.   Regarding ideas—one is not to accept hypotheses (alternatives to the parsimonious null outlook) except in the face of reasonably compelling evidence.

PARTICULARISTIC   Specific to a particular time and/or place (as opposed to abstract-general).

PARTICULARISTIC STUDY   A study whose ultimate object is particularistic (administrative, rather than scientific).

PERCENTILE   Centile (q.v.).

PHENOMENON   A state or event.

PMR   See PROPORTIONATE MORTALITY RATIO.

POINT ESTIMATE   See ESTIMATE.

POLYCHOTOMOUS   Misnomer for polytomous.

POLYTOMOUS   Divided in several categories (cf. DICHOTOMOUS and TRICHOTOMOUS).

POPULATION   See COHORT, DYNAMIC POPULATION, and CROSS-SECTIONAL POPULATION.

POPULATION ATTRIBUTABLE RISK   Etiologic fraction (q.v.).

POPULATION-BASED STUDY   Misnomer for study with primary base (q.v.).

POPULATION CROSS-SECTION   See CROSS-SECTIONAL POPULATION.

POPULATION TIME   The amount of population experience in terms of the integral of population size over the period of observation (cf. CANDIDATE TIME).

POSITIVE CONFOUNDING   Confounding that exaggerates the empirical relation (cf. NEGATIVE CONFOUNDING).

POSITIVE STUDY   A study that supports the hypothesis at issue (cf. INCONCLUSIVE STUDY and NEGATIVE STUDY).

POSTERIOR PROBABILITY   Credibility in light of the evidence from the study (cf. PRIOR PROBABILITY).

POTENTIAL CONFOUNDER   An extraneous characteristic that, in a priori terms, cannot be deemed not to be a confounder (q.v.).

POWER OF TEST (statistical)   Probability that the P-value will be less than the chosen level of the test conditionally on a particular (nonnull) value of the parameter at issue.

PRACTICE (of health care)   Activity undertaken on the presumption that it preserves or promotes health (rather than for learning whether it does) (cf. PRACTICE EVALUATION and PROCESS EVALUATION).

PRACTICE EVALUATION   Research (administrative) aimed at description (classification) of practice in terms of a scale of quality (cf. PROCESS EVALUATION).

PRAGMATIC STUDY (of exposure or intervention)   Study that addresses the effect of the exposure/intervention in terms of its operational definition, without regard to the particular agent(s) involved (cf. EXPLANATORY STUDY).

PRECISION   Reproducibility; that is, degree of lack of random error (as opposed to bias) in quantification; that is, degree of constancy of error in quantification.

PRECURRENCE PERIOD   The waiting time until the occurrence of the event at issue.

PREMISE EVALUATION   Research (scientific) into the tenability of a premise (scientific) of health care.

PREVALENCE   The existence (as opposed to the inception or termination) of a particular state among the members of a population.

PREVALENCE RATE   The proportion of a population that is in a particular state.

PREVALENT CASES   Cases that exist (as of given point in time).

PREVENTIVE

1. A category of a determinant, in relation to a particular reference category, incapable of completing a sufficient cause in some instances in which the reference category is capable of it (particularly if these instances are more common than those of causation); that is, the reference category of a cause.

2. A category of a determinant, in relation to a particular reference category, capable of blocking ("neutralizing," or "frustrating") a sufficient cause in some instances in which the reference category is incapable of it (particularly if these instances are more common than the converse ones).

PREVENTIVE FRACTION   Of the hypothetical total rate of occurrence (total load of cases) that would obtain were the preventive to be totally absent, the proportional reduction that is attributable to the preventive (cf. ETIOLOGIC FRACTION).

PRIMARY BASE   A base defined directly (rather than indirectly through a series of cases) (cf. SECONDARY BASE).

PRIMARY DIAGNOSIS   Diagnosis related to the reasons for, or causes of, the patient's coming to attention.

PRIMARY INFORMATION   Information in the sense of elementary data (as opposed to derived data or information).

PRIMARY OBJECTIVES (of a study)   Objectives that justify the study (as opposed to those that the study justifies, i.e., secondary objectives).

PRINCIPLE (of research)   A guideline for decision-making in research (ontologic as well as epistemologic or methodologic).

PRIOR PROBABILITY   Credibility in the absence of the evidence from the study (cf. POSTERIOR PROBABILITY).

PROBABILITY

1. Relative frequency, as in "the probability that a 95% confidence interval will cover the value of the parameter is 95%."

2. Credibility, as in "the prior probability of the hypothesis."

PROBABILITY SAMPLE   A sample resulting from probability sampling (q.v.).

PROBABILITY SAMPLING   Sampling in such a way that each member of the sampled population has a known and independent probability (chance) of selection into the sample.

PROCESS EVALUATION (of health care)   Practice evaluation (q.v.). [Note: quality scales have to do with process, not outcome, so that outcome evaluation (q.v.) addresses premises of practice rather than practice (health care) itself, except indirectly.]

PROGNOSIS   Expected future course in the sense of expected utility (disutility). (It is determined by the utilities of the various possible outcomes together with their respective probabilities.)

PROGRAM   A regimented undertaking of indefinite duration (cf. PROJECT).

PROJECT   A regimented undertaking of a priori limited duration (cf. PROGRAM).

PROPORTIONAL RATE   Proportionate rate (q.v.).

PROPORTIONATE MORTALITY RATIO   Ratio of proportionate rate for mortality between two categories of a determinant.

PROPORTIONATE RATE   The proportion that (the rate for) a given type of state or event represents out of (the rate for) two or more types of state or event.

PROSPECTIVE BASE   A study base whose experience is concurrent with the execution of the study.

PROSPECTIVE EXPERIENCE (of a cohort)   The experience subsequent to the time as of which the cohort is defined (zero time).

PROSPECTIVE STUDY   A study with a prospective base.

PROTOCOL OF STUDY   A written documentation of a study plan.

PUBLIC HEALTH
  1. The health of a community of people.
  2. Care for the health of a community of people.
  3. Social medicine; that is, public (social) aspects of health and health care (personnel, organization, finance, program policy, etc.).

QUALITATIVE SCALE   A nominal scale.

QUALITATIVE STUDY   A study whose objective is modification of the credibility of a hypothesis.

QUANTITATIVE SCALE   A scale that provides not only for ranking but also for quantification of differences (interval scale) and/or ratios (ratio scale).

QUANTITATIVE STUDY   A study whose object is the magnitude of a parameter (e.g., of relation) in a general way (rather than in the limited sense of a qualitative study).

QUANTITATIVE METHODS   Statistical methods (a recent euphemism).

QUASI-EXPERIMENTAL   Nonexperimental.

QUASI-QUANTITATIVE (scale)   Ordinal, with scores assigned to categories.

RANDOM ERROR   The difference between error and its average (in quantification).

RANDOM SAMPLE   A probability sample (q.v.).

RATE (of occurrence)   Frequency in population experience (empirical or theoretical).

RATE DIFFERENCE   Difference of rate between two categories of a determinant, especially the rate in an index category expressed as its difference from that in a reference category.

RATE RATIO   Ratio of rate between two categories of a determinant, especially the rate in an index category expressed as its ratio to that in a reference category. (cf. RELATIVE RATE.)

RD   Rate difference (q.v.).

REALIZATION   Value or category occurring in a particular instance.

REFERENCE CATEGORY   The category (of a determinant) that is viewed as the alternative to a category of direct interest; that is, the category that provides comparative, or reference, information for the experience in the index category (often about the null value of the outcome parameter), as in "the rate ratio for the heavily exposed, with 'never exposed' as the reference category."

REFERENCE GROUP/POPULATION   The group/population representing the reference category (in the study base).

REFERENCE SAMPLE   A series of individuals (units of observation) enrolled to supply reference information for a case series; that is, a sample of the study base (in a case-referent study).

REFERENT   That to which something refers, as in "the referent of the empirical occurrence relation, in direct, technical terms, is the study base."

REGRESSION   The relation of a parameter to its determinant(s).

REGRESSION COEFFICIENT (in linear regression)   The ratio of the "effect" of a unit increase in a determinant (on the dependent parameter) to that unit increase.

REGRESSION TOWARD THE MEAN   A tendency of a repeat observation, after an appreciable period of time, to be closer to the mean than the original one.

RELATION   See OCCURRENCE RELATION.

RELATIVE RATE   The magnitude of a rate (an index rate) expressed in terms of its ratio to a reference rate.

RELATIVE RISK   The magnitude of a risk (an index risk) expressed in terms of its ratio to a reference risk; also a misnomer for relative rate (q.v.).

RELIABILITY   Misnomer for reproducibility.

REPRESENTATIVE OF THE STUDY BASE   A member of the base sample.

REPRESENTATIVE SAMPLE
1. Unbiased sample.
2. Sample whose distribution conforms to that of the sampled population.

REPRODUCIBILITY   Precision (q.v.).

RESEARCH   Activity aimed at the advancement of knowledge (scientific or nonscientific).

RESISTANT   Not susceptible (q.v.).

RESPONSIVENESS   Susceptibility.

RESTRICTED   See CONDITIONAL.

RESULT OF STUDY
1. A product of data analysis; that is, a statistic, as in "the result section of a paper."
2. A consequence of a study (change in view).

RETROSPECTIVE BASE   A study base whose exprerience is antecedent to the implementation of the study.

RETROSPECTIVE EXPERIENCE (of a cohort)   The experience preceding the time as of which the cohort is defined (zero time).

RETROSPECTIVE STUDY   A study with a retrospective base. (Some use the term, as a misnomer, for a case-referent study).

RISK   The probability that an event (untoward) will occur.

RISK FACTOR   Causal risk indicator; also used (as a misnomer) as a synonym for risk indicator (q.v.).

RISK FUNCTION   A formal (mathematical) expression of risk in relation to its determinants (indicators of risk).

RISK INDICATION   Realization of risk indicator (q.v.).

RISK INDICATOR   A characteristic on which risk depends; that is, a determinant of risk; that is, a determinant of expected (theoretical) incidence for people of the type at issue.

RISK RATIO   Ratio of risk between two categories of a determinant, especially in the sense of relative risk (q.v.).

RR   Rate ratio (q.v.) or risk ratio (q.v.).

SAMPLING DISTRIBUTION (of a statistic)   Distribution in hypothetical replications of the study, infinite in number.

SAMPLING FRAME   A list of the members of a population, used as a basis for sampling.

SCALE   A set of mutually exclusive and all-inclusive categories.

SCIENCE (natural)
1.   Scientific knowledge—a systematized body of theoretical knowledge (about a particular category of natural phenomena), as in "the insights of the science of neoplasia (oncology)."
2.   Scientific research—activity aimed at the advancement of *theoretical* knowledge (about nature), and conforming to the rules of logic, as in "good science."

SCREENING   Routine (particularly mass) examination of individuals for indications of illness or of high risk for illness.

SECONDARY BASE   A base defined, indirectly, as the population experience, the entirety of it, from which each potential case, had it occurred, would have been enrolled in the case series of the study.

SECONDARY DIAGNOSIS   Diagnosis unrelated to the reasons for the patient's coming to attention.

SECONDARY OBJECTIVES   Objectives that the study justifies (as opposed to those that justify the study, i.e., primary objectives).

SENSITIVITY OF INDICATION
1.   The proportion (theoretical) of instances in which the indication is manifest when the state at issue is present, or when the event at issue has taken place (cf. SPECIFICITY and FALSE NEGATIVE RATE).
2.   The proportion (theoretical) of instances in which an indication comes about (the indicator turns positive) as a reflection of the event at issue.

SENSITIVITY OF STUDY   See POWER OF TEST.

SIGNIFICANCE LEVEL   See LEVEL OF TEST.

SIGNIFICANT (statistically)   See LEVEL OF TEST.

SIMPLE RANDOM SAMPLING   Probability sampling with identical selection probabilities (cf. STRATIFIED SAMPLING).

SINGLE BLINDED   Blinded with respect to the observers or the subjects but not both.

SIZE EFFICIENCY   See EFFICIENCY.

SOCIAL MEDICINE   See PUBLIC HEALTH.

SMR   See STANDARDIZED MORTALITY RATIO.

SOURCE POPULATION   A population from which the base population is selected (by the use of exclusions).

SPATIOTEMPORAL   Having to do with place and time.

SPECIFICITY (of indication)
   1. The proportion (theoretical) of instances in which the indication is absent when the state at issue is absent, or the event at issue has not taken place (cf. SENSITIVITY and FALSE POSITIVE RATE).
   2. The degree to which the indication, when present, is indicative of the state or event at issue.

SPURIOUS
   1. Apparent (as against real).
   2. Misnomer for confounded (as against causal/preventive).

STANDARD DEVIATION   Square root of variance (q.v.).

STANDARD ERROR   Estimate (point) of the standard deviation of the sampling distribution (of a point estimator of a parameter).

STANDARDIZED RATE   A rate adjusted to a structure (distribution, set of weights) viewed as a standard (common structure) for the purpose of comparison(s).

STANDARDIZED RATE DIFFERENCE/RATIO   Difference/ratio of two mutually standardized rates. (This defines an *internally* standardized rate difference/ratio; two or more *mutually* standardized measures of association involve a common internal standard.)

STANDARDIZED MORTALITY RATIO   Empirical rate ratio for mortality involving incidence density of death and standardization according to the distribution of the index experience; that is, O/E ratio of deaths, with E estimated with allowance for some covariates (usually age, gender, and calendar time).

STATIONARY POPULATION   A dynamic population whose profile is invariant over time.

STATISTIC   A measure summarizing (some aspect of) the evidence in the data.

STATISTICAL SCIENCE   Scientific research concerned with frequency of occurrence of a phenomenon (as is epidemiologic research within various medical sciences); it is not a science unto itself.

STATISTICS
1. The discipline that deals with collecting, summarizing, and interpreting data (demographic statistics).
2. The branch of mathematics that deals with random variates (mathematical statistics).

STRATIFIED ANALYSIS   Analysis in which elementary comparative information (about the studied relation) is abstracted within subdomains (strata) of some covariates, with such information then accumulated over the strata (in the form of summary statistics).

STRATIFIED SAMPLING   Sampling designed to have unequal sampling fractions among subdomains (strata) of the sampled population.

STUDY (in science)   A project designed to yield evidence for the advancement of knowledge (q.v.).

STUDY BASE   The population experience (particularistic) captured in a study (as a basis for inference about nature in the abstract); that is, the direct referent of the empirical result of a study; specifically, in occurrence research, the study base is the population experience manifesting the occurrence under study, but the relevant realizations of its determinants may be previous to the time segment that the base represents.

STUDY DESIGN
1. A plan as to the type of evidence a study is to yield, and as to the approach to obtaining and summarizing such information.
2. The process of developing a study plan.

STUDY POPULATION   The population whose experience constitutes the study base.

STUDY SUBJECT   A member of the study population, especially one on whom information is obtained and incorporated in the analysis.

SUBJECT-MATTER   The phenomenon under study and related phenomena (as opposed to the principles or methods of studying it).

SUBJECTIVE   Not objective (q.v.); involving view(s).

SUBSTANTIVE   Having to do with subject-matter (rather than principles or methods of studying it).

SUPERPOPULATION   An abstract population of infinite size, viewed as the source of the studied (base) population, and also as the target population of inference.

SURVEY   A particularistic and descriptive study.

SUSCEPTIBLE (person or unit of observation)
1. Causally susceptible—the event at issue would/does develop conditionally on the index but not the reference category of the determinant at issue.
2. Preventively susceptible—the event at issue would/does develop conditionally on the reference but not the index category of the determinant at issue.
3. Responsive to the index, but not the reference, category of the determinant.

SYNERGISM   Cooperative action between two factors; the effect of one is enhanced by the other (and conversely).

TARGET POPULATION   The population of interest in a particularistic study.

TEST (statistical)
1. Frequentist—computation of *P*-value.
2. Bayesian—computation of likelihood ratio, or likelihood ratio function, and then the posterior probability corresponding to a particular prior probability (or its distribution).

THEORETICAL
1. Having to do with principles (general) rather than subject-matter knowledge, as in "theoretical epidemiology."
2. Without specificity as to time or place; that is, abstract or abstract-general, as in "the theoretical proposition that smoking causes lung cancer," and "theoretical rate."

THEORETICAL EPIDEMIOLOGY   The discipline, or principles, of studying epidemiologic problems, that is, (frequency of) occurrence of phenomena of health care interest in population experiences. See EPIDEMIOLOGY.

THERAPEUTIC   Having to do with treatment of cases of illness (as opposed to prevention or rehabilitation).

TRACKING   Incomplete regression toward the mean; that is, correlation between repeat observations. (This concept has meaning in quantitative terms only.)

TRICHOTOMOUS   Divided in three categories (cf. DICHOTOMOUS and POLYTOMOUS).

TYPE I ERROR   The "rejection" of a correct "null hypothesis."

TYPE II ERROR   The "acceptance" of an incorrect "null hypothesis."

UNIT OF OBSERVATION   A member of the study population.

VALIDITY OF MEASUREMENT (quantitative)   Lack of bias (q.v.).

VALIDITY OF STUDY   Lack of median bias (q.v.).

VARIABLE
1. Subject to variation.
2. Variate.

VARIANCE   Average of squared deviations from the mean.

VARIATE   A characteristic as represented in a statistical model, potentially taking on differing realizations among the units of observation (the members of the study population).

ZERO TIME (of a cohort)   The time (individual or calendar) as of which the criteria of membership are satisfied; that is, the boundary between the retrospective and prospective experiences of a cohort.

References

Armitage, P. (1975). *Sequential Medical Trials*, 2nd ed. Blackwell Scientific Publications, Oxford.

Axelson, O., Andersson, K., Hogstedt, C., et al. (1978). A cohort study on trichloroethylene exposure and cancer mortality. *JOM*, **20**, 194–6.

Axelson, O., Dahlgren, E., Jansson, C-D., et al. (1978). Arsenic exposure and mortality: A case-referent study from a Swedish copper smelter. *Br. J. Ind. Med.*, **35**, 8–15.

Barnard, G.A. (1947). Significance tests for 2 × 2 tables. *Biometrika*, **34**, 123–38.

Barndorff-Nielsen, O. (1976). Nonformation. *Biometrika*, **63**, 567–71.

Birch, M.W. (1964). The detection of partial association. *J. R. Stat. Assoc.*, **26**, 313–24.

Birnbaum, A. (1962). On the foundations of statistical inference (with discussion). *J. Am. Stat. Assoc.*, **57**, 269–326.

Borow, K. M., Green, L. H., Castaneda, A. R., et al. (1980). Left ventricular function after repair of tetralogy of Fallot and its relationship to age at surgery. *Circulation*, **61**, 1150–8.

Boston Collaborative Drug Surveillance Program (1971). A relation between breast cancer and S blood-antigen System. *Lancet*, **1**, 301–5.

Boston Collaborative Drug Surveillance Program (1972). Excess of ampicillin rashes associated with allopurinol or hyperuricemia. *N. Engl. J. Med.*, **286**, 505–7.

Breart, G. L., Miettinen, O.S., Peckam, G. J., et al. (1985). Effect of maternal glucocorticoid administration on pulmonary and ductal maturation of the fetus. To be published.

Breslow, N. E. and Day, N. E. (1980). *Statistical Methods in Cancer Research*. Vol. 1. The analysis of Case-Control Studies. International Agency for Research on Cancer, Lyon.

Bronshtein, I. N. and Semendyayev, K. A. (1973). *A Guide Book to Mathematics*. Verlag Harri Deutsch, Frankfurt/Main, pp. 161–3.

345

Campbell, D. T. and Stanley, J. C. (1966). *Experimental and Quasi-Experimental Designs for Research*. Rand McNally College Publishing Company, Chicago.

Chiang, C. L. (1968). *Introduction to Stochastic Processes in Biostatistics*. John Wiley & Sons, New York, Chapter 12.

Cochran, W. G. (1954). Some methods for strengthening the common chi-square tests. *Biometrics*, **10**, 417–51.

Cole, P. T., Monson, R. R., Haning, H., et al. (1971). Smoking and cancer of the lower urinary tract. *N. Engl. J. Med.*, **284**, 129–34.

Cornfield, J. (1951). A method of estimating comparative rates from clinical data. Applications to cancer of the lung, breast and cervix. *J. Natl. Cancer. Inst.*, **11**, 1269–75.

Cornfield, J. (1956). A statistical problem arising from retrospective studies. In: Neyman, J. (Ed.), *Proceedings of the Third Berkeley Symposium on Mathematical Statistics*, Vol. IV. University of California Press, Berkeley, pp. 135–48.

Cornfield, J. (1966). A Bayesian test of some classical hypotheses—with applications to sequential clinical trials. *J. Am. Stat. Assoc.*, **61**, 577–94.

The Coronary Drug Project Research Group (1970). Initial findings leading to modifications of its research protocol. *JAMA*, **214**, 1303–13.

Cox, D. R. and Hinkley, D. V. (1974). *Theoretical Statistics*. Chapman and Hall, Ltd., London.

De Vita, V. T., Simon, R. M., Hubbard, S. M., et al. (1980). Curability of advanced Hodgkin's disease with chemotherapy. Long-term follow-up of MOPP-treated patients at the National Cancer Institute. *Ann. Intern Med.*, **92**, 587–95.

Diamond, G. A. and Forrester, J. S. (1983). Clinical trials and statistical verdicts: Probable grounds for appeal. *Ann. Intern. Med.*, **98**, 385–94.

Elandt-Johnson, R. C. (1975). Definition of rates: Some remarks on their use and misuse. *Am. J. Epidemiol.*, **102**, 267–71.

Esping, B. and Axelson, O. (1980). A pilot study on respiratory and digestive tract cancer among woodworkers. *Scand. J. Work Environ. Health*, **6**, 201–5.

Fieller, E. C. (1944). A fundamental formula in the statistics of biological assay, and some applications. *J. Pharm.*, **27**, 117–23.

Fisher, R. A. (1925). *The Design of Experiments*. Oliver and Boyd, Edinburgh.

Flodin, U., Andersson, L., Anjou, C-G., et al. (1981). A case-referent study on acute myeloid leukemia, background radiation and exposure to solvents and other agents. *Scand. J. Work Environ. Health*, **7**, 169–78.

Folks, J. L. (1981). *Ideas of Statistics*. John Wiley & Sons, New York.

Friend, J. W. and Feibleman, J. (1937). *What Science Really Means*. George Allen and Unwing Ltd., London, pp. 110–1, 141, 177.

Gabbay, K. H., Hasty, K., Breslow, J. L., et al. (1977). Glycosylated hemoglobins and long-term blood glucose control in diabetes mellitus. *J. Clin. Endocrinol. Metab.*, **44**, 859–64.

Galton, F. (1889). *Natural Inheritance*. Macmillan, London.

Gart, J. (1970). Point and interval estimation of the common odds ratio in the combination of 2×2 tables with fixed marginals. *Biometrika*, **57**, 471–5.

Gersony, W. M., Peckham, G. J., Ellison, R. C., et al. (1983). Effects of Indomethacin in premature infants with patent ductus arteriosus: Results of a national collaborative study. *J. Pediatr.*, **102**, 895–906.

Greenland, S. (1979). Limitations of the logistic analysis of epidemiologic data. *Am. J. Epidemiol.*, **110**, 693–8.

Hänninen, H., Eskelinen, L., Husman, K., et al. (1976). Behavioral effects of long-term exposure to a mixture of organic solvents. *Scand. J. Work Environ. Health*, **4**, 240–55.

Hernberg, S., Partanen, T., Nordman, C-H., et al. (1970). Coronary heart disease among workers exposed to carbon disulphide. *Br. J. Ind. Med.*, **27**, 313–25.

Hill, A. B. (1953). Observation and experiment. *N. Engl. J. Med.*, **248**, 995–1001.

Illich, I. (1976). *Medical Nemesis*. Pantheon, New York.

International Agranulocytosis and Aplastic Anemia Study (1983). The design of a study of the drug etiology of agranulocytosis and aplastic anemia. *Eur. J. Clin. Pharmacol.*, **24**, 833–6.

Jick, H. and Slone, D. (1969). Venous thromboembolism and ABO blood type. *Lancet*, **i**, 539–42.

Katz, D., Baptista, J., Azen, S. P., et al. (1978). Obtaining confidence intervals for the risk ratio in cohort studies. *Biometrics*, **34**, 469–74.

Khosla, T. and Lowe, C. R. (1967). Indices of obesity derived from body weight and height. *Br. J. Prev. Soc. Med.*, **21**, 122–8.

Koopman, J. S. (1981). Interaction between discrete causes. *Am. J. Epidemiol.*, **113**, 716–24.

Lancaster, H. O. (1952). Statistical control of counting experiments. *Biometrika*, **39**, 419–22.

MacMahon, B., Yen, S., Trichopoulos, D., et al. (1981). Coffee and cancer of the pancreas. *N. Engl. J. Med.*, **304**, 630–3.

Mantel, N. (1963). Chi-square tests with one degree of freedom; Extensions of the Mantel–Haenszel procedure. *J. Am. Stat. Assoc.*, **58**, 690–700.

Mantel, N. and Haenszel, W. (1959). Statistical aspects of the analysis of data from retrospective studies of disease. *JNCI*, **22**, 719–48.

Matroos, A., Magnus, K., and Strackee, J. (1979). Fatal and nonfatal coronary attacks in relation to smoking in some Dutch communities. *Am. J. Epidemiol.*, **109**, 145–51.

McMichael, A. J. (1976). Standardized mortality ratios and the healthy worker effect: Scratching beneath the surface. *JOM*, **18**, 165–8.

McNemar, Q. (1947). Note on the sampling error of the difference between correlated proportions or percentages. *Psychometrika*, **12**, 153–7.

Miettinen, O. S. (1968). The matched pairs design in the case of all-or-none responses. *Biometrics*, **24**, 339–52.

Miettinen, O. S. (1969). Individual matching with multiple controls in the case of all-or-none responses. *Biometrics*, **25**, 339–55.

Miettinen, O. S. (1970a). Estimation of relative risk from individually matched series. *Biometrics*, **26**, 75–86.

Miettinen, O. S. (1970b). Matching and design efficiency in retrospective studies. *Am. J. Epidemiol.*, **91**, 111–8.

Miettinen, O. S. (1972a). Components of the crude risk ratio. *Am. J. Epidemiol.*, **96**, 168–72.

Miettinen, O. S. (1972b). Standardization of risk ratios. *Am. J. Epidemiol.*, **96**, 383–8.

Miettinen, O. S. (1974a). Confounding and effect-modification. *Am. J. Epidemiol.*, **100**, 350–3.

Miettinen, O. S. (1974b). Proportion of disease caused or prevented by a given exposure, trait or intervention. *Am. J. Epidemiol.*, **99**, 325–32.

Miettinen, O. S. (1974c). Comment. *J. Am. Stat. Assoc.*, **69**, 380–2.

Miettinen, O. S. (1976a). Estimability and estimation in case-referent studies. *Am. J. Epidemiol.*, **103**, 226–35.

Miettinen, O. S. (1976b). Stratification by a multivariate confounder score. *Am. J. Epidemiol.*, **104**, 609–20.

Miettinen, O. S. (1979). Public health policy on coronary heart disease. *Hart Bull.*, **10**, 165–7.

Miettinen, O. S. (1980). Efficacy of therapeutic practice: Will epidemiology provide the answers? In: Melmon, K. L. (Ed.), *Drug Therapeutics: Concepts for Physicians*. Elsevier-North Holland, New York.

Miettinen, O. S. (1982a). Causal and preventive interdependence. Elementary principles. *Scand. J. Work Environ. Health*, **8**, 159–68.

Miettinen, O. S. (1982b). Design options in epidemiologic research. An update. *Scand. J. Work Environ. Health* **8** (Suppl. 1), 7–14.

Miettinen, O. S. (1982c). The "healthy worker effect" and the design of occupational mortality studies. In: von Berger, J. and Hohne, K. H. (Eds.), *Methoden der Statistik und Informatik in Epidemiologie und Diagnostik*. Jahrestagung der DMDS, Hamburg, 1982 Proceedings, p. 27. In: Koller, S., Reichertz, P. L., and Uberla (Eds.), *Medizinische Informatik und Statistik*, No. 40. Springer-Verlag, Berlin and New York.

Miettinen, O. S. (1983a). Philosophy in a learned profession. Observations and thoughts. *K. Neth. Acad. Wet.*, C **86**(4), 517–23.

Miettinen, O. S. (1983b). The need for randomization in the study of intended effects. *Stat. Med.*, **2**, 267–71.

Miettinen, O. S. (1985). The "case-control" study. Valid selection of subjects. *J. Chr. Dis.* **38**, 543-8.

Miettinen, O. S. and Cook, E. F. (1981). Confounding: Essence and detection. *Am. J. Epidemiol.*, **114**, 593–603.

Miettinen, O. S., Ellison, R. C., Peckham, G. J., et al. (1983). Overall prognosis as the primary criterion of outcome in a clinical trial. *Contr. Clin. Trials*, **4**, 227–37.

Miettinen, O. and Nurminen, M. (1985). Comparative analysis of two rates. *Stat. Med.* **4**, 213-26.

Miettinen, O. S., Slone, D., and Shapiro, S. (1977). Current problems in drug-related epidemiologic research. In: Colombo, F., et al. (Eds.), *Epidemiological Evaluation of Drugs*. Elsevier/North Holland Biomedical Press, Amsterdam.

Miettinen, O. S. and Wang, J. D. (1981). An alternative to the proportionate mortality ratio. *Am. J. Epidemiol.*, **114**, 144–8.

Moore, F. E. (1960). Committee on design and analysis of studies. *Am. J. Publ. Health*, **50**, 10–9.

Morris, J. N., Chave, S. P. W., Adam, C., et al. (1973). Vigorous exercise in leisure-time and the incidence of coronary heart-disease. *Lancet*, i, 333–9.

Morrison, D. E. and Henkel, R. E. (Eds.) (1970). *The Significance Test Controversy*. Aldine Publishing Co., Chicago.

Nadas, A. S. and Fyler, D. C. (1972). *Pediatric Cardiology*, 3rd ed. W. B. Saunders Company, Philadelphia, pp. 136–7.

Panayotou, P. P., Kaskarelis, D. B., Miettinen, O. S., et al. (1972). Induced abortion and ectopic pregnancy. *Am. J. Obstet. Gynecol.*, **114**, 507–10.

Patel, R., Fox, K., Taylor, J. F. N., et al. (1978). Tricuspid atresia. Clinical course in 62 cases (1967–74). *Br. Heart J.*, **40**, 1408–14.

Pearson, S. E. (1947). The choice of statistical tests illustrated on the interpretation of data classed in a 2 × 2 table. *Biometrika*, **34**, 139–67.

Pike, M. C. and Morrow, R. H. (1970). Statistical analysis of patient-control studies in epidemiology: Factor under investigation an all-or-none variable. *Br. J. Prev. Soc. Med.*, **24**, 42–4.

Prentice, R. (1976). Use of the logistic model in retrospective studies. *Biometrics*, **32**, 599–606.

Radhakrishna, S. (1965). Combination of results from several 2 × 2 Contingency tables. *Biometrics*, **21**, 86–98.

Rothman, K. J. and Keller, A. Z. (1972). The effect of joint exposure to alcohol and tobacco on the risk of cancer of the mouth and pharynx. *J. Chronic. Dis.*, **25**, 711–6.

Samuels, M. L. (1981). Matching and design efficiency in epidemiological studies. *Biometrika*, **68**, 577–88.

Schilling, R. S. F. (Ed.) (1973). *Occupational Health Practice*. Butterworths, London.

Schlesselman, J. J. (1982). *Case-Control Studies*. Oxford University Press, New York.

Slone, D., Shapiro, S., Rosenberg, L., et al. (1978). Relation of cigarette smoking to myocardial infarction in young women. *N. Engl. J. Med.*, **298**, 1273–6.

Slone, D., Shapiro, S., Kaufman, D. W., et al. (1981). Risk of myocardial infarction in relation to current and discontinued use of oral contraceptives. *N. Engl. J. Med.*, **305**, 420–4.

Strom, B. L., Miettinen, O. S., and Melmon, K. L. (1983). Post marketing studies of drug efficacy: When must they be randomized? *Clin. Pharm. Ther.*, **34**, 1–7.

Thomas, D. G. (1975). Exact and asymptotic methods for the combination of 2 × 2 tables. *Comput. Biomed. Res.*, **8**, 423–46.

Tocher, K. D. (1950). Extension of the Neyman–Pearson theory of tests to discontinuous variates. *Biometrika*, **37**, 130–44.

Tola, S., Koskela, R. S., Hernberg, S., et al. (1979). Lung cancer mortality among iron foundry workers. *JOM*, **21**, 753–60.

Truett, J., Cornfield, J., and Kannel, W. (1967). A multivariate analysis of the risk of coronary heart disease in Framingham. *J. Chronic. Dis.*, **20**, 511–24.

University Group Diabetes Program (1970). A study of the effects of hypoglycemic agents on vascular complications in patients with adult-onset diabetes: II. Mortality results. *Diabetes*, **19** (Suppl. 2), 789–830.

Veterans Administration Cooperative Study Group on Antihypertensive Agents (1970). Effects of treatment on morbidity in hypertension. II. Results in patients with diastolic blood pressure averaging 90 through 114 mmHg. *JAMA*, **213**, 1143–52.

Wahrendorf, J. and Brown, C. C. (1980). Bootstrapping a basic inequality in the analysis of joint action of two drugs. *Biometrics*, **36**, 653–7.

Walker, A. M. (1982). Anamorphic analysis: Sampling and estimation for covariate effects when both exposure and disease are known. *Biometrics*, **38**, 1025–32.

Wang, J. D. and Miettinen, O. S. (1982). Occupational mortality studies. Principles of validity. *Scand. J. Work Environ. Health*, **8**, 153–8.

Wilson, E. B. (1927). Probable inference, the law of succession, and statistical inference. *J. Am. Stat. Assoc.*, **22**, 209–12.

Woolf, B. (1955). On estimating the relation between blood group and disease. *Ann. Human Genet.*, **19**, 251–3.

World Health Organization (1958). Classification of atherosclerotic lesions—Report of a study group. Technical Report Series No. 143, Geneva.

Ziel, H. K. and Finkle, W. D. (1975). Increased risk of endometrial carcinoma among users of conjugated estrogens. *N. Engl. J. Med.*, **293**, 1167–70.

Index

Definitions of terms are not indexed, as they are given in a **glossary**, pp. 317–344.

351